NEUROLOGICAL CLASSICS

NEUROLOGICAL CLASSICS

Compiled by

Robert H. Wilkins, M.D.
Chairman, Dept. of Neurosurgery
Scott and White Clinic
Temple, Texas

and

Irwin A. Brody, M.D.
Associate Professor of Neurology
Duke University
Durham, North Carolina

JOHNSON REPRINT CORPORATION

NEW YORK AND LONDON

1973

Library of Congress Cataloging in Publication Data:

Wilkins, Robert H   comp.
  Neurological classics.

  Articles originally published in the Archives of neurology,
Sept. 1967-Jan. 1972.
  Bibliography: p.
  1. Neurology—Addresses, essays, lectures. I. Brody, Irwin A., 1934-
joint comp. II. Archives of neurology. III. Title. [DNLM: 1. Neurology—
Collected works. WL 5 W685n 1973]
RC360.W55   616.8'08   72-13750
ISBN 0-384-68503-X

This book is dedicated to

Dr. Guy L. Odom

and

Dr. Albert Heyman

in appreciation of their role in our training

Preface

This book was planned in 1965, shortly after the publication of its companion volume, *Neurosurgical Classics* (Johnson Reprint Corporation, 1965). Our purpose was to make available in English some of the outstanding original descriptions of neurological diseases.

After compiling the first several issues in the projected series, we consulted Dr. H. Houston Merritt, who was then Chief Editor, requesting that they be published in the *Archives of Neurology.* Dr. Merritt and the other members of the Editorial Board supported our proposal, and with their encouragement, 41 issues were published in the *Archives* between September 1967 and January 1972. Permission to republish the entire set in the present volume was then kindly granted by Dr. Merritt and by Mr. Robert W. Mayo, Executive Managing Editor of the American Medical Association.

Along the way we received help from several other individuals and organizations. Our expenses were met by grants from the National Institute of Neurological Diseases and Blindness, and the General Research Support Fund of the Duke University Medical Center, as well as by smaller amounts from the neurosurgical budget at the Durham Veterans Administration Hospital and the Duke University Medical Center. Mr. Wayne C. Williams helped with the job of translating, and the typing was done by Miss Nancy Seagroves, Mrs. Jo Grimes, and Mrs. Nadine Dennis. Dr. Lawrence C. McHenry, Jr. kindly supplied for our dust cover the drawing of Jean Martin Charcot by Édouard Brissaud that first appeared in *Nouvelle Iconographie de la Salpêtrière* in 1898, and which was republished as Fig. 105 in Dr. McHenry's revision of *Garrison's History of Neurology* in 1969.

As with the *Neurosurgical Classics,* we have included only works published before 1940. The emphasis has been on descriptive clinical neurology, rather than on basic science, diagnostic procedures, or treatment. Many pioneering neurologists are not represented in the collection of Classics because their major contributions were not made in written form. Other contributions of prime importance were not included because of their length or because of their recent republication in the *Neurosurgical Classics* or elsewhere.

In some areas of neurology it was difficult to find single outstanding works suitable for reproduction. To correct this deficiency in part, a list of references has been included in the Appendix, which also contains a number of other supplementary references, most of which are in the English language.

We hope that the present volume will be of value to those with an interest in the historical basis of neurology and also to students seeking an authoritative description of a neurologic disease. The commentaries and references that accompany each of the Classics, and the additional references in the Appendix, have been complied in such a way that they can readily be used as a starting point for the review of various neurological topics.

Robert H. Wilkins, M. D.
Irwin A. Brody, M. D.
Durham, North Carolina
May, 1972.

Contents

NEUROLOGICAL
CLASSICS

I   Huntington's Chorea

ADVANCES in neurology have not been made only by the laboriously documented treatises of academicians. George Huntington was a general practitioner from East Hampton, Long Island, who was 22 years old when he described hereditary chorea. The description was made possible by the fact that Huntington, his father, and his grandfather had practiced medicine in the same town and had observed several generations of afflicted families. Huntington's report is written in a vivid, personal style and is eminently readable. William Osler said of this paper: "In the history of medicine there are few instances in which a disease has been more accurately, more graphically, or more briefly described."[1] The unpretentiousness of Huntington's article is matched by the modesty shown in later years when he referred to its acclaim as an "unsought, unlooked for honor."[2]

Despite its brevity, little has been added to Huntington's original description. The trait is attributable to an autosomal dominant gene with complete penetrance.[3,4] Although Huntington stated that the onset is always in adulthood, rare cases have since been described in children.[5] Variations of the classical clinical picture have been observed, and the rigid and akinetic forms are particularly noteworthy.[6] Pathologic changes in the brain, consisting primarily of degeneration in the basal ganglia and the frontal cortex, were identified by Marie and Lhermitte.[7] The social history of the disease has also been investigated,[8,9] and it is evident that many persons burned as witches in England and America were victims of Huntington's chorea. The ancestry of Huntington's cases in East Hampton has been traced to a "young man of Bures [England], by the name of Jeffers, and not of choreic strain, [who] fell in love with the daughter of a choreic and wished to marry her. His family stoutly objected, and so to obtain his end, he, in 1630, had to marry her and take her to America."[2]

Huntington begins his article with a review of the well known Sydenham's chorea. He concludes with the description that made him famous.

References

1. Osler, W.: Historical Note on Hereditary Chorea, *Neurographs* 1:113-116, 1908.
2. Stevenson. C.S.: A Biography of George Huntington, M.D., *Bull Instit Hist Med* 2:53-76, 1934.
3. Entres, J.L.: Geneologische Studie zur Differentialdiagnose zwischen Wilsonscher Krankheit und Huntingtonscher Chorea, *Z Ges Neurol Psychiat* 98:497-509, 1925.
4. Pleydell, M.J.: Huntington's Chorea in Northamptonshire, *Brit Med J* 2:1121-1128, 1954.
5. Jervis, G.A.: Huntington's Chorea in Childhood, *Arch Neurol* 9:244-257, 1963.
6. Bittenbender, J.B., and Quadfasel, F.A.: Rigid and Akinetic Forms of Huntington's Chorea, *Arch Neurol* 7:275-288, 1962.
7. Marie, P., and Lhermitte, J.: Les lésions de la chorée chronique progressive: La dégénération atrophique cortico-striée, *Ann Med* 1:18-48, 1914.
8. Vessie, P.R.: On the Transmission of Huntington's Chorea for 300 Years—the Bures Family Group, *J Nerv Men Dis* 76:553-573, 1932.
9. Critchley, M.: "Huntington's Chorea: Historical and Geographical Considerations," in *The Black Hole and Other Essays*, London: Pitman Medical Publishing Co., Ltd., 1964, pp 210-219.

ON CHOREA*

By George Huntington, MD, Of Pomeroy, Ohio

Essay read before the Meigs and Mason Academy of Medicine at Middleport, Ohio,
February 15, 1872

And now I wish to draw your attention more particularly to a form of the disease which exists, so far as I know, almost exclusively on the east end of Long Island. It is peculiar in itself and seems to obey certain fixed laws. In the first place, let me remark that chorea, as it is commonly known to the profession, and a description of which I have already given, is of exceedingly rare occurrence there. I do not remember a single instance occurring in my father's practice, and I have often heard him say that it was a rare disease and seldom met with by him.

The *hereditary* chorea, as I shall call it, is confined to certain and fortunately a *few* families, and has been transmitted to them, an heirloom from generations away back in the dim past. It is spoken of by those in whose veins the seeds of the disease are known to exist, with a kind of horror, and not at all alluded to except through dire necessity, when it is mentioned as *"that disorder."* It is attended generally by all the symptoms of common chorea, only in an aggravated degree, hardly ever manifesting itself until *adult* or *middle* life, and then coming on gradually but surely, increasing by degrees, and often occupying years in its development, until the hapless sufferer is but a quivering wreck of his former self.

It is as common and is indeed, I believe, *more* common among *men* than women, while I am not aware that season or complexion has any influence in the matter. There are three marked peculiarities in this disease: 1. Its hereditary nature. 2. A tendency to insanity and suicide. 3. Its manifesting itself as a grave disease only in adult life.

1. Of its hereditary nature. When either or both the parents have shown manifestations of the disease, and more especially when these manifesta-

tions have been of a *serious* nature, one or more of the offspring almost invariably suffer from the disease, if they live to adult age. But if by any chance these children go through life *without* it, the thread is broken and the grandchildren and great-grandchildren of the original shakers may rest assured that they are free from the disease. This you will perceive differs from the general laws of so-called hereditary diseases, as for instance in phthisis, or syphilis, when *one* generation may enjoy entire immunity from their dread ravages, and yet in another you find them cropping out in all their hideousness. Unstable and whimsical as the disease may be in *other* respects, in *this* it is firm, it never skips a generation to again manifest itself in another; once having yielded its claims, it never regains them. In all the families, or nearly all in which the choreic taint exists, the nervous temperament greatly preponderates, and in my grandfather's and father's experience, which conjointly cover a period of 78 years, nervous excitement in a marked degree almost invariably attends upon every disease these people may suffer from, although they may not when in *health* be over nervous.

2. The tendency to insanity, and sometimes that form of insanity which leads to suicide, is marked. I know of several instances of suicide of people suffering from this form of chorea, or who belonged to families in which the disease existed. As the disease progresses the mind becomes more or less impaired, in many amounting to insanity, while in others mind and body both gradually fail until death relieves them of their sufferings. At present I know of two married men, whose wives are living, and who are constantly making love to some young lady, not seeming to be aware that there is any impropriety in it. They are suffering from chorea to such an extent that they can hardly walk, and would be thought, by a stranger, to be

*Reprinted from *The Medical and Surgical Reporter* 26:317-321, 1872.

intoxicated. They are men of about 50 years of age, but never let an opportunity to flirt with a girl go past unimproved. The effect is ridiculous in the extreme.

3. Its third peculiarity is its coming on, at least as a grave disease, only in adult life. I do not know of a single case that has shown any marked signs of chorea before the age of thirty or forty years, while those who pass the fortieth year *without* symptoms of the disease, are seldom attacked. It begins as an ordinary chorea might begin, by the irregular and spadmodic action of certain muscles, as of the face, arms, etc. These movements gradually increase, when muscles hitherto unaffected take on the spasmodic action, until every muscle in the body becomes affected (excepting the involuntary ones), and the poor patient presents a spectacle which is anything but pleasing to witness. I have never known a recovery or even an amelioration of symptoms in this form of chorea; when once it begins it clings to the bitter end. No treatment seems to be of any avail, and indeed nowadays its end is so well-known to the sufferer and his friends, that medical advice is seldom sought. It seems at least to be one of the incurables.

Dr. WOOD, in his work on the practice of medicine, mentions the case of a man, in the Pennsylvania Hospital, suffering from aggravated chorea, which resisted *all* treatment. He finally left the hospital uncured. I strongly suspect that this man belonged to one of the families in which hereditary chorea existed. I know nothing of its pathology. I have drawn your attention to this form of chorea gentlemen, not that I considered it of any great practical importance to you, but merely as a medical curiosity, and as such it may have some interest.

II   Babinski's Sign

IN a series of short publications which began in 1896, Joseph François Félix Babinski described one of the most significant signs in clinical neurology—the pathological cutaneous plantar reflex.[1-8] A similar reflex of the extensor hallicus longus had been mentioned earlier by Remak,[9] but the astute observations of Babinski established its importance and stimulated many subsequent investigators to study its relation to dysfunction of the pyramidal system.

Babinski, a Parisian of Polish parentage, was a thorough and methodical physician who made his greatest contributions in the area of clinical neurology. In his first two publications on the pathological plantar reflex, Babinski mentioned only the dorsiflexion of the toes,[10,11] but in 1903 he added the "signe de l'éventail", or fanning of the toes.[12,13] To illustrate the latter, Babinski cleverly demonstrated the sign of fanning of the toes in a photograph showing the shadow of the toes against the opposite leg.[12]

Numerous other pathological responses characterized by dorsiflexion of the toes have been described, including the Chaddock,[14] Oppenheim,[15] and Gordon[16] signs, but the Babinski sign has proven to be the most useful in current neurological practice.

References

1. Hall, G.W.: Neurologic Signs and Their Discoverers, *JAMA* **95**:703-707, 1930.

2. Fulton, J.F., and Keller, A.D.: *The Sign of Babinski: A Study of the Evolution of Cortical Dominance in Primates,* Springfield, Ill: Charles C Thomas, Publisher, 1932.

3. Fulton, J.: Joseph François Félix Babinski, *Arch Neurol Psychiat* **29**:168-174, 1933.

4. Wartenberg, R.: "Joseph François Félix Babinski (1857-1932)," in Haymaker, W. (ed.): *The Founders of Neurology,* Springfield, Ill: Charles C Thomas, Publisher, 1953, pp 234-236.

5. Walshe, F.: The Babinski Plantar Response, Its Forms and Its Physiological and Pathological Significance, *Brain* **79**:529-556, 1956.

6. US National Institute of Neurological Diseases and Blindness: *Great Names in Neurology: Bibliography of Writings by Joseph Babinski, Victor Horsley, Charles Sherrington, and Arthur van Gehuchten,* Bethesda, MD: US Public Health Service, 1957, pp 3-22.

7. Glowacki, J.: The Role of Jozef Babinski in the Development of Neurosurgery, *Bull Pol Med Sci Hist* **5**:40-41, 1962.

8. Babinski and the Plantar Reflex, editorial, *JAMA* **183**:281, 1963.

9. Remak, E.: Zur Localisation der spinalen Hautreflexe der Unterextremitäten, *Neurol Centralbl* **12**:506-512, 1893.

10. Babinski, J.: Sur le réflexe cutané plantaire dans certaines affections organiques du système nerveux central, *C R Soc Biol* **48**:207-208, 1896.

11. Babinski, J.: Du phénomène des orteils et de sa valeur sémiologique, *Sem Med (Paris)* **18**:321-322, 1898.

12. Babinski, J.: De l'abduction des orteils, *Rev Neurol* **11**:728-729, 1903.

13. Babinski, J.: De l'abduction des orteils (signe de l'éventail); *Rev Neurol* **11**:1205-1206, 1903.

14. Chaddock, C.G.: A Preliminary Communication Concerning a New Diagnostic Nervous Sign, *Interstate Med J* **18**:742-746, 1911.

15. Oppenheim, H.: Zur Pathologie der Hautreflexe an den unteren Extremitäten, *Mschr Psychiat Neurol* **12**:518-530, 1902.

16. Gordon, A.: A New Reflex: Paradoxic Flexor Reflex. Its Diagnostic Value. *Amer Med* **8**:971, 1904.

ON THE PHENOMENON OF THE TOES AND ITS SEMEIOTIC VALUE*
M. Babinski

In this lecture, I will discuss with you a phenomenon which I made known more than two years ago. I communicated a note on it to the Société de Biologie in February 1896, and I made it the subject of a recent communication to the Congress of Neurology held at Brussels in September of last year.[1] This phenomenon consists of a disturbance in the cutaneous plantar reflex.

Before giving you a description of it I must tell you something of the normal cutaneous plantar reflex in adults with whom I shall concern myself here. You should know that stimulation of the sole of the foot ordinarily provokes reflex movements, such as flexion of the foot toward the leg, of the leg toward the thigh, of the thigh toward the pelvis; however, I call your attention particularly to the flexion of the toes on the metatarsal bone. There are normal individuals whose toes appear to stay immobile following stimulation of the sole of the foot, but—and this is the essential point—there is never any movement of extension. This applies principally to the great toe, which we should have particularly in mind.

In certain pathological states, stimulation of the sole evokes extension of the toes, particularly the great toe. I refer to this modification in the form of the reflex movement as the *phenomenon of the toes*.

It is not only in the *direction* of movement that the normal reflex differs from the pathological; usually the extensor response is executed more slowly than the flexor. Furthermore, flexion is ordinarily stronger when one stimulates the inner part of the sole than when the stimulus is applied to the outer part, and it is the opposite with the extensor response. Finally, while flexion predominates generally in the last two or three toes, it is in the first one or two toes that extension is usually the most pronounced.

The phenomenon of the toes may show itself in "formes frustes", that is, the plantar reflex may exhibit characteristics partly pathological and partly physiological. Here are some examples: in certain subjects, stimulation of the sole of the foot evokes extension only in the big toe or in the first two toes and flexion of the last toes; in others, the toes are extended when one stimulates the outer part of the sole and are flexed when the inner part is stimulated. In still other subjects, the plantar reflex, no matter which part of the sole is stimulated, manifests itself now by flexion and now by extension of the toes. In this last case, the first stimulations are the ones which produce flexion.

This said, I will acquaint you with the technique one must employ in order to observe adequately the reflex movement of the toes. It is important that the muscles of the foot and leg not be in a state of contraction. To ensure this it is well not to forewarn the subject of the test which one intends to carry out, and to have him close his eyes. The leg should be slightly flexed toward the thigh, and the foot should be resting on the bed by its outer edge. Preferably the foot should be deprived of all support by having the leg lifted and held by the one doing the test. When the lower limb is placed in this attitude, one should await before proceeding with the stimulation until the muscles appear well relaxed.

It makes a difference whether the stimulation is light or vigorous, whether it is simply tickling or whether it is pricking the sole of the foot. This last mode of stimulation is necessary in certain subjects in order to cause a reflex movement of the toes to appear; but, on the other hand, it evokes in other individuals such vigorous movements of the various segments of the lower limb that it is difficult to analyse them. When this occurs the direction of the movement of the toes may be impossible to determine, and, when one perceives it,

---

*Translation of Du phénomène des orteils et de sa valeur sémiologique, *La Semaine Médicale*, 18:321-322, 1898.

[1]M. van Gehuchten has published several works confirming the facts which I have reported (*J Neurol*, April 5, June 20, and July 5, 1898).

he should ask himself if it is really a reflex movement or a voluntary movement. This is an important question to resolve, for it is scarcely necessary to call to your attention that while the normal cutaneous plantar reflex never manifests itself by an extension of the toes, this movement can be executed voluntarily when the sole of the foot is pricked. It is necessary, in such cases, to repeat the stimulus lightly.

There is still another source of error in observation that I would like to point out to you. The toes necessarily follow the foot in the movement which it executes toward the leg following stimulation of the sole. If the flexor movement on the metatarsal bone fails, as sometimes happens, the toes, drawn passively toward the anterior part of the leg, may give to the inattentive observer the illusion that they are executing a movement of extension on the metatarsal bone. To avoid this error, one must examine the region of metatarsophalangeal articulation of the great toe in order to see how the phalanx and the metatarsal bone behave in relation to each other.

I present to you first several normal individuals, taken at random, whom you may examine yourselves at your leisure and on whom you will be in a position to verify my assertion about that which concerns the cutaneous plantar reflex in the physiological state.

Here now are some subjects in whom one observes the phenomenon of the toes. . . .

[Eight patients are then presented]

Relying on these few facts and many others which I have collected since this phenomenon caught my attention, I will review methodically the disorders in which one can observe the toe phenomenon.

First, there is adult or infantile hemiplegia due to an organic lesion of the brain, whether the cause is hemorrhage, softening, or neoplasm.

In the subjects I have shown you, we are dealing with hemiplegia of long duration accompanied by contractures and exaggeration of the tendon reflexes. But I have also noticed this phenomenon in many cases of recent flaccid hemiplegia where the tendon reflexes were normal, diminished, or even absent on the paralysed side. I observed this in the second patient that I presented to you. The first examination was made 24 hours after the onset of the hemiplegia. At that time the tendon reflexes were of approximately the same intensity on both sides. In another patient with organic hemiplegia, examined by me an hour after the onset of apoplexy, the toe phenomenon was very marked, and the tendon reflexes of the hemiplegic side were very weak. Generally, extension of the toes has seemed even more marked in recent hemiplegia than in hemiplegia of long duration.

I have also observed the presence of this sign in two subjects with flaccid hemiplegia of long duration with absence of the patellar reflexes. One of them had a left hemiplegia for three years. The paralysis was flaccid in the lower extremity; the left upper extremity was slightly spastic; the patellar and Achilles reflexes were absent on both sides; the reflex of the brachial triceps was normal on the right side, exaggerated on the left. The patient had had lancinating pains and his right pupil was smaller than the left. It seemed that one dealt with an association of posterior root lesions and an organic lesion of the right hemisphere with secondary degeneration. The second patient was a woman with obvious tabes, characterized by shooting pains, bladder difficulties, Robertson's sign, and absence of the patellar, Achilles, and brachial triceps tendon reflexes. She was suddenly stricken with a left hemiplegia. The toe phenomenon existed at the onset of the paralysis, and three months later, the paralysis having remained flaccid and the tendon reflexes having remained absent, stimulation of the sole provoked, as on the first day, extension of the toes.

The phenomenon of the toes is not in direct relation to the intensity of the paralysis. It may be very marked in certain cases where the hemiplegia is slight and where voluntary movement of the toes is not markedly reduced. On the other hand, it may be very marked, weak, or even absent in cases where the paralysis is very pronounced.

In general, on the side which is not paralysed, the cutaneous plantar reflex is normal. However, sometimes I have observed the sign of the toes on this side, although less accentuated than in the paralysed foot.

In a woman who experienced spastic hemiplegia several years previously I have noticed the following curious sign. Stimulation of the sole of the paralysed foot resulted in an extension of the toes on this side. Stimulation of the sole of the normal foot provoked, besides a flexion of the toes on this foot, a flexion of the toes of the paralysed foot.

I have seen the phenomenon of the toes in several cases of diffuse meningo-encephalitis. There was a marked weakness of the lower extremities, and the tendon reflexes were exaggerated. The patient that I presented to you last is the exception to the rule, since, as you have seen, the lower extremities were only slightly weakened and the tendon reflexes were absent. Indeed, this is a case of diffuse meningo-encephalitis associated with tabes.

In one case of focal epilepsy, I had the occasion to observe the following phenomenon. A man subject to Jacksonian epilepsy had convulsions on the left side of the body. Having examined the patient immediately after a seizure, I observed that stimulation of the left sole resulted in extension of the toes. At other times, the cutaneous plantar reflex was normal and the left side did not present any disorder of movement.

I have also observed the sign of the toes in an individual with cerebro-spinal meningitis, and in a woman who had ingested a toxic dose of strychnine. In both patients the lower extremities were subject to spasms, exaggeration of the tendon reflexes and clonus of the foot. The poisoned subject got well quickly, and approximately 48 hours after the onset of the morbid disorder the cutaneous plantar reflex had returned to normal.

In spastic spinal paralyses, no matter what the cause, whether a traumatic lesion, compression of the cord by Pott's disease, meningomyelitis, transverse myelitis, sclerotic plaques, syringomyelia, or amyotrophic lateral sclerosis, one often observes the toe phenomenon, and it is generally more pronounced than in hemiplegia of cerebral origin.

This sign can also exist in certain flaccid paraplegias with diminished or absent tendon reflexes. I have observed it on the side of the paralysis in a case of hemiplegia with crossed anesthesia due to a traumatic hemisection of the spinal cord in the mid-dorsal region, 15 hours after the accident. The paralysed side was flaccid, and the tendon reflexes were abolished there.

Finally, I have observed the toe phenomenon in many cases of Friedreich's disease.

I now must mention several types of nervous system disorder in which the toe sign will not be present. I have never observed it in a case of hysteria, where the neurosis manifested itself as a motor disturbance in the form of hemiplegia, paraplegia, flaccid paralysis, or contracture. It did not exist in the cases of classic progressive myopathy or peripheral neuritis that I have had the opportunity to observe. I have not been able to observe it in anterior poliomyelitis nor in a subject with completely atrophied flexor muscles of the toes, but this was a very special case, since the toes, due to amyotrophy, were unable to perform voluntary or reflex movements. The toe phenomenon is also absent in pure cases of tabes; yet it can exist, as you have seen, in tabes associated with another nervous system disorder, such as organic hemiplegia or meningo-encephalitis.

In two cases of complete traumatic severance of the spinal cord, which were observed by my intern Mr. Cestan, stimulation of the sole did not produce any toe movements. In one of the subjects, the lesion was situated at the level of C7, and the examination was performed nine hours after the accident. In the other case, the lesion was situated in the upper dorsal cord, and the examination was performed three hours after the trauma. However, one may not conclude from these two cases that the toe phenomenon is always absent in paraplegia secondary to a complete transsection of the spinal cord.

If we now look at the facts which I have enumerated and attempt to determine the cause of the toe phenomenon, we see immediately that this inversion in the form of the cutaneous plantar reflex is associated with a variety of different disorders of the brain and spinal cord. Since all of these different cases have as a common characteristic a permanent or temporary disorder of the pyramidal system, this is the disorder responsible for the phenomenon under discussion. I cannot at present state that this relationship is a necessary one; but I can say that in all the cases in which I have diagnosed the toe phenomenon, this relationship was established either as incontestable, as very probable, or at the very least as possible, by the entire clinical picture or by a later autopsy. To the present, I have not observed this sign a single time in a subject whose pyramidal system was completely sound.

My observations have demonstrated that the toe phenomenon can be caused by a disturbance of the pyramidal system, whatever its duration, intensity, and extent. I have observed it in very old as well as in rather recent cases of hemiplegia, in cases where the nerve fibers of the pyramidal tract had been destroyed and in others (due to sclerotic plaques, for instance) where the alteration was only slight or the axis cylinders of this tract were preserved. In some subjects the lesions of the tract were very extensive and in others the lesions were limited.

It is worthwhile to note that this sign, although it indicates the presence of a pyramidal system disturbance, does not denote its severity. It can exist in cases of very slight paralysis or curable paralysis, and can disappear after recovery. It can manifest itself in a temporary fashion in focal epilepsy and in strychnine poisoning. At times it even can be the only sign indicating such a disturbance. On the other hand, it can be absent in patients with profound alteration of the pyramidal system. This paradox leads one to ask whether there are certain areas of the pyramidal system that produce the toe phenomenon when altered; but we are not in a position to be precise on this point.

From the preceding, it can be said that the phenomenon of the toes is associated with exaggeration of the tendon reflexes and spinal epilepsy which in turn are often dependent upon a lesion in the pyramidal system, but this association is by no means constant. Frequently one observes this association, as in the majority of the patients that I have presented to you. Nevertheless, I could show you that at times the toe phenomenon is absent in a limb afflicted with spastic paralysis with exaggeration of the tendon reflexes and clonus of the foot. Furthermore, one can clearly observe this sign in cases where, despite the existence of a pyramidal system lesion, the tendon reflexes are normal, weak or absent, be it because of a recent lesion, or because there is an associated alteration of the posterior roots.

I cannot emphasize the importance of the toe phenomenon from the diagnostic point of view without repeating the description of the facts which I have previously stated.

I only want you to note that its diagnostic value is very great in cases where the state of the tendon reflexes does not permit one to determine the state of the pyramidal system. As you know, the tendon reflexes in recent organic hemiplegia are generally normal or weak, and it is often impossible to distinguish the first stage of hysterical hemiplegia from organic hemiplegia. In such cases the existence of the toe sign is particularly valuable because it permits one to discard the hypothesis of hysteria. The same is true of early paraplegia. The tendon reflexes are generally absent in a lesion of the pyramidal system associated with an alteration of the posterior roots, and the presence of the toe phenomenon in a case of tabes would be important in revealing a disorder in the pyramidal system, which, without this sign, would remain unknown.

At the beginning of this paper I told you that I would occupy myself only with the cutaneous plantar reflex in adults. Before finishing, however, I want to say a word about the reflex in the newborn. Tickling the sole of the foot normally provokes extension of the toes in newborns. However, if one considers that the pyramidal system is not yet developed at birth, this observation confirms the idea that the toe phenomenon is related to a disorder of the pyramidal system.

ON ABDUCTION OF THE TOES*
by M. J. Babinski

Stimulation of the sole of the foot sometimes provokes, among other reflex movements, an abduction of one or more toes. This response has been described incidentally by other authors who did not attach any semeiotic value to it.

For a long time my attention has been directed to this phenomenon, which I have observed in the normal as well as in the pathological state (Fig 1 and 2). Healthy subjects show this response rarely, and when it exists it is slight. However, in patients with a disorder of the pyramidal system it is much more common, without always including

extension of the great toe, and it is sometimes very marked. It seems to me particularly pronounced in congenital spastic paralyses accompanied by athetosis, which includes abductor movements of the toes. I would like to add that in newborns, in whom the pyramidal system is not fully developed, tickling of the sole of the foot generally causes an abduction of the toes and at the same time an extension of the big toe.

The fact that this phenomenon can exist in the normal state prevents me from attributing to it the fundamental importance of extension of the great toe, which is indicative of a disturbance of the pyramidal system. Nonetheless, when this phenome-

*Translation of De l'abduction des orteils, Revue Neurologique 11:728-729, 1903.

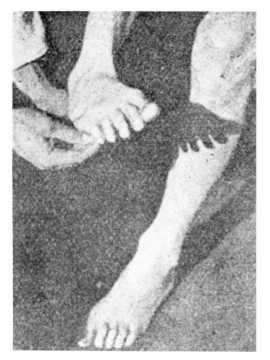

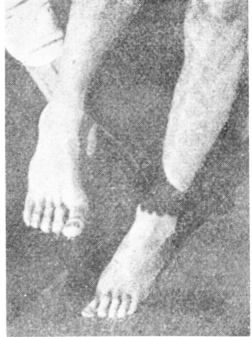

Fig 1.—Foot at rest.

Fig 2.—Foot at the moment of stimulation. Abduction of the toes of moderate intensity.

non is very marked, it seems to me to have definite significance. Recently, in a case of crural paraplegia due to trauma, which motivated a medico-legal evaluation, the physicians charged with the examination were of the opinion that they were dealing with hysteria or malingering because the classical objective signs of organic disease of the nervous system were absent. Having observed in this patient a very distinct abduction of the toes, I gave a contrary opinion. About three weeks after my first consultation, a second examination permitted me to demonstrate an extension of the toes which had not been found previously and which confirmed my view.

I therefore regard toe abduction, in conditions that I will specify, as constituting a sign of probability in favor of a disturbance of the pyramidal system. This can be valuable in certain doubtful cases.

THE TRADITIONAL EXAMINATION

So far as the traditional examination goes . . . the successful candidate need possess neither common sense nor common honesty, neither courage nor adequate physique, nor even an original mind. It is the kind of examination in which Shakespeare and Cromwell, and almost certainly Mr. Winston Churchill, would have ignominiously failed. For in early years the possession of a strong character or original mind only too often served as a sort of non-conductor for the ideas of other people . . . —Lord Elton, debate in House of Lords, May 1948. House of Lords: Official Report, May 26, 1948, col 1054.

III   Charcot-Marie-Tooth Disease

THE credit for discovering a "new disease" is often given not to the one who describes it first but to the one who describes it when the time is ripe. Thus, Virchow,[1] Schultze,[2] and others had reported cases of peroneal atrophy previously, but in 1886 medical knowledge had advanced sufficiently to accept this entity as a nosologic addition. The simultaneous publications by Charcot and Marie in France and by Tooth[3] in England do not attest to coincidence but to the fact that the medical world was ready to appreciate the finer clinical distinctions existing within the large group of progressive muscular atrophies.

Jean Martin Charcot and his pupil Pierre Marie carefully studied the multitude of infirm and paralytic inmates at the Salpêtrière, an asylum in Paris, and left a scientific discipline where there had been a muddle.[4] Their description of peroneal atrophy is only one of the many contributions of Charcot's school to our basic conceptions of the neuromuscular diseases.

Howard H. Tooth, whose paper was a thesis for the MD degree at Cambridge University, was aware of the work by Charcot and Marie, which had been published earlier the same year. In a footnote he justified his own paper as follows: "Since this thesis has been commenced, and some months after the lines, on which it was intended to work, had been laid down, there has appeared in the *Rev. de Médecine* for Feb. 1886, a paper by MM. Charcot and Marie on the same subject, illustrated by five cases."

To Tooth belongs the credit for emphasizing the early atrophy of the peroneal muscles and introducing the term "peroneal type of progressive muscular atrophy." Tooth's description is otherwise similar to Charcot and Marie's, but the former author, referring to the postmortem examinations of others, including Virchow,[1] proposed that the condition is a peripheral neuropathy, whereas Charcot and Marie favored the possibility of a myelopathy. Subsequent autopsy studies have shown degenerative changes in peripheral nerves, thus confirming Tooth's idea. Degeneration seen in the dorsal columns may be secondary to involvement of dorsal nerve roots, but the possibility of primary disease of the spinal cord cannot be completely excluded in certain cases (see the discussion by England and Denny-Brown[5]).

The finding of decreased nerve conduction velocities in patients with Charcot-Marie-Tooth disease is further evidence of a peripheral neuropathy, and conduction studies may even be used to detect genetic carriers of the disease.[6] The report of a primary myopathic change in this condition[7] must be reconsidered in view of the demonstration that such changes in muscle biopsy specimens may occur in chronic denervation.[8]

Although variants of Charcot-Marie-Tooth disease have been described[9] and families have been reported in which some members show the features of Friedreich's ataxia and some the features of peroneal atrophy,[10] nevertheless, peroneal muscular atrophy is usually encountered as the pure and characteristic form defined by Charcot, Marie, and Tooth.

References

1. Virchow, R.: Ein Fall von Progressiver Muskelatrophie, *Arch Path Anat Physiol* 8:537-540, 1855.
2. Schultze: Ueber eine Eigenthümliche Progressive Atrophische Paralyse bei Mehreren Kindern derselben Familie, *Berlin Klin Wschr* 21:649-651, 1884.
3. Tooth, H.H.: *The Peroneal Type of Progressive Muscular Atrophy*, London: H. K. Lewis, 1886.

4. Garrison, F.H.: Charcot, *Int Clin* 4:244-272, 1925.

5. England, A.C., and Denny-Brown, D.: Severe Sensory Changes, and Trophic Disorder, in Peroneal Muscular Atrophy (Charcot-Marie-Tooth Type), *Arch. Neurol. Psychiat.* 67:1-22, 1952.

6. Dyck, P.J.; Lambert, E.H.; and Mulder, D.W.: Charcot-Marie-Tooth Disease: Nerve Conduction and Clinical Studies of a Large Kinship, *Neurology* 13:1-11, 1963.

7. Haase, G.R., and Shy, G.M.: Pathological Changes in Muscle Biopsies From Patients With Peroneal Muscular Atrophy, *Brain* 83:631-637, 1960.

8. Drachman, D.B., et al: "Myopathic" Changes in Chronically Denervated Muscle, *Arch Neurol* 16:14-24, 1967.

9. Symonds, C.P., and Shaw, M.E.: Familial Claw-Foot With Absent Tendon-Jerks: A "Forme Fruste" of the Charcot-Marie-Tooth Disease, *Brain* 49:387-403, 1926.

10. Spillane, J.D.: Familial Pes Cavus and Absent Tendon-Jerks: Its Relationship With Friedreich's Disease and Peroneal Muscular Atrophy, *Brain* 63:275-290, 1940.

CONCERNING A SPECIAL FORM OF

PROGRESSIVE MUSCULAR ATROPHY

OFTEN FAMILIAL

STARTING IN THE FEET AND LEGS

AND LATER REACHING THE HANDS.*

By J. M. Charcot and P. Marie

I

Progressive muscular atrophy seems to subdivide into secondary groups, which increase in number as clinical observation becomes more attentive and more precise.

The form of muscular atrophy that constitutes the subject of this work seems to present characteristics sufficiently definite and stable to merit a special description and a place of its own in nosology.

During the past year, we had occasion to observe five patients with this affliction. It is from their symptoms that we shall describe the disease. We shall also have recourse, when necessary, to analogous observations published by other authors.

[Five case reports follow.]

II

Now we can try to assemble all the information furnished by these five cases and group them and coordinate them so that a nosologic description emerges containing the main traits of the clinical picture, always so similar in each case. These are the essential points that, in our opinion, distinguish this form of muscular atrophy:

Always, and this is an important characteristic, the disease starts in the lower limbs, and in their lower segments. In most cases it begins in the extensor of the big toe, or the common extensor of

*Translation of: Sur une forme particulière d'atrophie musculaire progressive souvent familiale débutant par les pieds et les jambes et atteignant plus tard les mains, *Revue de Médecine* 6:97-138, 1886.

the toes, or the lateral peroneals. This is, at least, the first sign that attracts the attention of the patient or of his parents. But is is very possible that the true beginning is not in the leg muscles but in the foot muscles proper, just as in the upper limbs, as we shall see later, the intrinsic muscles of the hand are the first affected. If this period generally goes unnoticed, it is probably because the functional symptoms caused by the atrophy of the intrinsic muscles of the feet are too slight for the patient to appreciate.

In any event, all the muscles of the lower limb are reached little by little. The gemellus muscles seem to be preserved a little longer than the others, but they too are finally involved by the degeneration. In all these muscles, weakness and atrophy seem to progress in parallel fashion. At an advanced enough stage, the weakness is such that there is no longer the slighest trace of voluntary contraction.

The thigh muscles seem to retain their strength and volume for a certain time, although, as we shall mention in respect to the electrical examination, this integrity is often more apparent than real. Among these muscles, the one first affected always seemed to us to be the vastus internus. This is the muscle, in any case, which has constantly been found to be the most atrophied. The other portions of the triceps femoris are reached later. The adductors, however, are well preserved, and the flexor muscles of the leg on the thigh seem almost unimpaired. Perhaps the biceps femoris was weak in one case. For the latter muscles it would be well to be able to examine them in cases more advanced than ours.

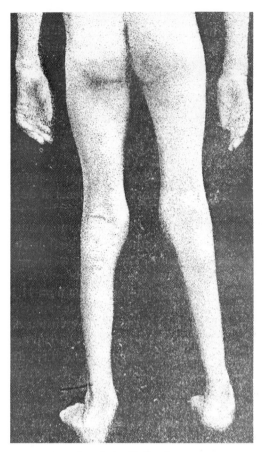

A patient with the disease.

The hand muscles become affected only after those of the lower limbs (on an average of 2 to 5 years). It would seem, from a case observed by Eichhorst (case of Jules), that this interval may become much more considerable and that the atrophy of the hands may never appear (?).

This atrophy of the upper limbs always starts in the hand muscles proper (interosseous, thenar eminence, hypothenar), and then it reaches the forearm muscles. It is difficult to say exactly which are the first muscles affected, since the order does not seem the same in all patients. Moreover, there often exists a dissociation for analogous muscles or for different bundles of the same muscles. Thus, for example, all the interosseous muscles are not equally affected. The deeper interossei still retain their contractility when it has disappeared in the superficial interossei. Similarly in the forearm, the flexors seem weaker in some patients, while in others, it is the extensors. It is not rare, either, for the bundle of the common flexor going to the index finger to be much more affected than other bundles of the same muscle. Yet, after these reser-

vations, we would have to admit that the extensors are generally reached after the hand muscles proper, and this especially for the extensor and the long abductor of the thumb. As for the other muscles of the forearm, the pronators and supinators are affected much later, if at all. We call attention to the fact that in no case did we see any alteration of the long supinator.

All the other muscles of the body, especially those of the trunk, shoulders, neck, and face, are absolutely unimpaired, as are the respiratory muscles. We must note, though, that in his report E. H. Wetherbee maintains that he could neither cough nor sneeze energetically.

It is well to remark again that, although the atrophic process evolves in an evidently symmetrical way, it is not rare to observe some predominance on one side of the body. This predominance often manifests itself from the beginning and can persist in a more or less marked form during the entire course of the disease.

The ailment is characterized chiefly by weakness and atrophy of the involved muscles. These two symptoms seem to be closely related and to advance in parallel.

If one examines more particularly the phenomena presented by the involved muscles, one observes the following:

In most of the muscles undergoing atrophy there are very distinct fibrillary contractions. They cannot be found when the destructive process has arrived at its final phase. Generally they are observed most easily and most distinctly in the thenar and hypothenar muscles. However, they never appear with the same intensity as in amyotrophic lateral sclerosis, for example.

Idiomuscular excitability to percussion is not augmented. On the contrary, it diminishes and even disappears in muscles involved early and thus precedes, by a rather long time, the loss of function and the atrophy. The tendon reflexes behave in the same way. They are first diminished in regions of the affected limbs, and then finally disappear. . . .

Moreover, it seems that all the modes of muscular excitability behave in a similar way since the same phenomenon is found for electrical contractility. In fact it is not rare to see a muscle almost healthy in appearance show a considerable diminution of faradic excitability and sometimes even a complete disappearance. It is especially at the level of the triceps femoris that one can observe a phenomenon of this kind. . . .

Another interesting characteristic of this affliction is the absence of fibrous contractures of the affected articulations. It is curious to see these joints retain enough mobility for passive movements while they are, in consequence of the absolute powerlessness of the muscles inserted in them, in a permanent state of repose. In some of our patients (especially Henri X . . .), we noticed a marked laxity of the tibio-tarsal articulation, allowing the foot to place itself in either varus or valgus. Although very noticeable, this laxity did not seem to us as pronounced as in some cases of infantile atrophic paralysis. In a word, it is not completely "jambe de polichinelle."[1]

Vasomotor disturbances are usually very intense in the affected parts, especially in the lower limbs. In all our patients the feet and legs presented a bluish or reddish coloration with widespread mottling. The general shape of the foot is slightly altered; not that there is, properly speaking, an edema or a volume augmentation, but the contours are less distinct, less well drawn. It looks somewhat like a foot that has remained some time in an immovable apparatus. We should also note that a few of our patients, especially the two women, had considerable subcutaneous adiposity of the affected parts, completely analogous to that studied specifically by M. L. Landouzy in various cases of atrophic paralysis.

Finally, the temperature is much reduced in the affected limbs. A hand applied to the feet and legs perceives a marked sensation of cold. In all our patients, and especially in the two women, this lowering of temperature is very clearly localized to these parts. Immediately above the knee, the skin is noticeably less cold, and the mid-thigh has almost normal heat. This lowering of temperature is, as we said, considerable. In one of the women patients the difference between the temperature of the mid-arm and the mid-leg was not less than 6 ° C.

The vasomoter and trophic disturbances just described also exist in the hands, but incomparably less marked than in the lower limbs.

We now reach the study of sensation. In four of our patients it is absolutely intact in all modalities. Only one (Sultz, Case V) is markedly affected. In the cases of Ormerod, Hammond, and in most of Eichhorst's, there were no sensory disturbances either; nevertheless, in one patient, the latter author noted hyperesthesia on the dorsum of the foot. In another patient he noted diminution of sensation of the legs. In view of these facts, we

believe that sensory disturbances are not an integral, indispensable part of the clinical picture but that in certain cases they may appear, even with some intensity. Their role is always non-essential.

In our patient (Case V) the sensory disturbances were multiple. This woman had anesthesia to pin prick and temperature, which was absolute on the sole of the foot, equally pronounced on the leg, and less marked on the thigh. Deep pain was also absent in the foot. Considerable delay of the sensations was noted, and they persisted for several minutes. Muscle sense also seems to be a little affected in the most involved parts.

Another phenomenon pertinent here is the presence of pain in this patient. However, this occurred only about two years after the onset of the weakness and muscle atrophy. It affected both lower limbs almost equally, although only one was distinctly atrophied. The pain lasted about two years and only reappeared later at rare intervals. It never appeared in the upper limbs, where there were only momentary mild sensations of numbness. . . .

Although pain can exist in the affliction we are studying, we cannot conclude that it is a principal and fundamental characteristic. Far from it, in the large majority of cases, pain, as well as other sensory disorders, do not exist at all, and even when it appears it seems to be completely non-essential. Thus, in our Case V the pain only appeared two years after the beginning of the atrophy in the feet and legs. It never reached the upper limbs, even though these were the sites of obvious lesions for a long time.

There is another phenomenon that is more or less painful but is evidently of another type and manifests itself in a completely different way. We refer to cramps. They occurred in almost all of our patients with a characteristic frequency and intensity such that they never failed to attract our attention. These cramps appear preferentially in the thigh muscles, especially on brisk voluntary movement and on electrical stimulation.

After this discussion of each particular symptom, it will be useful to say a few words about the general appearance of these patients since it is very special and completely typical.

The individuals affected usually enjoy perfect health, and their general nutrition leaves nothing to be desired. There is a singular contrast between the proportions of the distal extremities and those of the trunk and roots of the limbs. Thus it is understandable that one could (Eulenburg) consider

---

1. A French phrase referring to the leg of a marionette that dangles uncontrollably (translation note).

the thigh muscles as hypertrophied, although in our opinion this view is not exactly right. Foot-drop is present. There is little or no deviation of the feet when not on the floor, but they place themselves in varus or valgus when they support the weight of the body. The calf-less legs are almost cylindrical, at the most slightly conical. The internal condyles make a considerable bulge, and when the legs are placed together there is contact only at the malleoli and the most internal part of the condyles. Above and below, large empty spaces can be seen. The upper space comes from the flattening of the internal part of the thigh due to atrophy of the vastus internus. The lower part of the thigh above the patella is not in proportion with the upper part as a consequence of the greater atrophy at this level. Concerning the hands, it will suffice to recall, without wishing to repeat ourselves, that at a certain period they have the distinct appearance of the interosseous claw.

Moreover, the functional disturbances are not less characteristic. One finds a most marked step-page gait owing to the paralysis of the foot extensors. The steppage gait is such that a similarity to the walk of horses is very striking. Furthermore, even while resting in the standing position, the patient cannot stay immobile and is constantly obliged to stamp in place to keep his balance. All these functional disorders are evidently due to the wasting of the leg muscles. Eventually the tibio-tarsal articulation is no longer fixed, and the malleoli are in a state of pronounced instability with respect to the foot. Balance is compromised and can be maintained only by moving the whole leg into a more suitable position. Thus, one sees that the comparison with stilts, which naturally comes to mind and which Eulenburg has already made, is not really exact since it is not the poor function of the knee but of the tibio-tarsal articulation that is the main cause of these functional disturbances. It is for the same reason that walking becomes more difficult barefoot than when boots hold the foot and prevent it from turning.

So far we have dealt with the symptomatology of this affliction. We have still to discuss its onset and progression.

The onset is usually in childhood or adolescence. This has been true in the five cases we observed. Among the 19 cases that we could gather from different authors, in 14 the disease appeared before age 22. During childhood it is especially likely to appear at the age of 4 years; during adolescence at 15 or 16. In one of Eichhorst's cases (Ernest) it was perhaps congenital. It seems,

though, that it can appear later. One of Eichhorst's patients was 36, and two members of the Wetherbee family were stricken at the age of 39.

Another important fact concerning etiology is the influence of heredity. It is found in all the cases of the various authors. The patients of Eulenburg are twin brothers; ten members of the family studied by Eichhorst had the affliction, without counting the distant ancestors; in the Wetherbee family the great-grandfather, his two sons, his two daughters, E. H. Wetherbee's father, himself and his sister were equally affected. . . . From the preceding, it is evident that hereditary influence is indisputable and that, in some cases, the disease has the distinct appearance of a familial malady.

Is it always so? From the facts we have observed, we can confidently answer: no. In our cases I, IV, V, none of the members of the family was affected, and we could verify this ourselves in some. Of course, it cannot be asserted that it will not begin later in some of them, but, in the ancestors at least, it is certain that nothing similar occurred. On the other hand, it is true that a distinct familial factor was found in our cases II and III, which were two brothers, Henri and Gonzalo X. . . . We may add that their 9-year old sister is still completely normal, as we ascertained by a thorough examination.

We conclude that a familial factor, although very evident in a large number of cases, is missing in others and that even in families where several members are stricken, others are completely spared. This is a fact already noted in the cases of Eichhorst and Hammond. Can we say that the girls are affected less often than the boys? The facts do not seem to be numerous enough to allow a definite statement.

Concerning the causes of this disease, we know nothing for certain. . . .

Neuropathic heredity in its largest sense seems to deserve some attention here. For example, the father of our patients Henri and Gonzalo X . . . , who did not present any muscular atrophy, was so affected mentally that he was placed in a mental hospital.

There is still the matter left of the nature of this affliction. In the absence of an autopsy it is impossible to assert anything on this subject. However, one can, reasoning by analogy, arrive at hypotheses, which, if not certain, are at least very probable.

In the presence of muscular atrophy having the

appearance of a familial disease, occurring during childhood or adolescence, and having a slowly progressive course one can and must ask if it is not a myopathy.[1]

We do not think this is the case here, for the following reasons. All that we know about the localization of the affected muscles in simple progressive myopathy is completely contrary to what exists in the disease we are studying. In the former it always starts either in the trunk muscles or in the proximal muscles of the limbs. In the latter, on the contrary, it always starts in the muscles of the distal extremities (feet, legs, later the lower part of the thigh muscles, the intrinsic hand muscles), and the trunk muscles are not affected. This is a clinical fact of great importance. The two diseases are, therefore, completely different in localization, and it could almost be said that one attacks those muscles which the other spares. The Leyden-Möbius form seems at first to come close to our cases because of the predominance of atrophy in the lower limbs. However, after careful examination, this form is seen to be much further from our cases than from the different forms of simple progressive myopathy. Moreover, our patients show some signs that are in contradistinction to those we commonly meet in myopathy. Definite fibrillary contractions occur, which are never found in the latter. Also, there is a reaction of degeneration, whereas in the latter there is only a diminution of excitability without inversion of the formula.

It seems to us that these are serious arguments against the indentity or at least the similarity of these two diseases. As to the hereditary character, it is well to remember that this is not peculiar to myopathies and that it can be present in diseases of an established myelopathic nature. This occurs,

for example, in the hereditary ataxia of Friedreich, which as we know, is a familial disease associated with very gross lesions of the cord.

Are we, therefore, in the presence of a myelopathy? Is it a peripheral polyneuritis? Here, we must confess, the question becomes much more delicate, especially in the presence of the cases where there is pain or various sensory disturbances. Up to a certain point the hypothesis of a myelopathy appears preferable to us, but it seems difficult to make an absolute statement.

We thought it would be of some interest to gather similar cases from the medical literature. It will be seen that all these are similar to ours and in reality concern the same disease. It is quite strange that none of the authors who observed these patients has described them objectively and completely. Most of them noted only one aspect of the matter, especially heredity. Considering the time of publication, it is readily understandable that Eichhorst considered his patients simply an example of hereditary progressive muscular atrophy, as did Eulenburg and Hammond. It has, therefore, been necessary to affirm the existence of this clinical entity and to give a complete description of the disease, since no author had yet done so. This has been our aim.

To summarize all the documentation of this work, the principal characteristics of the form of muscular atrophy that we have attempted to isolate and describe seem to be the following:

Progressive muscular atrophy, first invading the feet and legs and only appearing in the upper limbs (hands first, then forearms) several years later; thus, slow evolution.

Relative integrity of the proximal muscles of the limbs, or at least much longer preservation than the distal muscles. Integrity of the muscles of the trunk, shoulders, and face.

Existence of fibrillary contractions in the muscles undergoing atrophy.

Vasomotor disturbances in the affected segments of limbs.

No notable tendinous contractures on the side of articulations where the muscles are atrophied.

Sensation most often intact, though sometimes altered in various ways.

Frequency of cramps.

Reaction of degeneration in the muscles undergoing atrophy.

Beginning of the disease usually during childhood, often among several brothers and sisters; sometimes it exists not only in collateral relatives but also in the forebears.

---

1. Messrs. Landouzy and Dejerine (Concerning Progressive Atrophic Myopathy, *Revue de Médecine*, 1885, p. 354 and following), commenting on Eichhorst's, Hammonds's and Ormerod's cases, considered them myopathic and classified them in their outline of muscular atrophies as Eichhorst's femoral-tibial type. This point of view seemed warranted by the interpretation of symtomatology and of evolution reported by Eichhorst as well as by the hereditary character of the atrophies. We explained above why the examination of cases at the Salpêtrière does not allow us to accept the nosologic interpretation proposed by Messrs. Landouzy and Dejerine. As for the word femoral-tibial, it seems inadequate to characterize the clinical aspects of this affliction in which the alteration of the femoral musculature is, as a whole, quite secondary, while that of the foot and hand muscles deserves special notice. We also think that the name of Eichhorst should not be retained, since Eulenburg's observation precedes Eichhorst's by 17 years and is not inferior in the study of the affected muscles. Moreover, the idea of heredity is also mentioned by Eulenburg.

IV   Encephalitis Lethargica

BARON Constantin von Economo was a man of varied background and interests.[1,2] Of Greek descent, von Economo was born in Rumania in 1876, studied in Austria, France, and Germany, and worked in Vienna until his death in 1931. In addition to his medical accomplishments, von Economo was a pioneering balloon and airplane pilot and enthusiastically promoted international aviation meetings.

His work in psychiatry and neurology was carried out in the clinic of Julius Wagner von Jauregg at the University of Vienna, and it was there that he detected encephalitis lethargica. As an outgrowth of his interest in encephalitis, von Economo also made important contributions to the study of the cerebral control of sleep. In all, 27 of his publications concerned encephalitis lethargica, including a book published in his last years.[3]

Von Economo's disease was the first epidemic of encephalitis to be clearly recognized and described. It raged in Europe and North America between 1916 and 1926, and when it receded into history its etiology had not yet been established. Because the influenza pandemic was nearly concurrent with the epidemic of encephalitis lethargica, some authors have tended to confuse the two diseases. However, von Economo made the distinction as follows:

When I described this new disease of encephalitis lethargica during the winter of 1916-17 in Vienna, I called the condition, on account of its slight febrile prodromal state, and in consequence of the role of the nasopharynx as the "gateway" of the infection, a "gripp-like" disease, and remarked on the likeness between its early stages and those of epidemic meningitis. But I should like here to emphasize the fact that, though there were many cases of "colds" in Vienna at that time, there was not any particularly notable increase in those influenza-like cases which are always a constant feature during the winter; certainly there was no epidemic of such a kind (i.e. at the time of my first encephalitis lethargica publication). . . . Only a year and a half later grippe, i.e. influenza—(Spanish grippe as it was then called)—appeared and took its heavy toll as a pandemic; in its wake encephalitis soon flared up again. . . . But the first cases of encephalitis, as was afterwards historically ascertained, had already appeared in some European countries a year before I recognized this disease as a new entity. Cruchet claimed to have observed several cases in the winter of 1915-16 amongst the French soldiers in Verdun, while a few cases are said to have been seen in Rumania by Urechia as early as the spring of 1915, and even though the observers failed to recognize the appearance of a hitherto unknown disease their descriptions were sufficiently accurate to identify their cases a few years later as our encephalitis. . . .[3]

The importance of von Economo's disease lies mainly in its legacy of postencephalitic parkinsonism. A large number of individuals who contracted encephalitis lethargica subsequently developed parkinsonism, though there was often a latent period of many years. More recent epidemics of encephalitis have occurred, but they probably differ from von Economo's disease since they have not had this sequela.[4]

References

1. von Economo, K., and von Wagner-Jauregg, J.: *Baron Constantin von Economo: His Life and Work*, R. Spillman (trans.), Burlington, Vt: Free Press Interstate Printing Corp., 1937.

2. Kolle, K.: Genealogie der Nervenärzte des deutschen Sprachgebietes, *Fortschr Neurol Psychiat* 32:512-538, 1964.

3. von Economo, C.: *Encephalitis Lethargica, Sequelae and Treatment*, K.O. Newman (trans.), London: Oxford University Press, 1931, pp 2-3.

4. Duvoisin, R.C., and Yahr, M.D.: Encephalitis and Parkinsonism, *Arch Neurol* 12:227-239, 1965.

From the Psychiatric Clinic in Vienna (Director:
Hofrat Prof. J. Wagner v. Jauregg.)

Encephalitis lethargica*

by Priv.-Doz. C. v. Economo, Assistant to the Clinic

Since Christmas, we have had the opportunity to observe a series of cases at the psychiatric clinic that do not fit any of our usual diagnoses. Nevertheless, they show a similarity in type of onset and symptomatology that forces one to group them into one clinical picture. We are dealing with a kind of sleeping sickness, so to speak, having an unusually prolonged course. The first symptoms are usually acute, with headaches and malaise. Then a state of somnolence appears, often associated with active delirium, from which the patient can be awakened easily. He is able to give appropriate answers and to comprehend the situation. He can follow commands correctly and is able to walk and stand, but if left by himself, he falls back into his somnolent state. This delirious somnolence can lead to death, rapidly, or over the course of a few weeks. On the other hand, it can persist unchanged for weeks or even months with periods, lasting hours or days or even longer, of fluctuation of the depth of unconsciousness, extending from simple sleepiness to deepest stupor and coma. It is also possible for a gradual improvement to take place, but the patients are psychically weakened for a long time thereafter. In the mildest cases, the sleepiness persists only briefly and quickly disappears, so that the clinical picture is dominated by possible coexisting paralysis, which we will discuss later.

In the very beginning, during the first days of illness, isolated signs of meningeal irritation appear, but never in a very pronounced way (a slight stiffness of the neck or just sensitivity to pressure in the neck, sensitivity to tapping the skull, pressure sensitivity of the eyes, and rarely an indication of a Kernig's sign).

The disease can run its course with or without fever. The temperature curve does not have a particular pattern. The appearance of fever and its intensity do not seem to have any effect upon the course and the signs of the disease. Even the depth of the somnolent-delirious state is completely independent of the fever, and we have

seen one febrile patient who in fever-free moments was even more delirious than before.

As a rule, these general symptoms are joined by paralysis in the distribution of the cranial nerves as well as in the extremities. The ocular muscles are affected particularly often. A slight ptosis, which can be interpreted as physiological heaviness of the eyelids due to the somnolence and which can be overcome with vigorous effort by the patient, gradually becomes a paralytic ptosis, often combined with a partial or total paralysis of the other branches of the oculomotor nerve. Paresis of the other ocular nerves, as well as paresis of other cranial nerves and paralysis of the extremities with reflex disturbances, can occur also. The disturbance of the ocular muscles can be the first sign of this clinical picture, and somnolence in a more or less pronounced form, may appear only later or may even be totally absent.

One gets the impression that one is dealing in these cases with one and the same disease process—an encephalitis—differing only in localization. Its recent increase in incidence suggests that we are dealing with a small epidemic of encephalitis. . . .

[Seven case reports follow.]

After the suspicion of tuberculous and other types of meningitis was dispelled by frequent lumbar punctures, by observation of the clinical course, by the recoveries, and by the post-mortem findings, a different diagnosis had to be considered. The slight signs of meningeal irritation, the paralysis of ocular muscles and extremities, and the subsequent disappearance of the signs made the diagnosis of encephalitis (polioencephalitis) seem justified in all these cases. This supposition was confirmed by the post-mortem findings.

Reviewing the individual symptoms, we find in most cases an acute onset with dizziness, headaches, and possibly fever. Only cases 4 and 6 started insidiously.

The most striking symptom of this disease is the sleepiness of the patients, which at times is associated with delirium and at times is not. This somnolence can vary from light sleep, entirely

---

*Translation of: Encephalitis Lethargica, *Wien Klin Wschr*, 30:581-585, 1917.

resembling physiological sleep, to the deepest stupor, independent of any fever. Case 3 was most remarkable in this respect. Usually one could awaken him by simply talking to him, but at other times he could not be awakened even by shaking. As a rule, delirium is present, but in case 1 it was absent throughout the entire illness. Its presence and intensity, however, are totally independent of the depth of the sleep and the severity of the fever. Case 1, who was never delirious, did not even have delirium when the fever climbed to 39°. Cases 3 and 5 were very actively delirious without fever. In the presence of these symptoms, one automatically thinks of a disease that raged through northern Italy during the 1890's. It was called nona in the vernacular, and, because of its puzzling nature, it was discussed frequently in the newspapers. This disease appeared at the time of the great influenza epidemic in the form of a lethargy with delirium, and it developed a malignant character. At that time, it was debated whether the grippe or typhus could be the cause of this somnolent state. The first report of such an epidemic was made in 1712. At that time, there was supposed to have been an epidemic in Tübingen, characterized by sleepiness and marked cerebral symptoms. . . .

I did not find anything about nona in the Italian medical journals available to me except the above mentioned remarks in Epstein's work.[2]

As far as the fever in our cases is concerned, we find that nearly every case is different. Malaise and chills usually were given as the first symptoms, but whether there also was fever could not be determined. Only in cases 2 and 4 could fever be detected at the onset with certainty. In case 2 the fever even became typhoid-like with daily variations from 38° in the morning to 40° in the evening and finally a lytic termination. In case 4 the fever increased throughout the entire illness to reach a height of 39.8° immediately before death. In the other cases, the fever was only significant periodically or was not even present at all (cases 3 and 7 and, even though it terminated with death, case 5).

Aside from the topor, slight meningeal symptoms are part of the clinical picture. Some cases were even brought to the clinic with the diagnosis of meningitis. However, these symptoms usually are not very pronounced. Only case 2 exhibited a meningitic picture for a few days. Most frequently one can find sensitivity of the eyes to pressure, sensitivity of the skull to percussion, and tenderness of the neck. Nuchal stiffness is present less frequently. Often a Kernig sign and hyperesthesia of the soles of the feet are present.

In all cases the spinal fluid was examined carefully and repeatedly by Dr. Schacherl. The fluid showed increased pressure usually at the beginning of the illness, as in cases 1, 2, 4, and 5. It later decreased in spite of persistent somnolence. The Nonne-Apelt reaction was negative in all cases. The total protein content was below the normal upper limit of 2.2 given by Nissl. The colloidal gold reaction showed no typical curve. The number of cellular elements in most cases was at the upper limit of normal. Only in cases 1 and 2 was there a distinct increase in cellular elements: in case 1, 43 cells/mm^3, in case 2, 19 cells/mm^3. Remarkable in these two cases was the strong predominance of polymorphonuclear leukocytes over lymphocytes. Repeated examinations for microorganisms was negative in every case.

The Wassermann reaction in the serum and spinal fluid was always negative.

A relatively constant sign is ocular muscle disturbance, especially in the distribution of the oculomotor nerve. The bilaterality and symmetry of the disease and the fact that the oculomotor palsy is only external, with the pupillary reaction and accommodation remaining undisturbed, speak against a pure neuropathy and for a central disease. The most remarkable sign of the oculomotor disturbance, and frequently one of the very first signs of the disease, is bilateral ptosis. Because of the existing lethargy, it is often hard to differentiate a slight palsy from a physiological relaxation of the levator palpebrae, particularly since the ptosis can vary from the slightest degree to a complete closure of the eyelids. In cases 1 and 6 we also found all the other branches of the oculomotor nerve paralyzed except the internal. Abducens paralysis (case 2) also occurs as well as gaze palsies and nystagmus (cases 3 and 7). Paresis of other cranial nerves, such as VII and IX, we saw in case 3 and in case 4, where singultus appeared unilaterally (!) as an early symptom and persisted throughout the 3-week illness until death. Here we have to consider an irritation of the phrenic nerve by the disease process.

The paralytic and irritative signs in the extremities also belong to the characteristic signs of this clinical picture. We often have, from the beginning, a unilateral increase in reflexes, a Babin-

---

[2]B. kl. W. 1891 Nr. 41—Some remarks on the so-called "nona."

ski phenomenon or even a slight paresis of the upper and lower extremities, which can progress to a paralysis (cases 1 and 4). As the residual of such a paresis, spasms, increased reflexes, or the Babinski phenomenon can persist for a long time, even long after the ocular muscle paralysis and somnolence have receded (cases 2, 7). Aside from the paralysis of the extremities, one often finds, as a rather obvious sign, a peculiar rigidity of the extremities (cases 1, 2 and 4). Like most of the signs, this rigidity disappears later.

Besides these signs of paralysis and irritation, we frequently find (cases 1, 2, 3, 4, 7) ataxic disturbances that make one think of involvement of the cerebellum. In case 1 the peculiar unsteady gait was noted the first day. Then it was joined by an ataxic tremor of the right upper extremity. Case 7 demonstrated these disturbances most obviously, with severe ataxic tremor not only of the lower and upper extremities, but also of the trunk and head. When the patient left the hospital improved and most of her symptoms had disappeared, one would have diagnosed multiple sclerosis because of the persistent ataxia and tremor and history of nystagmus and compulsive laughing, if one did not know of the stuporous phase of the illness. Such encephalitides that particularly affect the brain stem and cause only a few general symptoms are very hard to distinguish from acute multiple sclerosis except by observation of the course of the disease.[3] With reference to this pontine encephalitis I would like to describe briefly several cases that have been seen in the emergency room during the same period of time (January to March). . . .

[Six case reports follow.]

All of these last cases of diseases of the ocular nerve nuclei, which have changed little as long as we have been able to follow them, permit the probable diagnosis of pontine encephalitis. They probably belong to the disease we have described except that in the latter cases the symptoms of giddiness and sleepiness, characteristic of the first seven cases, are missing because of a different localization and smaller extension of the lesions.

We now ask ourselves what the cause of this disease might be. In the first place, one must think of an etiological factor from the group of microorganisms because of the increased incidence

of the disease. We also thought of the possibility, in the first cases, of a toxic process such as sausage poisoning, since this would be conceivable in view of the poor nutrition during the present war time. However, with the increased occurrence of these cases there was a total lack of gastrointestinal disturbances and we soon had to drop this idea. A possible common etiology through gas poisoning could not have been missed in the anamnestic questioning during repeated outbreaks of the illness. We never found any evidence for typhus which has been described in similar circumstances. Examination of the spleen and of the blood and the post-mortem findings permit one to exclude the possibility of typhus completely. The next suspicion was that this could be an influenzal encephalitis. This suspicion came readily to mind since Leichtenstern[4] and Oppenheim had emphasized the frequent occurrence of encephalitis with epidemics of influenza and since Nauwerk's study had demonstrated Pfeiffer's bacillus in foci of encephalomalacia. We therefore always examined the spinal fluid especially for influenza bacilli. These tests, however, as well as those on the material from the two autopsies, were negative. The negative findings in our cases, however, as with all negative results, do not exclude the possibility of an influenzal brain disease. The time of year when the disease occurred at least speaks for the idea that it could belong to the group of respiratory illnesses. The appearance of an influenzal encephalitis during epidemics of influenza is not rare. I would like to remind you, however, that we now have seen quite a lot of "grippe" in Vienna, but we have noted no influenza epidemic with proven Pfeiffer's bacillus any more than in other years. Recently, for instance, no fatal cases of influenza have come to the pathologic-anatomic institute for autopsy. We want to emphasize, however, that most of our cases started with the feeling of a cold, headache and general malaise and possibly joint pains. One could also think of a disease that at times can cause encephalitic symptoms, namely Heine-Medin poliomyelitis. The post-mortem finding in case 5 of a grayish-red discoloration of the spinal cord, and particularly of its gray substance, suggested this diagnosis on the dissecting table. However, recently we have heard or seen nothing of a poliomyelitis epidemic in Vienna. Of our cases, no two were from the same district of the city. Furthermore, we want to point out the regularly

---

[3]In this regard see Arch. f. Psych. 1914, 54. Simmerling and Räcke. "Beitr. z. Klin. und Path. d. mult. Scler." and also G. Henning, "Ueber seltenere Formen der akuten nicht eitrigen Enzephalitis", where the entire pertinent literature is to be found.

[4]D. med. W. 1890, pp. 509-642.

negative Wassermann reaction, which in many cases of early poliomyelitis is positive in the blood. Our cases were always tested immediately for this. Moreover, most of our cases, with the exception of case 4, had passed childhood.

The macroscopic autopsy findings of the fatal cases showed above all that in these two cases, and most likely in the others also, we are dealing with one and the same peculiar disease process, which is an acute inflammatory disease of the brain stem with involvement of the cerebrum. Tuberculosis could be excluded with certainty.

The microscopic findings, which are identical in both cases, prove indisputably that we are dealing with a single inflammatory process. There is a tremendous infiltration by small cells of the vessels in the gray matter of the third ventricle, the area of the ocular nuclei, around the aqueduct of Sylvius and the floor of the fourth ventricle. This infiltration at first is limited to the vascular sheaths. It extends caudally into the medulla oblongata. The vessels of the spinal cord are less affected. The vascular sheaths are congested with lymphocytes and plasma cells. Furthermore, the gray matter in individual areas appears to be strewn with mononuclear cells and to be somewhat edematous. These cells are distributed uniformly throughout the tissue. Such a focus in the medulla in the vagal nucleus probably caused death due to pulmonary edema in case 4, and in case 5 it must have caused the symptom of singultus due to irritation of the phrenic nerve. In the spinal cord of case 4, at the cervical as well as at the lumbar levels, we could demonstrate in the posterior horns small foci of inflammation with lymphocytic infiltration of the vascular sheaths and their adjacent areas. A predilection for the nerve cells cannot be observed in the spinal cord (in contrast to poliomyelitis of Heine-Medin), and signs of neuronophagia occur, but only rarely. In individual areas within the tissue of the medulla oblongata, one can find small aggregations of polymorphonuclear leukocytes, the meaning of which we do not know as yet.

We found the same alterations in the cerebrum, quite pronounced in individual areas. The blood vessels of the cortex were surrounded by a mantle of lymphocytes and plasma cells. Here, too, we found the peculiar nests of polymorphonuclear leukocytes, as well as much more distinct neuronophagia than in the other parts of the nervous system. These peculiar inflammatory alterations appear in spots. As far as our examinations show at present, the greater part of the cere-bral cortex appears to be free of severe inflammatory lesions. The cerebral white matter remains, for the most part, free of the disease process. Only close to the cortex are the vessels of the white matter also infiltrated at times. On the other hand, there exists a severe hyperemia of the cerebral cortex as well as of the spinal cord. All blood vessels are congested with blood, but bleeding generally does not occur. Only in a single area in the floor of the fourth ventricle (case 5) and in some isolated areas of the cerebral cortex (case 4) could we observe an extravasation of blood into the perivascular space. Otherwise, we could find no hemorrhage in these two cases and could detect thus far no bleeding into the tissue. We particularly stress this because influenzal encephalitis generally has a hemorrhagic character. Neither the meninges on the surface of the cerebral cortex nor on the spinal cord are severely altered. A small collection of lymphocytes in the pia can be found in the region of the brain stem. Here, too, they are seen particularly around individual vessels and not spread over a large area.

Therefore, we have the histologic picture of a *polioencephalitis cerebri, pontis et medullae oblongatae, with a slight poliomyelitis of a perivascular, inflammatory and diffusely infiltrative but not hemorrhagic and only slightly neuronophagic character.*

We therefore think that this encephalitis of somewhat epidemic occurrence, with the peculiar symptom of somnolence, and with characteristic anatomic-histologic findings is a specific disease sui generis and must be caused by a specific, living virus. We also think that the remarkable *paucity of the general symptoms of "grippe" and the severity of the cerebral symptoms indicate a specific affinity for the central nervous tissue, similar but not identical to the virus of poliomyelitis (Heine-Medin).*

In the staining experiments for bacteria, which we did with tissue sections, we found, in isolated areas of the meninges, coccus-like formations. We communicate this finding here only with the greatest reservations. The appropriate further bacteriologic examinations (inoculations, etc.) are being carried out by Prof. Wiesner of the pathologic-anatomic institute of Prof. Koliskos. If such cases of encephalitis lethargica should come to exitus in the care of other colleagues, it would be very much appreciated in the interest of research if the anatomical material could also be sent for examination to Prof. Wiesner in the pathologic-anatomic institute.

V   Guillain-Barré-Strohl Syndrome

IN the midst of World War I, Georges Guillain, J. A. Barré, and A. Strohl made an important contribution to neurology by reporting an illness in two French soldiers. The significance of their observation did not lie in the description of a new disease. Landry,[1] in 1859, had reported a similar condition, characterized by acute ascending paralysis, which was mainly motor and which usually led to complete recovery. Following this original description, Landry's paralysis had become a well-known clinical entity. The contribution of Guillain, Barré, and Strohl was made possible by Quincke's introduction of the technique of lumbar puncture in 1891[2] and consisted in the observation of increased protein in the spinal fluid without cellular reaction. The pathologic identification of the disease as a radiculopathy was not made by Landry, who observed no abnormality in the nervous system at autopsy, nor by Guillain, Barré, and Strohl, who had no autopsy material. Walter[3] and later Haymaker and Kernohan[4] found that the primary lesion is in the region where the motor and sensory roots join to form the spinal nerve.

The etiology of the condition was unknown to Landry and to Guillain, Barré, and Strohl, and is still undetermined. An infectious cause is possible, but there is much evidence in favor of an immunologic basis for the disease (see the review by Wiederholt et al[5]). It is interesting that Guillain, Barré, and Strohl's cases had no apparent antecedent illness, whereas Landry noted the onset of the condition during convalescence from an acute illness in two of the ten cases that he reviewed. Haymaker and Kernohan[4] found upper respiratory infection as a prodromal symptom in 58% of cases, and the condition has been reported to occur following or in association with a great variety of disorders.[5] It seems possible that the pathogenesis may differ in different cases.

Attempts have been made to establish rigid criteria for the diagnosis of Guillain-Barré-Strohl syndrome.[6,7] However, the clinical phenomena described by Guillain, Barré, and Strohl may more profitably be considered part of a wide spectrum of polyradiculoneuropathies that await further definition by the Neurological Classics of the future.

References

1. Landry, O.: Note sur la paralysie ascendante aigue, *Gaz hébdomadaire du médecine et de la chirurgie* 6:472-474, 486-488, 1859.

2. Quincke, H.: Die Lumbalpunction des Hydrocephalus, *Berlin Klin Wschr* 28:929-933, 965-968, 1891.

3. Walter, F.K.: Zur Frage der Lokalisation der Polyneuritis, *Z Ges Neurol Psych* 44:150-178, 1919.

4. Haymaker, W., and Kernohan, J.W.: The Landry-Guillain-Barré Syndrome: A Clinicopathologic Report of Fifty Fatal Cases and a Critique of the Literature, *Medicine* 28:59-141, 1949.

5. Wiederholt, W.C.; Mulder, D.W.; and Lambert E.H.: The Landry-Guillain-Barré-Strohl Syndrome or Polyradiculoneuropathy: Historical Review, Report on 97 Patients, and Present Concepts, *Mayo Clinic Proc* 39:427-451, 1964.

6. Guillain, G.: Radiculoneuritis With Acellular Hyperalbuminosis of the Cerebrospinal Fluid, *Arch Neurol Psychiat* 36:975-990, 1936.

7. Osler, L.D., and Sidell, A.D.: The Guillain-Barré Syndrome: The Need for Exact Diagnostic Criteria, *New Eng J Med* 262:964-969, 1960.

CONCERNING A SYNDROME OF RADICULAR NEURITIS WITH
HYPERALBUMINOSIS OF THE CEREBROSPINAL FLUID WITHOUT CELLULAR
REACTION. NOTES ON THE CLINICAL AND GRAPHIC CHARACTERISTICS
OF THE TENDON REFLEXES.*

BY MESSRS. GEORGES GUILLAIN, J. A. BARRE AND A. STROHL.

In the present note, we call attention to a clinical syndrome that we observed in two patients. The syndrome is characterized by motor disorders, abolition of the tendon reflexes with preservation of the cutaneous reflexes, paresthesias with slight disturbance of objective sensation, pain on pressure of the muscle masses, marked modifications in the electrical reactions of the nerves and muscles, and remarkable hyperalbuminosis of the cerebrospinal fluid with absence of cytologic reaction (albuminocytologic dissociation).

This syndrome seemed to us to depend on a concomitant injury of the spinal roots, the nerves, and the muscles, probably of infectious or toxic nature. It must be differentiated from cases of simple radiculitis, pure polyneuritis, and polymyositis. Experimental research by the graphic method on the speed of reflexes and their latencies and on the modalities of muscular contraction show the involvement, in this syndrome, of the entire peripheral neuromuscular motor apparatus. We particularly emphasize the hyperalbuminosis of the cerebrospinal fluid without cytologic reaction—a feature which, to our knowledge, has not been mentioned in similar cases.

Case I.—Soldier D . . ., from the . . . hussars, 25 years old, entered the Neurology Center of the VIth Army on August 20, 1916 because of a motor disorder of the upper and lower limbs. The affection started about July 25 with formications in the feet and weakness in the lower limbs

*Translation of: Sur un syndrome de radiculo-névrite avec hyperalbuminose du liquide céphalo-rachidien sans réaction cellulaire. Remarques sur les caractères cliniques et graphiques des réflexes tendineux, *Bulletins et mémoires de la société médicale des hôpitaux de paris* 40:1462-1470, 1916.

obliging him to stop after a 200 to 300 meter walk. In the following days, formications appeared in the upper limbs and the lower part of the face, and muscle strength diminished in the upper limbs.

These various symptoms developed without any particular cause. The patient had not had any recent infectious disease, not even a slight sore throat. He had shown no symptom of alimentary intoxication. He had not been greatly fatigued. We will add that in his medical history no important fact could be found; the patient denied any syphilitic infection and any alcoholic habit.

The first examination on August 25 allowed us to establish the following:

Muscle strength is reduced in the upper and lower limbs in global fashion without, however, a total paralysis. This diminution of muscle strength is especially marked distally, where great weakness is noted in flexion and extension of the toes, of the foot on the leg, of the fingers, and of the hand on the forearm.

The trunk muscles are weak. Thus, the patient lying down cannot sit up spontaneously without reaching for support.

He can only walk a few steps before some instability is noted. He cannot maintain himself standing on one foot.

There is no disorder of the facial musculature.

Electrical examination shows that in the upper limbs faradic excitability is normal and galvanic excitability is good for all muscles with strong shocks. There is no polar inversion. A slight hypoexcitability of the common extensor of the fingers is noted. In the lower limbs, faradic excitability is slightly diminished. Galvanic excitability is also diminished for the trunk of the sciatic nerve, the internal popliteal nerve, the semitendinosus, and the extensor of the toes. Sometimes when the shock is slowly reduced polar inversion is noted for the external gemellus, but the reaction of degeneration is very incomplete.

The patellar, achilles, and medio-plantar reflexes, tested with the percussion hammer, are abolished, as are the antibrachial, radial-and ulnar-pronator and olecranon reflexes.

The plantar reflex elicits frank flexion of the toes with distant contraction of the tensor fasciae latae. The cremasteric and cutaneous abdominal reflexes are normal. No defense reflex is observed either by pinching the instep or by hyperflexion of the toes.

Neuromuscular excitability to the percussion hammer is preserved.

The patient complains incessantly of formications in both feet to above the ankles and in both hands to above the wrists. There are no clearly appreciable disorders of objective sensation except a slight decrease to touch, temperature, and pain in the feet and hands. The muscle masses of the upper and lower limbs are painful on pressure.

The pupils are equal in size and react to light and accommodation.

There are no sphincteric disorders.

There is no fever and no respiratory or gastrointestinal disorder. The pulse is normal.

The urine, examined at the Laboratory of Bacteriology and Chemistry of the Army, contains no sugar, albumin, or indoxyl. Chemical elements are in their normal proportions.

The lumbar puncture reveals clear cerebrospinal fluid, not under increased pressure. The fluid is hyperalbuminous (2.5 grams of albumin per liter) without leucocytic reaction (2 to 4 lymphocytes per field).

The Wassermann reaction in the blood is negative.

Culture of the pharynx and nasal mucus shows the absence of any diphtheria bacillus.

Treatment consists of absolute bed rest, massage of the upper and lower limbs, injections of strychnine, salicylate of soda and salol.

On August 27, the formications are diminished in the lower limbs.

On Sept. 2, some improvement of muscle strength is noted and there are no more formications in the feet. Formications persist in the hands. Tendon reflexes are still absent. A new lumbar puncture shows, as had the previous one, a very marked hyperalbuminosis without appreciable leucocytic reaction.

On Sept. 19, the motor disturbance is very much improved. The patient can walk for an hour and can maintain himself on one foot. The paresthesias have disappeared completely in the lower limbs; they persist, though attenuated, in the hands. Tendon reflexes are clinically absent. Defense reflexes are nil; cutaneous reflexes are normal. Neuromuscular excitability to the percussion hammer seems normal in the upper and lower limbs and in the face.

The patient, progressively improving, was sent to convalesce on Sept. 30.

.   .   .

The two cases we have described are entirely similar. In these two patients a clinical syndrome developed without apparent cause. As we said at the beginning, the syndrome is characterized by a motor disturbance affecting all the muscles of the upper and lower limbs but predominantly the distal muscles; loss of the tendon reflexes; with preservation of all the cutaneous reflexes; paresthesias with slight impairment of objective sensation; pain on pressure of the muscle masses; minimal change in the electrical reactions of nerves and muscles; and an unusual abnormality of the cerebrospinal fluid, characterized by a marked hyperalbuminosis without cytologic reaction.

The striking hyperalbuminosis of the cerebrospinal fluid without cellular reaction is a feature that seems to us to be of signal importance. This albuminocytologic dissociation (Sicard and Foix) is observed most often in some spinal-cord compressions, in Pott's disease, and in some cases of syphilis of the neuraxis, but it has not been described, it seems to us, in case of pure radiculitis and polyneuritis.

.   .   .

All the disorders observed in these two patients are attributable to simultaneous pathology of the spinal roots, peripheral nerves and muscles. The considerable hyperalbuminosis of the cerebrospinal fluid is evidence of meningeal involvement. The character of the paralytic difficulty, predominant in the distal portions of the extremities, and the pain in the muscle masses on pressure show involvement of muscle and nerve. Moreover, it seems to us that the distinction between polyneuritis and polymyositis is too schematized in neurology. In a large number of cases of infectious or toxic polyneuritis, the intramuscular nerve terminals and the muscle fibers themselves can be involved. In reality, it may very often be more a matter of polyneuromyositis than pure polyneuritis.

.   .   .

Therefore, while the simple clinical examination allows us only to ascertain the loss of tendon reflexes, the detailed analysis of the myographic curves reveals which elements of the reflex have undergone alteration. The following remarks are worthy of interest. The complete disappearance of the reflex portion of the myographic curve, or, when it remains, its morphologic character of extremely reduced amplitude, great slowness, and considerable delay, almost double the normal, show the profound and predominant alteration of the nerve conductors or of the central part of the reflex. Moreover, the direct response of the muscle also seems modified, diminished in amplitude, slowed, and delayed in appearance. It leads us to think that the muscular element has also been af-

fected by the toxic process. Finally, the comparison of the curves obtained after percussion of the patellar and achilles tendons allows us to describe a different evolution for these two reflexes. While the first was lost rapidly and showed no tendency to reappear until the patient left the hospital, the second, although it seemed lost clinically, could be recorded with characteristics progressively approaching normal. We stress the important fact that the graphic method allows a much more precise understanding of the state of the tendon reflexes than does examination with the percussion hammer.

The pathogenesis of the syndrome of radicular neuritis observed in our patients could not be determined precisely. Infection or intoxication must doubtless be considered, but we could not find them. The prognosis does not seem very grave if we judge by the evolution of the affection in our two patients. The first was almost cured and the second on the way to improvement when they were evacuated from the Army.

VI Ramsay Hunt Syndrome

R AMSAY HUNT'S original description of geniculate herpes zoster is a model of thoughtful analysis applied to a clinical observation. From an eruption in the ear, Hunt was able to define the concept of inflammation of cranial nerve ganglia and deduce the sensory distribution of the facial nerve. Hunt, who was an American neurologist, saw in geniculate herpes not only a new syndrome but also a unique neuroanatomical demonstration, and he elaborated his ideas on the functions and dysfunctions of the seventh cranial nerve in a series of articles over a period of 30 years. One significant contribution of the later papers was the description of oral eruptions in geniculate herpes.[1] A major review of the subject was published by him in 1937,[2] the year of his death.

Additions to Hunt's clinical picture have been made by other authors, and involvement of the ninth and tenth cranial nerves, along with the seventh nerve, has been observed in some cases of herpes zoster (see the review by McGovern and Fitz-Hugh[3]).

Although Ramsay Hunt's syndrome is recognized today just as he described it in 1907, his concept of the pathogenesis has not gone unchallenged. Hunt insisted that the geniculate ganglion is the site of the inflammation in herpes associated with facial palsy, but in his only postmortem study the geniculate ganglion was lost in prosection and was hence unavailable for examination. Later studies by others have failed to establish Hunt's thesis. Denny-Brown, Adams, and Fitzgerald[4] examined a case of cranial herpes zoster with facial palsy at autopsy and found inflammatory reaction and degeneration in the seventh nerve but no pathologic change in the geniculate ganglion. Nevertheless, the term "geniculate herpes" is generally retained and serves as a tribute to Ramsay Hunt's skill at lucid and logical interpretation.

References

1. Hunt, J.R.: The Sensory Field of the Facial Nerve: A Further Contribution to the Symptomatology of the Geniculate Ganglion, *Brain* **38**:418-446, 1915.
2. Hunt, J.R.: Geniculate Neuralgia (Neuralgia of the Nervus Facialis): A Further Contribution to the Sensory System of the Facial Nerve and its Neuralgic Conditions, *Arch Neurol Psychiat* **37**:253-285, 1937.
3. McGovern, F.H., and Fitz-Hugh, G.S.: Herpes Zoster of the Cephalic Extremity, *Arch Otolaryng* **55**:307-320, 1952.
4. Denny-Brown, D.; Adams, R.D.; and Fitzgerald, P.J.: Pathologic Features of Herpes Zoster: A Note on "Geniculate Herpes." *Arch Neurol Psychiat* **51**:216-231, 1944.

ON HERPETIC INFLAMMATIONS OF THE GENICULATE GANGLION. A NEW SYNDROME AND ITS COMPLICATIONS.*

By J. Ramsay Hunt, MD, of New York.

Chief of the Neurological Clinic and Instructor
in Nervous Diseases in the Cornell University
Medical College.
(From the Pathological Laboratory of the Cornell
University Medical College.)

Heretofore the only recognized seat of an herpetic inflammation on a cranial nerve was that of the Gasserian ganglion of the trifacial. Herpes zoster in the distribution of one or more of its branches was the result. I believe, however, that the geniculate ganglion situated in the depths of the internal auditory canal at the entrance to the Fallopian aqueduct may be the seat of this specific inflammation. . . .

As was long ago pointed out by Bärensprung and is now definitely established by the elaborate clinical and pathological researches of Head and Campbell, the primary or infectious form of herpes zoster is dependent upon a specific inflammation of one or more of the posterior spinal ganglia. Head suggested the name, posterior poliomyelitis for the affection, and certain points of resemblance were drawn between it and acute anterior poliomyelitis. The ganglia involved are swollen by the products of inflammation and by extravasation of blood, and in some cases even the sheath and nerve roots may be involved in the inflammatory process. In very rare instances the anterior or motor root, resting upon the sheath of the ganglion may be implicated and paralysis result. . . .

*Reprinted from *Journal of Nervous and Mental Disease* 34:73-96, 1907.

Where the herpetic inflammation attacks the geniculate ganglion, palsies are of much more frequent occurrence than in any other localization of the disease. I have collected 56 cases from the literature to which I can add 4 personal observations, making a total of 60 cases in which palsies accompanied the inflammation in this situation. This I would attribute to the peculiar location and relations of the ganglion involved.

Clinically the cases of geniculate herpes resolve themselves into three groups. The simplest expression of the disease is a herpes of the auricle and external auditory canal. *Within this skin area is to be found the zoster zone for the geniculate ganglion.* In another group of cases there is added to the aural herpes a paralysis of the facial nerve. This I explain by pressure of the inflamed ganglion or in some cases by a direct extension of the inflammation to the nerve. The most interesting, as well as the most severe, type of disease occurs when the acoustic nerve is also involved. In this form there are with herpes auricularis and facial palsy, various auditory symptoms, ranging in severity from tinnitus aurium and diminution of hearing to the more severe forms of acoustic involvement as seen in Ménière's syndrome. In these cases I assume that the inflammatory process has extended to the auditory nerve which is envel-

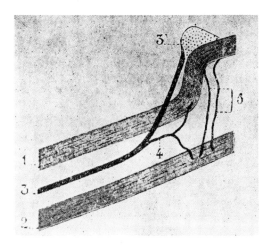

Testut.—Anastomoses of the facial and auditory nerves. I. Facial. 2. Auditory. 3. Nerve of Wrisberg. 3^1. Geniculate ganglion. 4. Internal anastomoses. 5. External anastomoses.

oped in the same sheath, and courses in the same canal as the facial nerve.

Each of these groups has separately been the subject of careful study by many observers; but their intimate clinical relationship to one another, their common pathology and their common seat of origin, the geniculate ganglion of the facial nerve, has not heretofore been recognized.

I have already expressed my belief that the geniculate ganglion has its cutaneous representation and zoster zone in the auricle and external auditory canal, and that herpes zoster in this region may have facial and auditory complications. In regard to the distribution of the zoster I wish to lay especial stress upon this fact, that while these neural complications occur in auricular herpes, they also accompany herpes facialis, herpes occipitalis and cervicalis. It will be observed that in these forms of zoster, the herpes facialis and herpes occipito-collaris, the zoster zones lie immediately in front of and behind that which I have indicated as the geniculate zoster zone. Thus the Gasserian, geniculate and 2d and 3d cervical ganglia may be regarded as forming a ganglionic series or chain, their cutaneous zones corresponding to the face, ear, head and neck.

An idea of the relative frequency of these neural complications and their associated herpetic eruptions may be obtained from the following statistics. In the 60 cases at my disposal for analysis, all had a facial palsy of the peripheral type. In 19 of these cases irritative or paralytic symptoms of acoustic origin were present. In 32 cases the cutaneous manifestation was herpes occipito-

collaris, in 12 cases herpes facialis, in 12 cases herpes auricularis, in 3 cases a combined herpes auricularis and occipito-collaris, in one case herpes facialis and occipito-collaris combined. I may also add that I have found but one case of herpes zoster with an associated facial palsy in which the eruption was not facial, auricular, or occipito-cervical. . . .

As the specific infection of herpes attacks only cells of the spinal ganglion type, the geniculate may very properly be brought within the sphere of its influence. Furthermore the intimate relations existing between the facial, the geniculate ganglion, and the terminal division of the acoustic would render all these structures liable to involvement when the seat of an inflammatory process; all the more because they are lodged in the depths of an osseous canal, within a common sheath, which would tend to resist expansion and increase the effect of pressure. (See Fig. 4.)

It may be added that the geniculate ganglion varies in size.

In some subjects it is scarcely visible to the naked eye; in others the swelling is double the caliber of the nerve. This may well have a certain influence in determining the severity of the case, anatomical peculiarities of the canal contributing.

The Zoster Zone for the Geniculate Ganglion.—Admitting the sensory nature of this ganglion, its analogy to a spinal ganglion and its probable involvement in cases of herpes zoster, it is still necessary to demonstrate the existence of a cutaneous area on the head or face to represent it. This area must be independent of other recognized zoster zones and in it should be found the zoster zone of the geniculate. This zone, I believe, is situated within the auricle and external auditory canal. My argument bearing on this part of the subject is briefly as follows: The peripheral innervation of the external ear is effected through the fifth nerve, branches of the cervical plexus, and *the auricular branch of the vagus.* The anterior half of the auricle and the superior and anterior walls of the external auditory canal are innervated by the auriculo-temporal branch of the trigeminus nerve. This nerve is a branch of the inferior division of the trigeminus, and I wish particularly to emphasize the neural connections existing between it and the geniculate ganglion through the otic ganglion and the small superficial petrosal nerve. The otic ganglion rests upon the inferior maxillary division of the fifth, just below its origin from the Gasserian. The posterior surface of the auricle receives its sensory innervation through the auricular branches of the superficial cervical plexus, which also overlap the rim and supply a posterior marginal area on its external surface. The inferior and posterior walls of the canal are supplied by the small auricular branch of the vagus, which also sends filaments to the interior of the concha. The ganglionic representations of sensation on the auricle and external auditory canal have been divided between the Gasserian in front and the second and third cervical ganglia behind. The anterior half of this region has been referred to the Gasserian and the posterior half to the cervical ganglion. An eruption of herpes in this area has been regarded as emanating from disease of one or other of these ganglia.

The error of the prevailing views will be shown by a study of the anesthesia produced by the extirpation of these ganglia for the relief of tic douloureux. In all of Krause's cases following extirpation of the Gasserian the sensation of the skin of the auricle and external auditory canal was found to be preserved and normal. In these operations during the tearing out of the ganglion, the connections existing between the fifth nerve, Meckel's ganglion, the otic ganglion, and the geniculate ganglion through the superficial petrosal nerves may be separated. This might cause confusion, by adding a geniculate anesthesia to that produced by removal of the Gasserian. This may have happened in some of Cushing's cases in which parts of the external auditory canal were found anesthetic after extirpation of the ganglion. The method of operation as practised by Frazier and Spiller is free from this disadvantage. It consists in cutting the sensory root of the fifth on the central side of the ganglion. In such a procedure as this there is no undue tension or tearing the neural connections between the geniculate, and the second and third divisions of the fifth are not implicated. No procedure could be more exact for protecting the ganglionic area of the Gasserian. Following this operation the sensation of the auricle and auditory canal was found to be normal. The ganglionic innervation of the second and third cervical ganglia has been studied in a case of extirpation for the relief of obstinate occipito-cervical neuralgia by Harvey Cushing. In outlining the anesthesia in this case Cushing found the posterior marginal area on its external surface anesthetic. The interior of the auricle and external auditory canal had normal sensation.

If we now bring together and carefully adjust these respective areas of anesthesia, produced by extirpation of the Gasserian and the cervical ganglia, there still remains the interior of the auricle, and the external auditory canal in which sensation is preserved. In this area, I believe, it is to be found the cutaneous representation of the geniculate ganglion and its zoster zone.

It will be recalled that the peripheral innervation of this skin area is furnished by the auriculo-temporal branch of the third division of the fifth, and the auricular branch of the vagus. That these fibers do not pass through the inferior division of the fifth to the Gasserian is demonstrated by the anesthesia resulting from section of the sensory root of the fifth, this area retaining its sensation. If their afferent course is not through the trigeminus, how do they reach the brain? The relation of these sensory fibers to the geniculate ganglion is established if we accept the occurrence of geniculate herpes with a zoster zone in the auricle. So that it seems probable that these afferent fibers passing from the auricle on their way to the geniculate follow one or other of two routes, i.e., from the skin of the auricle through the auriculo-temporal branch of the fifth, or the auricular branch of the vagus to the seventh nerve, the afferent fibers passing to the geniculate in the trunk of the facial nerve; or they may possibly be continued in the auriculo-temporal branch of the fifth to the otic ganglion and thence via the lesser petrosal nerve to the geniculate. Of these two routes, that through the facial is, in my opinion, the more likely one.

Clinical Types of the Disease

Herpes Auricularis.—The simplest manifestation is to be found in the characteristic and well-known picture of herpes zoster of the auricle. There are the usual slight prodromes in the initial stage of the infection, followed by fever and mild general symptoms. Then sharp, darting pains are felt in the ear, the preherpetic pains, sometimes reaching a high degree of intensity. The skin of the ear may assume a red, swollen, somewhat erysipelatous appearance, until on the third or fourth day typical patches of herpetic vesicles make their appearance. These are situated in the concha, on the lobule, the tragus, the marginal portion of the auricle (helix and antihelix), and within the auditory canal, indeed, as rarely happens, on the *membrana tympani* itself. With the appearance of the eruption the acute pains usually subside, the ear still remaining swollen and tender.

At this stage the orifice of the external auditory

canal may become constricted by the swollen soft parts, so as to interfere with the proper drainage and cleansing of the canal. The defect in hearing which may result from this temporary occlusion of the meatus, is purely mechanical and is not in any sense related to the disturbances of audition which accompany another group of cases and which is dependent upon involvement of the auditory nerve. In a few days the vesicles dessicate, the swelling and edema of the parts subside until at the end of a fortnight only a few scattered zoster scars remain to tell the tale. The sensory symptoms may, however, persist for a considerable time; burning pains, itching, paresthesia with impairment of the cutaneous sensation of the parts. In old people more especially the sharp neuralgic pains in the ear, the post-herpetic pains, may persist for a considerable time. (Herpetic otalgia.)

In this class of cases it will be observed that the herpetic pains and the herpetic eruption are localized within that skin area which retains its sensation after extirpation of the Gasserian and the second and third cervical ganglia. It was this area which I assigned to the geniculate ganglion as its cutaneous representation and zoster zone.

Remarks.—Idiopathic herpes zoster of the auricle has long been a recognized manifestation of zona. It is the herpes auricularis and herpes oticus of systematic writers. Dr. Anstie who was personally afflicted with the disease gave a very vivid description of his own case in "The Practitioner" of 1871. This localization of zoster has always been regarded as belonging to the trigeminal area, and due to disease of this nerve or its ganglion. If the observer favored the neuritic theory of herpes zoster, the skin lesions on the auricle were ascribed to a neuritis of the auriculo-temporal branch of the fifth nerve; if the ganglionic theory was accepted, the lesion was placed in the Gasserian. Some authors also speak of the auricular branches of the cervical nerves as playing a role in aural herpes, but no mention is made of the geniculate ganglion and its possible relation to this affection.

Compared with other manifestations of zona, the ear is an infrequent localization. Gruber records five typical cases as occurring in a series of 20,000 cases of ear disease.

To determine, if possible, the relative frequency of these cases, I examined the annual reports of several of our large hospitals for the eye and ear, with rather varying results. The total number of cases recorded is surprisingly small, so small indeed that it seems very possible that the affection not infrequently escapes recognition. It may be that when seen in the early stage of intense inflammation cases are regarded as perichondritis or inflammation of the auricle, or when seen later after dessication of the vesicles, as cases of eczema of the auricle. In the Manhattan Eye and Ear Dispensary during the past ten years, with a total of 47,600 cases, the diagnosis herpes of the auricle was made in only two cases. In the Brooklyn Eye and Ear Hospital, during the past five years, with a total of 15,000 cases, the diagnosis was made but once. The New York Eye and Ear Infirmary averages at the present time 10,000 out-patients a year, and is one of the largest institutions of its kind in the world. During the past twenty-three years this diagnosis was recorded but six times. The reports of the Massachusetts Eye and Ear Infirmary show a much larger proportion of these cases. In the past ten years with a total of 65,000 cases, the diagnosis was made 33 times. In these tabulations it was not possible to determine whether the cases were of the true infectious type, or merely of secondary origin, but the infrequency with which the diagnosis was made is worthy of note.

Herpes Auricularis with Facial Palsy.—In this manifestation of the affection, there is superadded to the herpes auricularis, as just described a peripheral facial palsy, which appears on the same side as the zoster. The time of the appearance of this palsy varies, coming on in some cases simultaneously with the eruption, in others it may be delayed a week or even longer. In the majority of instances it appears on the second or third day. Too much stress should not be given to the patient's statements in this respect as the onset is often insidious and unobserved.

The paralysis is complete and involves all three branches of the nerve, and has certain peculiarities. A conspicuous feature is the frequent evanescence of the symptom, evidences of paralysis lasting only a few days or a fortnight. Many of the palsies clear up within three weeks or a month. There still remains, however, a large group of cases in which the palsy is of a severe type, reactions of degeneration persisting for a long time, leaving permanent weakness and contractures of the face. It is also a striking fact that in an unusually large number of these cases the sense of taste is lost or altered. This is not surprising when one considers that the seat of the lesion is in the geniculate, a level where the taste fibers are still coursing with the facial.

I would explain the involvement of the nerve

in this group of cases by the pressure of an inflamed and swollen ganglion or by the direct extension of the inflammation to the sheath and connective tissue structures of the nerve. In light palsies probably inflammatory edema and pressure are the factors at play, whereas in the more severe forms inflammation and structural changes probably take place.

Remarks.—As has already been emphasized, a similar palsy may complicate herpes facialis and herpes occipito-collaris. I would explain the occurrence of the palsy in such cases by an herpetic inflammation of the geniculate ganglion, based on the well recognized tendency of this affection to produce inflammatory changes in a series of spinal ganglia. The Gasserian, geniculate and upper cervical ganglia constitute such a serial chain.

These cases of facial palsy complicating herpes of the ear, face, and neck, have long been the subject of study and controversy.

The old theories as to the origin of these palsies are as follows: The prevailing opinion is that the same exposure to cold produces both the herpes and the palsy, in which case the latter is regarded as rheumatic in nature, the common form of Bell's palsy. Another favorite theory was based on the infectious origin, the poison or toxin concerned in herpes zoster also producing a neuritis of toxic origin. A somewhat fantastic hypothesis which found great favor with certain observers was the following: The herpetic inflammation is supposed to have extended along the peripheral filaments of the trifacial nerve, this nerve having numerous points of inosculation with the terminals of the facial. The inflammatory process then passes by continuity of structure, directly from the peripheral filaments of the trifacial to the termination of the facial, in this way producing an ascending neuritis.

Herpes Auricularis with Facial Palsy and Auditory Symptoms.—This is the most interesting as well as the severest type of the affection. In this group to the herpetic eruption on the ear, face or neck and facial palsy, are added symptoms pointing to involvement of the auditory nerve. The proximity of the terminal divisions of the auditory nerve to the facial and its ganglia, the common sheath and narrow osseous canal in which they lie would render such an auditory complication not only possible but probable. Contributing factors may be severe forms of the inflammation or certain anatomical peculiarities such as a large ganglion or a narrow bony canal.

The auditory symptoms may be both irritative and paralytic in character and make their appearance about the same time as the facial palsy. First there is tinnitus aurium followed by progressive diminution of hearing. In the more severe cases the symptoms of Ménière's disease are also present. Disturbances of equilibrium, vertigo, nausea and vomiting, nystagmus. In the course of a few weeks the acute symptoms subside, the vertigo and disturbances of the gait and equilibrium disappear, but the tinnitus often persists for a considerable time and the hearing may be permanently impaired.

Remarks.—In this group of cases as in that previously described the auditory symptoms may complicate herpes on the neck and face as well as on the auricle. In my series of 60 cases, auditory symptoms of various degrees of severity occurred in 19 cases. Of this number the zoster was in the occipito-cervical distribution in 9 cases, on the face in 4 cases, and on the auricle and auditory canal in 6. . . .

Pathological Evidence.—Recorded below under Case II is the pathological report of a case of herpes occipito-collaris in which a complete facial palsy supervened on the fourth day. There were no symptoms referable to the auditory nerve. Evidences of facial paralysis and objective sensory disturbances in the occipito-cervical region were still present at the time of death, which occurred 87 days after the onset of the disease. Corresponding to the cervical distribution of the herpes, old inflammatory changes were found in the tip of the third cervical ganglion, with loss of nerve fibers and islets of sclerosis in the corresponding posterior root of the spinal cord. These could be traced through the 1st, 2d and 3d cervical segments, with evidences of myelin degeneration (granule cells and myelin droplets) in that portion of the posterior column, immediately adjacent to the posterior horns. Evidences of regeneration were also found in the branches of the superficial cervical plexus. Such pathological changes both in character and distribution are in accord with the findings in similar cases.

It is, however, to the facial nerve that I would particularly direct attention. The facial nerve, including the nerve of Wrisberg, from its exit at the medulla to its entrance at the internal auditory canal, was treated by the osmic acid method and cut in transverse sections. By this method the nerve of Wrisberg was found to have lost a large number of its nerve fibers, with a compensatory increase of connective tissue. . . . Fortunately that portion of the medulla which was treated by the Marchi method corresponded to the roots of the facial, auditory and nerve of Wrisberg, all of these structures taking their origin at the same level.

The nerve of Wrisberg (*pars intermedia*) lies between the origin of the other two nerves, sometimes it joins one, sometimes the other, as it enters the substance of the medulla. Sections through this level show distinct evidences of degeneration (myelin droplets and granule cells) along the course of the internal root of the auditory nerve, after its entrance into the medulla. . . . In other words, we find in the nerve of Wrisberg, which is the sensory root of the 7th and having its trophic centre in the geniculate ganglion, the same extra- and intra-medullary changes as were found in the spinal cord and posterior nerve root corresponding to the 3d cervical ganglia.

Unfortunately that portion of the facial nerve removed and which was supposed to contain the intumescentia ganglioformis consisted only of membrane, so that the changes in the ganglion itself cannot be given. But even in the absence of the geniculate ganglion, the existence of well-marked degenerations in the nerve of Wrisberg and its intrabulbar root is sufficient proof that this structure was involved. . . .

Concluding Remarks.—Briefly summarized my conclusions are as follows: The facial nerve like the trifacial is a mixed nerve. Its sensory ganglion is the geniculate. The motor root of the geniculate is the facial nerve proper and its sensory root is the nerve of Wrisberg. Below the ganglion the peripheral divisions are the facial nerve proper, the great and lesser superficial petrosal nerves, the external petrosal and the chorda tympani. This ganglion is of the spinal ganglion type and therefore in common with other ganglia of this type, comes within the realm of true herpes zoster.

The zoster zone for the geniculate is found in the interior of the auricle and in the external auditory canal.

The only neural connections existing between the geniculate ganglion and this cutaneous area are the auriculo-temporal branch of the 5th through the medium of the small superficial petrosal nerve and otic ganglion and through the fa-

cial nerve proper. One or both of these routes may be taken by the afferent fibers from the auricle in their central course; in my opinion the facial route is the more probable one.

The ear-zone of the geniculate is intercalated between the zone for the Gasserian in front and the cervical ganglion behind, so that the zoster zones of the cephalic extremity are represented by the Gasserian (face and forehead), the geniculate (ear), the 2d and 3d cervical ganglia (occiput and neck). The zoster inflammations while attacking chiefly one, not infrequently involve more than one ganglion, milder changes showing in a series of ganglia above and below, diminishing in intensity from the central focus. For the same reason zoster in any of the zones of the cephalic extremity, may be accompanied by inflammatory reaction in the other ganglia of this group.

The pathology underlying the affection is the specific hemorrhagic inflammation of the ganglion as found in zona. As the geniculate is lodged in a narrow bony canal and stands in close relation to the 7th and 8th nerves, the characteristic syndrome is produced.

This syndrome may be divided into three clinical groups:

1. Herpes zoster auricularis.

2. Herpes zoster in any of the zoster zones of the cephalic extremity (Herpes auricularis, herpes facialis, and herpes occipito-collaris) with facial palsy.

3. Herpes zoster of the cephalic extremity with facial palsy and auditory symptoms (Tinnitus, deafness, vertigo, vomiting, nystagmus and disturbances of equilibrium).

In the foregoing pages I have endeavored to outline as briefly as possible the anatomical, pathological and clinical facts upon which I have based the syndrome. For the sake of conciseness and clearness, I have eliminated as far as possible all material not absolutely necessary for a convincing argument. For the same reason but few direct personal references have been made to the work of the long list of able investigators, who were my predecessors in this field. In a subsequent communication I hope to be able to give the subject broader and more elaborate treatment. . . .

VII   Adie's Syndrome

MEDICAL men have seldom been shy in claiming paternity for orphaned syndromes and bestowing their names on them. William Adie's description of the tonic pupil with absent tendon reflexes is partly a dialectic to establish his priority. It is also an attempt to broaden the syndrome by defining incomplete forms. Although Adie's priority is dubious (see the review by Lowenstein and Loewenfeld[1]) and his inclusion of absent tendon reflexes *sine* tonic pupil as an abortive form has not been generally accepted, nevertheless the enthusiasm he brought to the subject has made his paper a classic. He succeeded in directing medical attention toward a pupillary abnormality often mistaken as a sign of a more serious disease.

The syndrome has stood substantially as described by Adie (1886-1935), who was an Australian neurologist working in England.

The only significant advance has been the pharmacologic study of Scheie,[2] which provided the clinically useful mecholyl test. This study suggested that the tonic pupil is due to a lesion in the ciliary ganglion or the ciliary nerve because the increased pupillary response to mecholyl may indicate postganglionic parasympathetic denervation. Recently it has been pointed out that the sudomotor system is impaired in some cases.[3,4] This observation may provide evidence of a widespread cholinergic defect in Adie's syndrome. The cause of the tendon areflexia is still unknown.

References

1. Lowenstein, O., and Loewenfeld, I.E.: Pupillotonic Pseudotabes (Syndrome of Markus-Weill and Reys-Holmes-Adie): A Critical Review of the Literature, *Survey Ophthal* **10**:129-185, 1965.

2. Scheie, H.G.: Site of Disturbance in Adie's Syndrome, *Arch Ophthal* **24**:225-237, 1940.

3. Petajan, J.H., et al: Progressive Sudomotor Denervation in Adie's Syndrome, *Neurology* **15**:172-176, 1965.

4. Hardin, W.B., and Gay, A.J.: The Phenomenon of Benign Areflexia: Review of the Holmes-Adie Syndrome With Case Reports and a Study of the Achilles Reflex, *Neurology* **15**:613-621, 1965.

TONIC PUPILS AND ABSENT TENDON REFLEXES: A BENIGN DISORDER SUI GENERIS; ITS COMPLETE AND INCOMPLETE FORMS*
By W. J. Adie.

. . .

Every experienced neurologist has seen a few patients with absence of the tendon reflexes for which no cause could be found. Acting on the suggestion of Dr. James Collier, I mention these cases here and submit that some of them are incomplete examples of this disorder. For proof I await a case in which a tonic pupil appears under observation.

If my views are correct the disorder I am describing may manifest itself in the following forms:—

(1) The complete form—typical tonic pupil and absence of reflexes.

(2) Incomplete forms: (*a*) tonic pupil alone; (*b*) atypical phases of the tonic pupil alone ("iridoplegia"; "internal ophthalmoplegia"); (*c*) atypical phases of the tonic pupil with absent reflexes; (*d*) absent reflexes alone.

*Reprinted from *Brain* 55:98-113, 1932.

THE TONIC PUPIL.

In its most characteristic form the tonic pupil is usually unilateral and almost always larger than its normal fellow; it is never miotic.

When the usual bedside methods are used the reaction to light, direct and consensual, appears to be completely or almost completely absent; after a sojourn in a dark room for an hour or so the pupils dilate to an equal size; thereafter, on exposure to bright diffuse daylight, the abnormal pupil, perhaps after a short delay, contracts slowly; this contraction may continue until the pupil becomes smaller than it was before it dilated in the dark; it then, again after a short delay, dilates to its original size. The most important feature of the tonic pupil is its behaviour on convergence. If the patient fixes a near object and continues to gaze at it intently the pupil, sometimes after a delay of several seconds, contracts slowly and with increasing slowness through a range often greatly in excess of the normal; contraction down to a pinhead size is not uncommon; the larger abnormal pupil then becomes smaller than its fellow. After the effort to converge is relaxed the pupil continues to contract, or remains fixed for a few seconds, or begins to dilate slowly again at once; dilatation once begun proceeds at a slower rate than contraction, so that many seconds or several minutes may elapse before it reaches its original size. Accommodation may be affected in the same manner; the defect is noticed most often during relaxation; after fixation of a near object some seconds elapse before distant objects become clear. There is no constant relation between the rate of contraction of the iris on convergence and of the ciliary muscle during accommodation in the same case (Axenfeld).

The same slow dilatation can sometimes be observed after the pupil has contracted on forcible closure of the lids (tonic lid-closing reaction).

The tonic pupil dilates fully and promptly to mydriatics and contracts under eserine.

In nineteen cases that I have examined myself, the abnormal signs were unilateral in fourteen.

There are very few exceptions to the rule that the abnormal pupil is the larger one. I have seen one example and I know of two others (Oloff, Domarus). It may be regularly or irregularly oval with its long axis vertical or horizontal. The pupil often varies in size through a considerable range during the day; it is often at its smallest in the morning; two patients said that a pupil, usually widely dilated, became quite small after they had been crying (probably a tonic lid-closing reaction). Behr states that he saw "ausgesprochener Hippus" confined to the abnormal pupil in three of his cases. In one of Oloff's cases the signs were found now in one eye, now in the other; the abnormal pupil was always the larger one. This is an unique observation. The findings, however, often vary considerably in the same eye at different examinations.

In most of my cases I have been able to confirm the observations that the pupil dilates in the dark (Dimmer), and then contracts in diffuse daylight (Lerperger), sometimes to a size smaller than it was before (Behr). In some of them, however, I obtained no response. In two of my cases with bilateral tonic convergence reactions the response differed in the two eyes on exposing them to light after an hour in the dark room. In one case one pupil contracted slowly and remained small; in another, one pupil contracted, but in this case the response was prompt and not maintained. In both instances the pupil that reacted to light was usually smaller than its fellow and it had varied in size from time to time.

Relaxation after convergence always proceeds much more slowly than the tonic contraction. In a large majority of the cases the pupil remains small for several or many seconds before it begins to dilate again. Contraction and relaxation are slowest, always I think, towards the end of the movement. I know of only one exception to the rule that both movements are always affected. In one of Marcus's patients, contraction on convergence was normal, but dilatation was very slow.

Some of these patients have difficulty in sustaining the act of convergence. If they are not encouraged to persist the presence of the tonic contraction may easily be missed. Repetition does not facilitate movement as it often does in myotonic muscles.

Tonic accommodation is mentioned in but a small proportion of the cases. It has never been observed as an isolated sign. . . .

The typical tonic pupil then appears to be inactive to light but reacts after a sojourn in a dark room; it contracts slowly on convergence through a wide range and dilates still more slowly. But we must be prepared to encounter many cases of the disorder in which the pupils do not conform strictly to this description. The pupil may contract feebly to light when ordinary methods are used. The reaction to light is often unobtainable by any method; or it may be found in one eye but not in the other when suitable tests are made. The contraction of the pupil may be normal on convergence, dilatation only being delayed. The tonic convergence reaction may be present in one eye while the other pupil is fixed. In unilateral cases the abnormal pupil may be fixed to light and on convergence. The pupil may be fixed at the time the patient is first seen and show tonic reactions later; or a pupil known to be tonic may suddenly dilate and become fixed. Whether such a pupil ultimately becomes tonic again I do not know, but I suspect that it does.

THE RELATION OF THE TONIC REACTION TO OTHER ABNORMAL PUPILLARY REACTIONS.

In so far as the tonic pupil is or seems to be inactive to light but contracts on convergence it conforms to the prevailing loose definition of the Argyll Robertson pupil. It is for this reason that patients with tonic pupils with and without loss of tendon reflexes are almost invariably thought to be suffering from syphilis of the nervous system.

The true Argyll Robertson pupil, as I have emphasized elsewhere, is an infallible sign of syphilis; its characters, as described by its discoverer, are that it is small, usually bilateral, constant in size, and unaltered by light or shade; it contracts promptly and fully on convergence and dilates again promptly when the effort to converge is relaxed; it dilates slowly and imperfectly to mydriatics. It thus differs from the tonic pupil in every essential particular and can hardly be confused with it by anyone who is familiar with the characteristic features of both anomalies.

Behr's view is that the tonic reaction differs essentially from the other well-known abnormal reactions: Argyll Robertson pupils, fixed pupils and ophthalmoplegia interna.

The tonic reaction was confined to one side in 80 per cent of the cases I have seen or analysed; the Argyll Robertson pupil, in my experience, is unilateral in about 5 per cent.; the fixed pupil in less than 10 per cent., and ophthalmoplegia interna in about 20 per cent.

The tonic pupil is almost without exception larger than its normal fellow; the unilateral Argyll Robertson pupil is always the smaller.

If we distinguish between small (under 3 mm.) and large pupils the tonic pupil is never small, whereas the Argyll Robertson pupil is small in 75 per cent., the fixed pupil in 9 per cent., and the pupil of internal ophthalmoplegia in 10 per cent. (Behr).

The tonic pupil varies in size from time to time

and may show hippus confined to the affected pupil. It often dilates in the dark and then becomes equal in size with its fellow. This never happens to the Argyll Robertson pupil.

The behaviour of the tonic pupil on subsequent exposure to bright diffuse light is peculiar to it. In other abnormal pupils a slight change may be detected in similar circumstances, but the range of the movement is very narrow and contrasts strongly with the full or even excessive movements of tonic pupils.

The tonic reaction on convergence differs from the contraction on convergence of the Argyll Robertson pupil in that in the latter it is typically prompt and dilatation after the act ceases is also prompt.

The fact that the tonic pupil contracts through a normal or wide range suggests that there is no true paralysis or paresis, but some qualitative change in its mobility. This also applies to accommodation: the movement is slow but not reduced in range; it always corresponds to the age of the patient (Axenfeld). This is essentially different from the findings in ophthalmoplegia interna where the narrow range of movement on accommodation is decisive for diagnosis.

Syphilis is an important factor in the production of other abnormalities of the pupil. Here it plays no part.

This evidence supports Behr's contention that the tonic reaction is distinct from all the other known forms and that it is a manifestation of a disorder *sui generis*. The fact that the extra-ocular nervous phenomena are unlike anything with which we are familiar also supports the view that we are confronted here by a hitherto unknown kind of perversion of nervous activity.

THE TENDON REFLEXES.

In the published reports on forty-four patients with tonic pupils, loss of one of more of the tendon reflexes is mentioned in nine; this is either passed over without comment or accepted as further evidence of the presence of syphilis of the nervous system.

All of these cases were described by ophthalmologists; it is almost certain therefore that the proportion with some defect in the reflexes is much higher than these figures indicate. Of nineteen patients with a tonic pupil that I have seen myself thirteen had abnormal reflexes.

Loss of one or both ankle-jerks is most frequent; I have never seen loss of any other jerks with both ankle-jerks still present. Sometimes one or more of the arm-jerks cannot be obtained at a time when the knee-jerks though sluggish can still be obtained on reinforcement.

Asymmetry is not uncommon. I have seen two cases with the knee and ankle jerks absent on one side and still present on the other. In one of these patients the remaining knee-jerk seemed to be abnormally brisk.

In one of Behr's cases the knee and ankle jerks were absent; three years later the ankle-jerks could be obtained on reinforcement. One of Axenfeld's patients was examined "repeatedly" over a period of nine years by expert neurologists; the triceps, knee, and ankle jerks were absent throughout. I suspect that jerks once lost do not return.

One of Oloff's patients had been in hospital five years before when the knee-jerks were present. At the second examination they were absent. The absence of reflexes therefore is probably not congenital.

General Features.

Of my own cases fifteen were females, four males. Including the cases described by others, the figures are forty-five females and eighteen males. The proportion of males thus rises when cases with pupillary abnormalities alone are taken into account. It may be that females are not only more susceptible but also that they are more likely to lose their tendon-jerks.

The age at which the signs appear has not yet been determined. Some patients state that the pupils have "always" been unequal. This was noticed in one of Foster Moore's patients at the sixth month; at the age of 5 years this patient presented typical tonic reactions.

Most of those who complain of sudden mistiness of vision and dilatation of the pupil are in the twenties and thirties; but this gives no indication of the age at which their pupils became tonic, because, as we have seen, a pupil known to be tonic may dilate suddenly at any time and cause visual symptoms.

Mackay examined Bramwell's case, a healthy unmarried woman, in 1894, and found normal pupils; in 1906 when she was about 38 years of age he found unequal pupils with "no apparent reaction to light in either." This is the only case I have been able to find where an expert has found normal pupils at one examination and tonic reactions at another, and this is not a proven case of our disorder.

My impression is that the abnormal pupillary reaction may appear at any age. The cases of Oloff and Axenfeld, already mentioned, suggest that this is true for loss of reflexes also.

In many cases, perhaps in a large majority the disorder is symptomless throughout life. In a few the onset appears to be sudden; in the course of a game perhaps, some discomfort is felt in and around the eye and vision becomes misty; when the eye is inspected it is found that one pupil is dilated and examination reveals defects in accommodation and in its reactions.

I have never heard of a case with symptoms that could be associated with the loss of reflexes in the lower limb. Repeated careful examinations by myself and by my assistants have failed to reveal any other evidence of disturbance of the functions of the muscles or nervous system in patients with absent reflexes.

There is nothing in the family history of these patients to indicate that they belong to a neuropathic or degenerate stock; nor does anything in the personal history recur with sufficient frequency to deserve mention as a possible aetiological factor. Their general health is remarkably good. They are not nervous; they do not conform to any special physical type.

Relation of the Disorder to Syphilis.

In 1921, when Behr discussed this subject, he had to contend with the fact that most of the writers who preceded him had attributed the tonic pupillary reaction to the effects of syphilis; they based this diagnosis on the ocular signs alone, believing that the tonic pupil was a form of the Argyll Robertson pupil and they made it with still greater confidence when absence of tendon reflexes seemed to confirm it. Nevertheless, from his study of twenty-one cases in the literature and eight cases of his own, Behr formulated the following cautious conclusion: the presence of pupillotonia alone does not justify the assumption that the patient is suffering from syphilis of the nervous system. Our position now, based on a study of over sixty cases, is much stronger.

The majority of the patients are healthy young females; the ocular signs they present are not observed in syphilitics; in many of them tendon areflexia persists for many years without the addition of any other sign or symptom referable to disease of the nervous system. A patient with evidence that this disorder was present in childhood has lived to the age of 75 without nervous troubles (Foster Moore).

I know of eighteen cases of tonic pupil with absent tendon reflexes in which the blood and cerebrospinal fluid were examined; the results were negative in all. In five more the blood alone was tested, with negative results.

Without making another search throughout all the published reports I cannot give the exact number of the cases of tonic pupil alone in which the blood and cerebrospinal fluid were examined, or the blood only, but tests were made in many cases with negative results in all but one (Barkan's case) in which the reaction in the blood was positive. In this case there was no other evidence of syphilis of the nervous system.

I think the following conclusions may now be drawn with safety: the tonic convergence reaction in pupils only apparently inactive to light is, in all probability, never a manifestation of syphilis of the nervous system. The combination of this sign with absent tendon reflexes and without other signs of organic nervous disease has never been observed in syphilis of the nervous system; it is not one of its manifestations.

DIAGNOSIS.

The diagnosis of this disorder in its complete form presents no difficulty; the combination of the tonic convergence reaction in a pupil apparently inactive to light, with absence of one or more of the tendon-jerks, is pathognomonic. . . .

It must be understood that slowness of movement by itself does not constitute a tonic reaction; that is seen in retinal disease, in traumatic iridoplegia and in many other dissimilar affections of the visual and oculomotor mechanism. The decisive diagnostic features of the true tonic pupil are delay as well as slowness in responding, the inactivity to light which is only apparent, its tendency to retain a new size after the stimulus is removed, and its much slower relaxation compared with the rate of contraction to light, on convergence and, when present, in accommodation. . . .

We have no proof at present that absence of tendon reflexes alone may be a manifestation of this disorder. This diagnosis might be entertained if the signs are of long standing, if other signs and symptoms of organic nervous disease are missing, and the family history is negative for familial nervous disorders and syphilis.

In the past syphilis of the nervous system was almost always diagnosed or suspected because the tonic convergence reaction in pupils apparently inactive to light was mistaken for the Argyll Robertson phenomenon. So long as the prevailing definition—the pupil reacts on accommodation but not to light—is supposed to define what Argyll Robertson described, the same regrettable mistake will continue to be made. The tonic pupil and the Argyll Robertson pupil have hardly anything in common and should not be confused. Syphilis is usually suspected too in the cases where the pupil appears on superficial examination to be fixed or partially fixed. If efforts to disclose tonic reactions have failed and a careful consideration of all of the features of the case leaves room for doubt, the appropriate tests to exclude syphilis must be made. . . .

NATURE OF THE DISORDER.

The tonic reaction seems to be the expression of a unique kind of perversion of pupillomotor activity. A stimulus is applied; for a time there is no response; then a contraction begins and continues at an ever diminishing rate but through a range in excess of the normal; once begun this contraction may continue after the stimulus is removed; or having reached its maximum it retains it long after the stimulus has ceased to act; relaxation then proceeds with even greater slowness than contraction.

The curious manner in which stimuli are stored in excess and slowly emitted points to some change in the activity of the cells in the vegetative portion of the oculomotor nucleus. We are driven to the viscera for analogous types of innervation.

The problem raised by the tendon areflexia is one that we have been forced to consider in relation to other disorders of the nervous system.

We are most familiar with this abnormality as a sign of disease of the spinal cord or peripheral nerves, but we encounter it in a number of conditions in which the central nervous system, apart from the vegetative nervous system, is intact.

In dystrophia myotonica and other myopathic atrophies absence of knee and ankle jerks is seen in patients with powerful unwasted lower limb muscles and intact sensibility. The extra-muscular phenomena in dystrophia myotonica point to a disorder of the vegetative nervous system.

In family periodic paralysis the tendon reflexes may be absent for hours or days. In the intervals there are no organic signs. During the cataplectic attacks in narcolepsy the tendon reflexes are completely abolished. In the cases where narcolepsy is symptomatic of encephalitis lethargica, the common association of obesity and the occasional oc-

currence of disturbances of sugar and water metabolism, vasomotor and heat regulation and the
like indicate the region of the brain whose functions are disturbed.

I have seen complete abolition of the tendon
reflexes in a patient with myasthenia gravis at a
time when there was no weakness in the limbs. . . .

Most of these diseases present ocular signs.
There can be little doubt that they are all related,
more or less closely.

SUMMARY.

The tonic pupillary reaction, under a number of
different names, has been known to ophthalmologists since 1902.

In some of their cases absence of one or more of
the tendon reflexes was noted, but this was mis-
construed as further evidence that the ocular signs
were due to syphilis.

My conclusions here are based on a study of
nineteen patients with tonic pupils, thirteen of
them with absent tendon reflexes, that have come
under my own observation, and forty-four published cases of tonic pupil, nine with absent tendon reflexes, that have been reported, almost all, in
journals of ophthalmology. . . .

The conclusion is reached that the symptoms
described are the manifestation of a disorder of
the vegetative nervous system. They are the expression of a kind of perversion of nervous activity of
which at present we can form no conception.

References.

[1] ADIE, W.J. *Brit. Med. Journ.*, 1931, 1, 928.

[2] *Idem Ibid.*, 1931, 2, 136.

[3] AXENFELD, T. *Klin. Monatsschr. f. Augenheilk.*, 1919, 62, 59.

[4] BARKAN, O. *Arch. f. Augenheilk.*, 1921, 87, 189.

[5] BEHR, C. *Klin. Monatsschr. f. Augenheilk.*, 1921, 66, 770.

[6] BRAMWELL, E., and SINCLAIR. *Scott. Med. and Surg. Journ.*, 1906, 526.

[7] DIMMER, F. *Klin. Monatsschr. f. Augenheilk.*, 1911, 49, 332.

[8] DOMARUS, A. *Münch. Med. Woch.*, 1919, 66, 987.

[9] GEHRCKE, *Neur. Centralbl.*, 1921, 40, 93.

[10] JESS, A. *Klin, Monatsschr. f. Augenheilk*, 1920, 64, 114.

[11] LERPERGER, O. *Ibid.*, 1914, 53, 241.

[12] MARCUS, C. *Trans. of the Ophth. Soc. of the U.K.*, 1906, 21, 50.

[13] MOORE, F. *Ibid.*, 1924, 44, 38.

[14] *Idem. Ibid.*, 1931, 51, 203.

[15] MORGAN, G. and SYMONDS, C.P. *Guy's Hosp. Rep.*, 1927, 77, 13.

[16] *Idem. Trans. Roy. Soc. of Med.*, 1931, 768.

[17] NONNE. *Neur. Centralbl.*, 1902, 21, 1000.

[18] OLOFF, H.: *Klin. Monatsschr. f. Augenheilk.*, 1914, 53, 493.

[19] REITCH, W. *Ibid.*, 1925, 74, 159.

[20] SAENGER, A. *Neurolog. Centralbl.*, 1902, 21, 837.

[21] STRASBURGER, J. *Ibid.*, 1902, 21, 738.

[22] WEILL, G., and REYS, L. *Rev. d'oto-neuro-ocu-list.*, 1926, 4, 433.

VIII   Romberg's Sign

MORITZ Heinrich Romberg is best remembered for the neurological sign that bears his name. Less widely recognized is his role as a founder of modern neurology.[1-5] One of the earliest physicians to specialize in the neurological disorders, Romberg had established an active neurology clinic at the University of Berlin by 1837 and wrote the first major textbook of neurology, published in segments between 1840 and 1846.[6]

In this outstanding work, which was translated into English in 1853,[7] Romberg presented his classical description of tabes dorsalis. Despite the fact that syphilis had been introduced into Europe in the 15th century, cases of true tabes dorsalis apparently had not been described in medical writings until the 19th century.[8] Romberg presented the first organized account of this disease, although he did not recognize its relationship to syphilis and he did not clearly distinguish ataxia from weakness.

In his account of tabes dorsalis, Romberg described a sign that he thought was pathognomonic of the disease—ie, the loss of balance demonstrated by the erect patient when his eyes are closed. This phenomenon, now known as Romberg's sign, has subsequently been found in other conditions, but some confusion has arisen because of failure to heed Romberg's original description.

Romberg stated that the patient *begins* to sway when he closes his eyes, implying that he does not sway when his eyes are open. Consequently, most patients with cerebellar ataxia cannot be said to have Romberg's sign, since they sway with the eyes open or shut.

Romberg's sign has value as an indicator of altered position sense, whether caused by tabes or some other neurological disease, and testing for its presence has become a routine part of the neurological examination.

References

1. Cobb, S.: One Hundred Years of Progress in Neurology, Psychiatry and Neurosurgery, *Arch Neurol Psychiat* 59:63-98, 1948.
2. Garrison, F.H.: "History of Neurology," in Dana, C.L. (ed.): *Textbook of Nervous Diseases for the Use of Students and Practitioners of Medicine*, ed 10, New York: W. Wood & Co., 1925, pp xv-lvi.
3. Riese, W.: History and Principles of Classification of Nervous Diseases: A Short History of the Doctrines of Nervous Function Under Pathological Conditions and a General Scheme of Classification of Nervous Diseases According to Function, *Bull Hist Med* 18:465-512, 1945.
4. Viets, H.R.: Neurology—Past and Present, *JAMA* 109:399-402, 1937.
5. Viets, H.R.: "Moritz Heinrich Romberg (1795-1873)," in Haymaker, W. (ed.): *The Founders of Neurology*, Springfield, Ill: Charles C Thomas, Publisher, 1953, pp 367-370.
6. Romberg, M.H.: *Lehrbuch der Nervenkrankheiten des Menschen*. Berlin: A. Duncker, 1846, pp 794-801.
7. Romberg, M.H.: *A Manual of the Nervous Diseases of Man*, E. H. Sieveking (trans.), London: Sydenham Society, 1853, vol 2, pp 395-401.
8. Merritt, H.H.; Adams, R.D.; and Solomon, H.C.: *Neurosyphilis*, New York: Oxford University Press, 1946, pp 235, 236.

TABES DORSALIS.*

The spinal cord viewed as a central organ, not only serves as an agent for the mutual transmission of stimuli, but also as a source of nervous power, of the principle of motor and sensory tension, by which the continuance and vigour of motion and sensation is secured, and a general stimulus for the entire organism provided. The disease, which is characterized by a diminution of this power, is termed tabes dorsalis.

*Reprinted from Romberg, M.H.: *A Manual of the Nervous Diseases of Man*, E.H. Sieveking (trans.), London: Sydenham Society, 1853, vol 2, pp 395-401.

The first symptom by which it is manifested is reduction of the motor power in the muscles, first and foremost in the inferior extremities; at the commencement one leg may be affected more than the other, but in the progress of the disease both suffer. The patient complains of weakness and inability to perform any movement or endure any position for a continuance. If he is required to attempt any act demanding a larger consumption of motor power, *e.g.* to bend down or to stand on one foot, his strength at once fails; the practised rider is unable to hold on to his horse as long as usual. Early in the disease we find the sense of touch and the muscular sense diminished, while the sensibility of the skin is unaltered in reference to temperature and painful impressions. The feet feel numbed in standing, walking, or lying down, and the patient has the sensation as if they were covered with a fur; the resistance of the ground is not felt as usual, its cohesion seems diminished, and the patient has a sensation as if the sole of his foot were in contact with wool, soft sand, or a bladder filled with water. The rider no longer feels the resistance of the stirrup, and has the strap put up a hole or two. The gait begins to be insecure, and the patient attempts to improve it by making a greater effort of the will; as he does not feel the tread to be firm, he puts down his heels with greater force. From the commencement of the disease the individual keeps his eyes on his feet to prevent his movements from becoming still more unsteady. If he is ordered to close his eyes while in the erect posture, he at once commences to totter and swing from side to side; the insecurity of his gait also exhibits itself more in the dark. It is now ten years since I pointed out this pathognomonic sign, and it is a symptom which I have not observed in other paralyses, nor in uncomplicated amaurosis; since then I have found it in a considerable number of patients, from far and near, who have applied for my advice; in no case have I found it wanting. Some patients mention the circumstance without being asked about it; one gentleman, a foreigner, whose eyesight was unimpaired, told me that he was at present unable to wash himself in his dark bedroom while standing; and that if he wished to keep his balance he was obliged to have a light while performing his toilet. Another, whose business rendered it necessary for him to go out at six o'clock in the morning, complained that he required some one to support him in the house and out of doors, but that he could dispense with assistance in full daylight. Independently of this peculiarity, there is also a difference in the movements themselves; the patient experiences a greater difficulty in executing forced and limited movements, than those in which he merely follows the impulse of his inclinations; he finds it much more laborious to walk slowly with a measured step in a given direction, than to let his feet take their own course; rising from the chair, or going up stairs, is more difficult than sitting down or descending; the most difficult matter is to turn round in walking. After prolonged rest, walking and standing are more laborious and insecure than when once begun. The loss of muscular power is also manifested in organs provided with a sphincter, and especially in the bladder. At the commencement of the disease, the desire to micturate occurs more frequently, and cannot be gratified soon enough, for the patient is unable to retain his urine till the utensil is brought to him. Enuresis not unfrequently occurs during sleep. The urine is not discharged in an arched jet, as in health, but falls more perpendicularly; nor is the bladder entirely emptied. Costiveness prevails almost universally; the patient feels that he is unable to strain as long and as forcibly as before. Painful sensations of different kinds almost invariably accompany the affection; the most common is a sense of constriction, which proceeds from the dorsal or lumbar vertebrae, encircles the trunk like a hoop, and not unfrequently renders breathing laborious. Several of my patients have described this sensation as particularly troublesome during sleep, causing them suddenly to start up and scream out. Others complain of a heavy weight pressing upon the rectum and the bladder, others again of colic and gastric pains; the majority suffer from pain shooting through the legs, and a sense of pricking, itching, burning, or cold in the skin of the lower as well as of the upper extremities; the face alone is an exception. Formication very rarely occurs in the back. These symptoms may endure for a considerable time, and at first they attract little attention. After an uncertain period the weakness of the legs diminishes visibly. The patient, owing to the threatening loss of balance, is obliged to evert his feet, and walk with his legs apart; he leaves his heels as long as possible in contact with the ground, and keeps his knees bent; he is still able to propel himself, (one of my patients stated to me, that he found it necessary to think of every one of his movements,) and to totter along the streets, but if arrested in his progress, he is unable to stand still without clinging to some support. The patient's own strength soon fails to support him, and he is obliged to have recourse to assistance. The necessity of employing his eyes becomes more and more urgent; if he closes his eyes, even while sitting, his body begins to sway to and fro; in one case the patient was unable to maintain himself erect in his chair, and slid down to the ground; when in an horizontal posture, the patient is no longer able to recognize the position of his own limbs, and cannot tell whether the right leg is crossed over the left or the reverse. A foreigner, who was a patient of mine, told me that in visiting the diorama he had not the slightest sensation of his progression when led from the light to the dark department. The condition of these unfortunate individuals is rendered the more distressing by the circumstances that amblyopia often supervenes; in many cases it is associated with the disease from the commencement. Even when the optic nerve was not implicated, I have repeatedly found a change in the pupils of one or both eyes, consisting in a contraction with loss of motion, which in one case, that of a man aged 45, attained to such a height that the pupils were reduced to the size of a pin's head. In one case, where there was no cerebral affection, a strabismus towards the inner angle took place, the patient at the same time being able to move his eye outwards at will. As the disease progresses, the loss of power also extends to the superior extremities, though they are not affected to the same degree as the inferior. The sphincter of the bladder becomes completely paralysed; erections cease, and the virile power becomes extinct. The intellect of these patients generally remains unimpaired; the majority do not complain much, and they are inclined to represent their condition, especially to the medical man, in a too favorable light; if they are members of the higher classes, they anxiously endeavour to conceal their loss of motor power, in order to avoid the evil reputation of being affected with tabes dorsalis. Nutrition is not impaired in a measure corresponding to the diminution of motor and sensory power. Such patients may even retain their embonpoint for a considerable time, so that the term tabes does not apply to this feature. At a later period the muscles become flaccid and atrophied, especially about the nates, the legs, and the back. Towards the termination of the disease the patient becomes utterly incapable of holding himself erect or moving; still he continues able to execute movements with his feet at will when the trunk is supported. Diuresis alternates with ischuria; the faeces pass off involuntarily. Gangrene at the sa-

crum and trochanters, accompanied by febricitations, ushers in death.

Tabes dorsalis is a chronic disease, which may extend over several—as many as ten and fifteen—years. It is only shortened by complication with other more rapidly fatal diseases, especially pulmonary and intestinal phthisis. Intercurrent diseases may also accelerate its progress.

Although the post-mortem records of this disease may present considerable variations, they almost without exception show the existence of partial atrophy of the spinal cord; the lumbar portion and the nerves given off from it are the parts generally affected. The loss of substance, which may amount to one half or two thirds of the healthy spinal cord, either affects the grey and the white substance, or only one of them. It would be well always to have a fresh, healthy specimen at hand for the sake of comparison, and to render the examination more satisfactory. As yet we possess no microscopic investigation of the atrophied portion. The contents of the cords of the cauda equina have often been found to have disappeared to such an extent that nothing but the empty nurilemmatous sheaths seemed to remain. The roots of nerves inserted at a higher segment of the cord also suffer from atrophy; and it is a point of especial interest to observe that the posterior, sensory roots, are occasionally alone affected in conjunction with the posterior columns of the spinal cord, the anterior motor columns and nerves retaining their normal structure. A remarkable instance of this occurred to me in the person of a medical practitioner of a provincial town, of 52 years of age; after violent emotions and severe colds, caught in the prosecution of his profession, he had in his fortieth year been attacked with partial paralysis of the lower extremities and amblyopia, for which, at the suggestion of myself and the late Professor Rust, he went through a course of the Marienbad waters, but to no purpose; the amblyopia passed into complete amaurosis, and tabes dorsalis became fully developed in spite of all the remedies employed. I did not see the patient again; but I ascertained that the insensibility of the skin was maintained to the last and that he correctly appreciated variations of temperature. I was present at the post-mortem examination which was made by Professor Froriep, and the spinal cord, compared with the fresh cord of a man of the same age, only amounted to two thirds of its normal size; I was not a little surprised to find that the atrophy was confined to the lower part of the posterior columns and nerves. The medullary tissue of the former had almost entirely disappeared, so that they were translucent, and of a greyish-yellow colour. The posterior roots of the nerves were deprived of their nerve matter, and presented a watery appearance. From the middle of the dorsal nerves upwards, the atrophy passed into a healthy condition. The anterior columns and roots of the nerves presented no abnormity. Froriep has observed the same in another case of tabes dorsalis. When the disease has been accompanied by amaurosis, we almost invariably find the optic nerve, the chiasma, and the optic tracts atrophied; one or both optic thalami are also either atrophied, or they exhibit changes of texture and colour. The other morbid changes found in tabes dorsalis vary; sometimes the white substance presents a coriaceous condensation, but it is more usual to find softening of the grey matter. In 1832, I examined a man, aged 42, who had been under my care for three years for tabes dorsalis, and found the lumbar, the cervical, and a portion of the dorsal region of the cord of an almost fluid consistency; it was traversed by a number of white longitudinal fibres, as if a delicate cauda equina passed through the cord. The meninges rarely retain their healthy condition; the arachnoid is thickened and beset with cartilaginous and osseous plates, and contains more or less serum. It is exceptional to meet with morbid changes in the osseous envelopes.

Two circumstances that have been shown with certainty to predispose to tabes dorsalis are the male sex and the period between the thirtieth and fiftieth year of life. Scarcely one eighth of the cases are females. The loss of semen has always been looked upon as one of the most fruitful sources of the complaint; but this in itself does not appear to be a matter of much consequence as influencing the disease, as patients who have been labouring under spermatorrhoea for a series of years, are much more liable to hypochondriasis and cerebral affection than to tabes dorsalis; but when combined with hyperstimulation of the nerves to which sensual abuses give rise, it not unfrequently favours the origin and encourages the development of the disease after it has com-

menced. When the strength is much taxed by continued standing in a bent posture, by forced marches, and the catarrhal influences of wet bivouacs, followed by drunkenness and debauchery, as is so often the case in campaigns, the malady is rife; this is the reason why tabes dorsalis was so frequent during the first decennia following the great wars of the present century. Rheumatism appears to be the morbid process which most frequently gives rise to it. The cases are not rare in which the most careful examination fails to establish an exciting cause.

There is no prospect of recovery for patients of this class; the fatal issue is unavoidable; the only consolation that can be offered to those fond of existence is the long continuance of the disease. If in any case the busy activity of the physician increases the sufferings of the patient, it is in tabes dorsalis. When one of these unfortunate individuals presents himself to us, we generally find his back seamed with cicatrices, he brings us a heap of prescriptions, and gives a long list of the watering-places he has visited in search of health. It is but common humanity to inform him at once that therapeutic interference can only injure, and that nothing but the regulation of his diet can retard the calamitous issue. Every unnecessary tax made upon the motor powers, as well as sexual excitement, ought to be strictly prohibited. The best remedy for the obstinate costiveness is to be found in cold water enemata; the careful use of cold water in washing the trunk and spinal cord, and in the shape of affusion to the latter, may be recommended. I have employed an ointment containing veratrine with benefit against the painful sensations in the back and extremities. The thing most to be avoided is the frequent application of cupping and issues; nor are long journeys to watering-places advisable, because the driving itself is injurious, and the baths will only afford temporary relief, which will disappear on the return of the patient. Incurable patients should be allowed to spend their lives quietly in their family circle, that their last moments may be soothed by the fond cares of those whom they love.

IX Wernicke's Encephalopathy

To CARL WERNICKE, mental disorders were diseases of the brain. Wernicke, a German psychiatrist and neuroanatomist, devoted his career to finding the morphologic bases for psychiatric disorders. His description of hemorrhagic superior polioencephalitis, which became known as Wernicke's encephalopathy, was characteristic in that he defined the new entity in both clinical and anatomical terms. The account appeared in Wernicke's three-volume tome *Lehrbuch der Gehirnkrankheiten,* published in 1881-1883.

Wernicke's encephalopathy, manifested by ophthalmoplegia, ataxia, and disturbance of consciousness, came to be so widely regarded as a complication of alcoholism that more recent authors have seen fit to emphasize its occurrence in nonalcoholics.[1,2] Wernicke's first case, however, was a 20-year-old seamstress who had pyloric stenosis as the result of sulphuric acid ingestion.

An important contribution to the pathology of Wernicke's encephalopathy was made by Gamper[3] who described involvement of the mammillary bodies in chronic cases. It is still not understood why the gray matter near the third and fourth ventricles and the cerebral aqueduct is selectively vulnerable in this disease. The pathogenesis of the vascular changes and the minute hemorrhages is also not known, and in many patients with Wernicke's encephalopathy the hemorrhagic component is completely absent.[4]

Wernicke had no clear idea of the cause of the condition. Malnutrition has since been accepted as the etiology, and the administration of thiamine has been found to produce rapid reversal of the ophthalmoplegia.[5,6]

Neurology and psychiatry have drifted apart since Wernicke's day, but Wernicke's encephalopathy remains a bridge between the two disciplines.

References

1. Neubuerger, K.: Ueber die nichtalkoholische Wernickesche Krankheit insbesondere ueber ihr Vorkommen beim Krebsleiden, *Virchow Arch Path Anat* **298**:68-86, 1936.

2. Drenick, E.J.; Joven, C.B.; and Swenseid, M.E.: Occurrence of Acute Wernicke's Encephalopathy During Prolonged Starvation for the Treatment of Obesity, *New Eng J Med* **274**:937-939, 1966.

3. Gamper, E.: Zur Frage der Polioencephalitis Haemorrhagica der Chronischen Alkoholiker: Anatomische Befunde beim Alkoholischen Korsakow und ihre Beziehungen zum Klinischen Bild, *Deutsch Z Nervenheilk* **102**:122-129, 1928.

4. Rosenblum, W.I., and Feigin, I.: The Hemorrhagic Component of Wernicke's Encephalopathy, *Arch Neurol* **13**:627-632, 1965.

5. Jolliffe, N.; Wortis, H.; and Fein, H.D.: The Wernicke Syndrome, *Arch Neurol Psychiat* **46**:569-597, 1941.

6. Phillips, G.B., et al: A Study of the Nutritional Defect in Wernicke's Syndrome: The Effect of a Purified Diet, Thiamine, and Other Vitamins on the Clinical Manifestations, *J Clin Invest* **31**:859-871, 1952.

ACUTE HEMORRHAGIC SUPERIOR POLIOENCEPHALITIS*

By Carl Wernicke

The medulla oblongata, as the borderland between the brain and spinal cord, has a double character even in pathologic states. On one hand, we have recognized in the medulla hemorrhages and malacia that completely resemble those in the rest of the brain. On the other hand, the medulla differs from the brain in that, like the gray substance of the anterior horns of the spinal cord, the gray floor of the fourth ventricle, and especially its motor nuclei, is the favorite site for independent disease processes of possible inflammatory origin, which are analogous only to poliomyelitis. As far as this analogy applies, one can speak of a polioencephalitis with the same variations of its course that are characteristic of poliomyelitis: viz.; a chronically progressive form, Duchenne's disease; an acute form, the so called acute bulbar paralysis; and a subacute, rarer form, which corresponds to a rare form of poliomyelitis.

These disease processes analogous to poliomyelitis extend far beyond the medulla upward into the gray substance of the midbrain and diencephalon. Here the affected nerve nuclei belong exclusively to the ocular musculature. Here too the spinal-cord character can be noticed, and from the standpoint of pathology, the homologous origin of the motor cranial nerves and the anterior roots of the spinal cord can be confirmed. On morphologic grounds, this fact could not be rejected previously. The upper area of the polioencephalitis extends from the posterior wall of the infundibulum in the third ventricle to the level of the abducens nucleus. Like poliomyelitis there is an acute and a chronic form. For practical purposes, we must differentiate between a polioencephalitis inferior and superior, according to the area affected. The border between the two, however, will be rather fluid, so that the distinct pathological process of one area will show, now and then, focal symptoms belonging to the contiguous area. . . .

A twenty year old seamstress was admitted to the Charité on December 5, 1876 because of sulphuric acid poisoning and discharged as cured on January 6, 1877. Soon after discharge she vomited but was otherwise healthy until February 3, 1877. Thereafter she was bedridden and re-

markably sleepy. She yawned much and had a staggering gait when she attempted to leave the bed. Furthermore, the patient noticed a decrease in vision, which was later joined by a persistent and very annoying flickering and a severe photophobia as well as by dizziness and a sensation of heaviness in the head. Since all symptoms increased and the vomiting continued, she was re-admitted to the Charité on February 11, 1877. A specific infection had never occurred.

On February 12 her status was as follows: The very pale, somewhat emaciated patient is lying with half-closed eyes. She opens her eyes only about 1 cm., and even in the shade she cannot open them further. On upward gaze, the eyes are opened somewhat more. The right palpebral fissure is narrower than the left generally and on looking up. The eyes can be closed completely but less energetically and without formation of wrinkles. Through the reflex elicited by touching the eye, a tighter closure is not possible. When looking straight ahead both eyeballs are steady and in slight convergence. On upward gaze, there are jerky movements with large excursions, but the movement can finally be performed fully. On downward gaze, the same can be observed. Movement of both eyes to the left is significantly decreased. Despite obvious efforts and jerky movements, the left eye cannot go beyond the midline. The right eye moves somewhat further medially; however, only momentarily can the inner corneal rim be brought near the caruncle. Usually the inner corneal rim only reaches the line of the lower lacrimal punctum. Movements to the right are affected similarly, i.e. the right eye can only be brought to the midline, while the left can be moved into the inner canthus but still is distinctly restricted. The same phenomenon occurs with convergence (fixation on the tip of the nose), the inward movement being better on the left than on the right. In the position of rest, the deviation of the ocular axes is not very apparent, even though there is an obvious convergence positioning. The pupils are equal, normal-sized, and react sluggishly to light. When the face is at rest the right corner of the mouth is somewhat deeper and the right half of the cheek is somewhat flatter. On the left side the nasolabial fold and the fold bordering the lower eyelid are very well formed. The right corner of the mouth is opened less than the

*Translation of "Die Acute Haemorrhagische Poliencephalitis Superior," in Wernicke, Carl: *Lehrbuch der Gehirnkrankheiten*, Kassel and Berlin: Fischer, 1881, vol 2, pp 229-242.

left. The facial expression is depressed, morose, and at the same time apathetic. When she laughs or opens her mouth widely, the same difference remains. However, on other voluntary movements there is no noticeable difference between the two sides of the face. There is no other paralysis detectable, although she has a feeling of great weakness. With assistance, the patient can walk. There is no disturbance in sensation. The extremities are cold. The patient complains of great fatigue, and her voice is tired, as if she were half asleep. During the course of the day she vomits repeatedly. Temperature is 37.0 to 37.4.

February 13. Somnolence continues. The patient moans at times or calls her fiance's name. Otherwise she is disoriented and seems not to know where she is. When she is awakened, for instance at mealtimes, she talks reasonably with the personnel but suddenly interrupts the conversation to complain about back pain and heaviness in the head. The urine, which she passes in small amounts, is of a peculiar oily consistency and contains peptones but no protein nor sugar. Cool extremities. Temperature is 36.4 to 37.2.

February 14. The patient has to be awakened before answering but remains disoriented. She complains of headache and neck stiffness. She appears extremely anxious. She is afraid of falling and wants to be carried. Frequent yawning and moaning. She only answers after repeated questioning. Pupils enlarged due to atropine. Ophthalmoscopically, there is bilateral optic neuritis with only moderate swelling and many streak-like hemorrhages. The abdomen is distended, very tense and painful. Temperature 37.3 to 37.5; pulse 120 and barely palpable. At night very restless, frequent crying out.

February 15. Stuperous with painful wimpering. No answer when spoken to. Death in the afternoon.

Autopsy. There is no flattening of the gyri. The cavities in the brain contain only a few drops of fluid. The choroid tela and plexus are bright red. On cross section through the basal ganglia one sees in the walls of the entire third ventricle, to a depth of about three to five mm., a pink discoloration of the brain tissue, in which numerous small punctate hemorrhages are apparent. The changes are present bilaterally with almost mathematical symmetry. This can be observed particularly well on cross sections in the region of the massa intermedia, which is well formed and also penetrated by hemorrhages. A similar alteration is not noted in the lamina quadrigemina, and noth-

ing is found in the cerebellum. The pia of the extended spinal cord has a smoky gray color. In the pons and medulla, no gross alterations are detectable. In the spinal cord, there are no macroscopic changes. Numerous hemorrhages in both retinas. Otherwise the residua of sulphuric acid poisoning.

Anatomical diagnosis: Hemorrhagic encephalitis of the gray matter of the third ventricle. Bilateral retinal hemorrhages. Pyloric stenosis and chronic, ulcerative gastric dilatation due to sulphuric acid poisoning. Examination after fixation showed that the hemorrhages were mostly around blood vessels. The punctate hemorrhages were of different sizes, and a few reached the size of a pinhead. The smaller vessels and capillaries were very dilated and congested. The vessel walls were without striking alterations. Only here and there the epithelial cells of the capillaries appeared to be swollen. Granule cells were present in the vicinity of the hemorrhages. These changes did not extend to the structures and fiber masses of the neighboring gray floor. Only in the inferior colliculus on the left side, there was, exactly in the center, an isolated pinhead size hemorrhage. Caudally, the same alterations of the gray floor extended with gradually decreasing intensity into the area of the striae acusticae. Arteries at the base appeared normal.

[The second case is omitted.]

A 33 year old man was admitted to the Charité on March 10, 1878 after delirium tremens appeared in the morning. Heavy whisky drinker, particularly for the past several months. Since the last military campaign, frequent complaints about pulling in the legs. In a previous campaign he had typhus. As a young man he was infected once. Poor gait at times for the last four weeks. Three weeks ago for eight days he had difficulty passing water. Eight weeks ago the patient allegedly fell off a wagon, possibly on his head; however, there were no sequelae. For four weeks dizziness and headaches at times and in the mornings also vomiting, especially after heavy drinking. During the last two days the patient complained about double vision, and during this time he was jaundiced. He never had a stroke or convulsions.

On March 11 his status was as follows: Very strong, well-nourished individual with slight icteric tint. . . . Since admission, the patient has behaved deliriously and is disoriented to place and surroundings. Now considerable motor restlessness; the hands constantly pick the bed clothes;

the patient throws himself about and twists his head in order not to fixate those persons present. He calls acquaintances and has terrifying hallucinations. During his vigorous gesticulations a severe tremor is present. Voice is hoarse; speech is fast, jumbled, somewhat tremulous without thickness and without dysarthria. Face is covered with sweat; respiration is very rapid, apparently due to psychic excitation; there is no cough. Face is slightly cyanotic with a swollen appearance. The lips and teeth have a barky film. The gait is staggering and interrupted by sudden ataxic and tremorous movements. Standing on one leg is possible for a short time. When asked, the patient complains about weakness in the legs. Straight posture of the trunk and head. Tongue is somewhat dry, without evidence of bites, and is extruded in midline, but with severe tremor. There is a suggestion of right facial paresis. The patient is not torpid. His attention can be obtained momentarily through questions. Pulse 110 to 120, regular, rather full, very soft; temperature 39.3. Urine free of protein and sugar. Thoracic organs normal. Liver dullness two finger breadths below the costal margin. There is bilateral complete abducens paralysis. Neither eye can be moved laterally beyond the midline. The remaining ocular movements appear intact. Pupils react to light and convergence; they are medium wide and without inequality. A prompt reaction follows pinprick on the face and hands. There is only a slight reaction on the feet. A deep pinprick on the right great toe is noticed by the patient only after a period of time; he then complains of a very severe burning. On the left great toe most pinpricks evoke no reaction. Percussion of the skull is not painful, nor is slight pressure on the spinal column and neck musculature. In the evening, the ophthalmoscope reveals intensive reddening without papilledema. The disc borders are not entirely sharp. No hemorrhages. . . .

March 14. Pulse 98 to 100, temperature 37.8. Pulse slow and very weak, but regular. The patient was delirious during most of the night. This morning, however, he is less confused than yesterday and begins to become oriented. Since the patient can fixate well, the ocular movements are examined more precisely. Lateral movement is as before. Internal movement appears today to be impaired too. Upward and downward movements are intact. When he sits up there is rather definite neck stiffness. . . .

March 16. Pulse 96, begins to become irregular, temperature 38.5. General condition is rela-

tively unchanged. The patient still is delirious at times but is, on the whole, quieter. Weakness has increased. The patient lies for the most part with half-closed eyes, only the white being visible. Frequent coughing, no sputum. When taken out of bed, the patient likewise exhibits increased weakness and goes onto his knees after a few staggering stiff steps. When called, the patient's consciousness is relatively good for a few moments. He is oriented and attempts to fixate presented objects. He complains of severe weakness. Ocular motility is further reduced and internal rotation is jerky and very defective bilaterally. Downward movements are likewise impaired. Upward movements are preserved the best, but also appear somewhat limited. Ophthalmoscopic findings: A pronounced picture of optic neuritis is present in the right eye. The disc is intensely reddened, possibly somewhat swollen, and the borders are indistinct. The arteries are not visible; the veins are very congested and filled in all branches. A small vessel directed toward the macula in the vicinity of the disc is surrounded by a spindle-shaped hemorrhage. Otherwise there are no hemorrhages. In the left eye, the disc is only hyperemic with somewhat hazy borders, and arteries and veins are very congested into the finest branches. Toward noon death occurred.

Autopsy: Pia of the convexity and base equally transparent, edematous to a very small degree. Dura not tense, without alterations; the pia also shows no alterations. The hemispheres themselves show nothing significant, except for slight reddening of the cortex. No changes at the base. After removing the roof of the third ventricle, one sees that the substance of the massa intermedia is penetrated by small punctate hemorrhages. After removal of the cerebellum, the areas that are most gray in the gray floor are also seen to be sprinkled with fine red dots, possibly containing capillary hemorrhages. Otherwise nothing remarkable. Spinal cord without findings. . . .

Anatomical diagnosis: Multiple punctate hemorrhages in the massa intermedia, third ventricle, and gray substance of the fourth ventricle. Edema and hyperemia of the lungs. Chronic endocarditis on the mitral valve. Splenic hyperplasia. Fatty infiltration of the liver. Ulceration on the vocal cords. Examination of the fixed preparations revealed the same findings as in the two cases already described; however, nowhere were the hemorrhages the extent of a pinhead. These alterations, which were indicative of inflammation, did not extend caudally beyond the gray floor of the fourth ventricle. In the third ventricle they were not so pronounced as in the previous case; however, they extended somewhat further downward into the upper region of the calamus scriptorius.

We are dealing with an independent, inflammatory, acute nuclear disease in the region of the ocular nerves, which leads to death within 10 to 14 days. The focal symptoms consist of the corresponding ocular muscle palsies, which develop rapidly, progress, and finally lead to almost total paralysis of the ocular musculature. But even then certain muscles are spared, such as the sphincter iridis and the levator palpebrae. The patient's gait becomes staggering and shows a combination of stiffness and ataxia, reminiscent of the ataxia of the alcoholic. The general appearance is very striking. It consists of impairment of consciousness, which is either somnolence from the onset or a terminal state of somnolence preceded by a longer period of agitation. In addition, involvement of the optic nerves by inflammatory changes

of the discs were characteristic of all three cases. There was always a severe injury before the onset of the disease. One patient had sulphuric acid poisoning followed by pyloric stenosis. The other two patients misused alcohol to an unusually high degree. The question of whether the appearance of delirium tremens in these last cases is to be regarded as a complication or as another one of the general symptoms of this disease can be asked but cannot be answered. In any case, there was not a simple delirium tremens, but one complicated by the symptoms of polioencephalitis. It might be pointed out that the characteristic disorientation could also be demonstrated in the first patient, whose appearance was very far from that of delirium. After the first case, which could not be understood at all during her lifetime, I was able in the second and third cases to make the diagnosis in spite of the variation in the general symptoms. This probably gives justification for presenting these cases as a specific disease picture.

X   Brown-Séquard Syndrome

THE BROWN-SEQUARD syndrome represents a turning point in the history of neurophysiology.[1-3] Before Charles Edouard Brown-Séquard performed his classical experiments in the mid-19th century, the doctrines of Sir Charles Bell were dominant and all sensory impulses were believed to ascend the spinal cord ipsilaterally in the posterior column. Crossing to the opposite side was believed to occur only when the sensory impulses reached the brain.

Brown-Séquard, the son of a Frenchwoman and an American sea captain, pursued his career as a physician and investigator mainly in Paris but also in the United States. By demonstrating that hemisection of the cord in animals produces sensory loss on the opposite side of the body with retention of sensation on the ipsilateral side, he challenged the idea that the posterior column is the sole sensory pathway and provided concrete evidence of sensory decussation in the spinal cord.

Observation of human cases of cord hemisection has confirmed Brown-Séquard's concepts. Position sense, which is conveyed by the ipsilateral cord, is indeed lost below the lesion on the same side, but pain and temperature sensations, which are carried by the contralateral spinothalamic tract, are diminished only on the opposite side. Tactile sensation is usually preserved since it ascends in crossed and uncrossed tracts. These neurologic signs, together with paralysis of the ipsilateral limbs, have come to be called the Brown-Séquard syndrome in commemoration of the man who recognized the complexity of fiber-tract organization in the spinal cord.

References

1. Olmsted, J.M.D.: "Charles Edouard Brown-Séquard (1817-1894)," in Haymaker, W. (ed.): *Founders of Neurology,* Springfield, Ill: Charles C Thomas, Publisher, 1953, pp 263-266.

2. Olmsted, J.M.D.: *Charles Edouard Brown-Séquard, A Nineteenth Century Neurologist and Endocrinologist,* Baltimore: Johns Hopkins Press, 1946.

3. Schiller, J.: Claude Bernard and Brown-Séquard: The Chair of General Physiology and the Experimental Method, *J Hist Med* 21:260-270, 1966.

ON THE TRANSMISSION OF SENSORY IMPRESSIONS BY THE SPINAL CORD*

By M. Brown-Séquard

Four years ago I announced in my inaugural thesis (*Research and experimentation on the physiology of the spinal cord,* pp. 22 and 26.—Paris, January 3, 1846) that section of a lateral half of

*Translation of De la transmission des impressions sensitives par la moelle epinière, *Compt Rend Soc Biol* 1:192-194, 1849.

the spinal cord does not destroy sensation in the parts of the body which receive their nerve supply from the portion of the cord separated from the brain. This finding was similar to those of Schoeps, Van Deen and Stilling and contrary to the statements of Kürschner, M. Longet and other physiologists. Since that time I have had occasion to do this experiment more than sixty times either in my courses, or particularly in the process of studying all the circumstances of the phenomenon, or finally to satisfy many peoples' curiosity. This is what I have seen:

1. Immediately after cutting a lateral half of the cord in the dorsal region of a mammal, sensation appears very diminished in the hindlimb on the side of the section. Feeling is completely lacking in the other hindlimb. Sometimes I have found sensation intact or nearly so in the lower limb corresponding to the side of the section, while the opposite hindlimb was either insensitive or very slightly sensitive.

2. After five to ten minutes of rest following the operation, one always finds the hindlimb corresponding to the side of the section very sensitive. In many cases, or even in most cases, this limb appears noticeably more sensitive than normal. This fact is certainly very curious; but there is another fact, even more unexpected: the hindlimb of the side opposite the section is insensitive or very slightly sensitive.

It follows from these facts that cutting a lateral half of the spinal cord, far from causing loss of sensation in the parts caudad to the section on the same side, renders them hyperesthetic. At the same time, a more or less complete anesthesia is produced on the other side of the body, caudad to the section.

Eighteen months ago, we showed to the Biological Society a healthy guinea pig in which we had cut a lateral half of the cord at the level of the eleventh dorsal vertebra. Everyone present could verify that the sensitivity of the hindlimb on the side of the section was very great. The animal was sent to M. Rayer, who had an autopsy performed by our late colleague, M. Désir. At the next meeting, M. Désir showed the Society the portion of the cord where the cut had been made. One could recognize that it was at the indicated place and really involved the designated half of the cord.

In the meeting of December 1, 1849, we showed a guinea pig in which the *right* lateral half of the cord had been cut before the eyes of several members of the Society. The section was at the tenth dorsal vertebra; the animal had lost much blood. The operation, carried out in half-darkness, had been long and very painful. In such circumstances, one ordinarily finds the two hindlimbs paralyzed for voluntary movement and sensation for some time after the operation. This is what occurred in this case. But at the end of five or six minutes, voluntary movement returned in the *left* hindlimb and sensation in the *right* hindlimb. About twelve minutes after the operation, sensitivity was extreme in the *right* hindlimb and nil in the *left*. An autopsy was then done by M. Claude Bernard, with the meeting still in progress. The Society verified that the *right* lateral half of the cord was cut transversely at the indicated level.

Schoeps Van Deen and Stilling have observed perfectly that the hindlimb on the same side as the section of a lateral half of the cord does not lose sensation. To this fact we add the following:

1. Generally this section leads to a momentary decrease in the sensitivity of the corresponding hindlimb.

2. At the end of a certain time (from three to fifteen minutes) after the section, the sensitivity of the corresponding hindlimb appears markedly increased.

3. The hindlimb of the side opposite to that where the section is made loses its sensitivity completely or in large part.

The spinal cord thus appears to have, at least in part, a crossed action with respect to the transmission of sensory impressions. This is so true that if, after having cut one lateral half of the cord in a mammal, one then cuts the other half some centimeters away from the first section, one finds the two hindlimbs insensitive or very slightly sensitive. We cannot examine here the questions that these experiments raise; we will make them the subject of an extensive report. Nevertheless, we believe it is necessary to say that if the transmission of sensory impressions occurs partly in the posterior columns of the cord, it occurs mainly in other areas of this nerve center. In fact, not only is sensation not lost after section of the posterior columns, but it is even markedly increased in the parts of the body which should be insensitive according to the erroneous theory that the systematic physiologists persist in supporting despite the contrary evidence and despite the retraction of Charles Bell.

Argyll Robertson Pupil

Robertson pupil has become an uncommon finding, but the research stimulated by Douglas Argyll Robertson's description has contributed greatly to our present knowledge of the optic reflexes.[6-10]

SOME CLINICAL phenomena may be viewed as experiments of nature and serve to stimulate investigation into the mechanisms of normal function. An example is Argyll Robertson's pupillary syndrome.

Douglas Argyll Robertson of Edinburgh was a pioneering ophthalmic surgeon who made several important contributions to our basic understanding of ocular mechanisms.[1,2] In 1869, the same year that Johann Friedrich Horner described his well-known form of miosis,[3] Robertson reported miosis of another type, characterized by absence of the pupillary light reflex with retention of pupillary contraction to near vision.[4,5]

Robertson noted the association between the pupillary syndrome and disease of the spinal cord. Later, the Argyll Robertson pupil was found usually to be the result of neurosyphilis, and it became a cardinal sign of the disease.[6]

Robertson reasoned that a lesion in the ciliospinal (sympathetic) nerves was responsible for the syndrome. The matter is still unsettled despite much disputation. Experimental production of the Argyll Robertson pupil has not been achieved, and current theories attribute its etiology to lesions in the periphery[7] or in the midbrain tegmentum rostral to the third-nerve nuclei.[6,8]

With decline of neurosyphilis, the Argyll

References

1. Leake, C.D.: "Douglas Moray Cooper Lamb Argyll Robertson (1837-1909)," in Haymaker, W. (ed.): *The Founders of Neurology*, Springfield, Ill: Charles C Thomas, Publisher, 1953, pp 364-367.

2. Bailey, H., and Bishop, W.J.: *Notable Names in Medicine and Surgery*, London: H. K. Lewis & Co., Ltd., 1959, pp 128-129.

3. Horner, F.: Ueber eine Form von Ptosis, *Klin Mbl Augenheilk* 7:193-198, 1869.

4. Robertson, D.A.: On an Interesting Series of Eye-Symptoms in a Case of Spinal Disease: With Remarks on the Action of Belladonna on the Iris, etc, *Edinburgh Med J* 14:696-708, 1869 (also in *Med Classics* 1:850-868, 1937).

5. Robertson, D.A.: Four Cases of Spinal Myosis: With Remarks on the Action of Light on the Pupil, *Edinburgh Med J* 15:487-493, 1869 (also in *Med Classics* 1:869-876, 1937).

6. Merritt, H.H., and Moore, M.: The Argyll Robertson Pupil: An Anatomic-Physiologic Explanation of the Phenomenon, With a Survey of its Occurrence in Neurosyphilis, *Arch Neurol Psychiat* 30:357-373, 1933.

7. Walsh, F.B.: *Clinical Neuro-Ophthalmology*, Baltimore: The Williams & Wilkins Co., 1957, pp 160-164.

8. Lowenstein, O.: The Argyll Robertson Pupillary Syndrome, *Amer J Ophthal* 42:105-121, 1956.

9. Ingvar, S.: On the Pathogenesis of the Argyll-Robertson Phenomenon, *Bull Hopkins Hosp* 43:363-396, 1928.

10. Langworthy, O.R., and Tauber, E.S.: The Control of the Pupillary Reaction by the Central Nervous System: A Review, *J Nerv Ment Dis* 86:462-475, 1937.

FOUR CASES OF SPINAL MYOSIS;
WITH REMARKS ON THE ACTION OF LIGHT ON THE PUPIL.*

By D. Argyll Robertson, MD, FRCSE,
Lecturer on Diseases of the Eye, Edinburgh.

George Smith, æt. 51, tailor, applied to me for advice on account of dimness of sight. He stated that he enjoyed good health until July last year, when one very hot forenoon, while crossing the North Bridge, he felt giddy and faint, but managed with some difficulty to walk home. The following day he experienced pain in his back, extending to his legs, increased while taking exercise. His back was also tender on pressure. He had, moreover, twitchings, and occasional numbness in his legs, especially the right, with want of power, so that in walking he staggered, and had to use a stick. He could not stand steadily in the dark, but had to grasp at some object for support. He at this time complained of dull pains in his forehead, and noticed that his water constantly dribbled away. These symptoms prevented him continuing more than a few hours daily at work. He did not observe his sight affected till the end of December, when he discovered that the sight in his right eye was dim. Since then the sight has neither improved nor deteriorated, while with his left eye he sees as well as he ever did, but he has noticed that objects appear darker than they used to do, and that he requires more light while working than formerly sufficed. He is not conscious that his face flushes more readily than natural.

On examination, I found that while walking his gait was unsteady, and that he could not plant his feet firmly on the ground. He also exhibited considerable awkwardness in turning. He stood erect with his eyes closed, but swayed a little from side to side. On looking at the eyes, the drooping of the lids and the small size of the pupils at once attracted attention. The drooping of the lids was more marked in the left than the right eye—the

left palpebral aperture at the widest point measuring only 3¾ lines, while the right measured 4 lines. Each pupil measured ¾ line in diameter; they were insensible to the influence of light, but contracted to ½ line during the act of accommodation for a near object. Under repeated instillations of a strong solution of sulphate of atropine, the right pupil became dilated to a little beyond medium size, so that it measured 2¾ lines in diameter, and was quite immobile.

With the right eye the patient was slightly myopic, but even with a suitable glass had difficulty in making out very large print (N. LXX. of Snellen) at 20 feet distance. With the left eye vision was normal (N. XX. at 20 feet).

With the ophthalmoscope a slight degree of atrophy, with shallow cupping, of the right optic nerve was discovered. From the very small size of the pupil, the interior of the left eye could not be examined. Under the use of iron, combined with small doses of strychnia, a considerable improvement occurred in most of the patient's symptoms, but the pupils remained contracted, and the sight in the right eye unaltered.

For notes of the history and general symptoms of the following case, and for bringing the patient under my notice, I am indebted to my friend Dr Sanders.

John Grey, æt. 35, a clerk, was admitted to the Royal Infirmary on the 11th of June 1869, complaining of weakness in his legs and right arm.

He always enjoyed good health until fifteen years ago, when he contracted syphilis. He has never had any eruption, nor sore throat, but suffered from a swelling over his right ulna, probably of periostitic nature, which disappeared under the use of iodide of potassium. He resided for a year in India, and shortly after his return, nine years ago, he had an attack of hemiplegia, which

*Reprinted from Edinburgh Medical Journal 15:487-493, 1869.

affected the left side of the face and right side of the body. Twelve months afterwards, when nearly convalescent, he consulted Dr. Christison for convergent squint of his left eye, and was ordered some mercurial pills, and, while taking them, he states that he caught cold, to which he refers the commencement of his present disease.

The patient is a man of middle height, somewhat emaciated; has large joints and florid cheeks. There is very marked contraction of pupils. They each measure half a line in diameter, are insensible to light, but contract during the act of accommodation for near objects. There is no drooping of the eyelids. The skin is cool, soft, and moist. The temperature of the inferior extremities, more especially the right leg, is below that of the body. There is diminution in the motor power of both legs, accompanied by a feeling of stiffness. He can move them in all directions, but not actively. He can stand pretty steadily, even when the eyes are closed; but when he does so, he bends his body forwards, while his legs are curved slightly backwards at the knee-joints. He walks with a peculiar straddling gait. The muscles of his right calf and thigh are smaller than those of his left. There is no atrophy of the deltoid. There is partial anæsthesia, without analgesia in the right iliac and inguinal regions, extending down the right leg. Reflex action is very marked in right leg—so much so, that it often starts up without any apparent stimulus. Motor power in the right arm and hand is diminished, so as to prevent the patient carrying on his occupation as clerk. He does not complain of headache, but considers his memory affected.

The patient's vision is very slightly affected. With either eye he is able to read fine print, and is able to distinguish colours perfectly. To permit of ophthalmoscopic examination, and to test the extent to which the pupil will dilate, a drop of a strong solution of atropine was introduced into the left eye. The following day the left pupil measured two lines in diameter. With the ophthalmoscope a slight degree of "cupping" and lighter colour of the optic disc, indicating a little atrophy of nerve substance, was the only pathological condition discovered.

Dr. G. W. Balfour directed my attention to the following two cases, and kindly supplied me with notes of their history and the results of examination into their general, and more especially their nervous, symptoms:—

John Dann, æt. 43, iron-turner, was admitted to the Royal Infirmary May 12, 1869, complaining of a staggering and inability to walk, a difficulty in making water, and dimness of sight after reading for a time.

About six years ago he was seized with pain in his bladder, which was so severe as to compel him to leave his work. This pain returned at intervals of a month or two, after which he noticed that he could not make his water freely, and eventually that it dribbled away at night. He applied to a local practitioner for relief, and was treated for paralysis of the bladder, and subsequently for stricture. He was next treated at the Newcastle Infirmary for stricture and diseased prostate, and after two months was discharged as cured. He soon thereafter felt that he staggered, and could not walk straight in the streets, and observed, while washing his face, that, on shutting his eyes, he could not help falling forwards on to the basin. He once more applied for advice at the Newcastle Infirmary, and was again treated for enlarged prostate; but obtaining no benefit from the treatment pursued, he was sent to the Edinburgh Royal Infirmary to the care of Dr Watson, because of supposed prostatic disease. Finding it to be a case of nervous affection, Dr Watson transferred the patient to the Medical House. The patient has for five years past had severe pains in the rectum, to allay which he used to employ laudanum injections, but has desisted from their use since January last.

Dr Balfour found, on careful examination, that the skin of the trunk and extremities was insensible to pain, except in a narrow zone extending round the body, its breadth corresponding to the distance between the sixth and twelfth dorsal vertebræ. Sensibility in this zone is not increased. Electro-mobility and electro-sensibility were unimpaired. He complained of the sensation of a tight cord round his waist. He walks somewhat feebly, and staggers on turning. He also sways considerably if he closes his eyes while standing, and would fall if he did not open his eyes, or grasp some object for support.

On examining his eyes I found the left pupil more contracted than the right; the left measuring ¾ line, the right 1 line in diameter. There is a tendency to divergent strabismus of the left eye, for when the patient looks fixedly at an object about a foot from the eye, the left eye is seen after a time to roll outwards. Vision in the right eye is perfect, but with the left only moderate-sized print can be read. The pupils are insensible to light, while atropine only occasions medium dilatation (to 2 lines). On ophthalmoscopic examination both optic nerves were found considerably inject-ed; while in the left eye there was a peculiar con-genital abnormality, a portion of the sheaths of the optic nerve fibres passing beyond the fascia cribro-sa, and extending over the retina upwards and out-wards from the optic disc for a distance about equal to the diameter to the optic disc. In other respects, the fundus of both eyes is normal.

Under the use of nitrate of silver in $\frac{1}{2}$ gr doses, the patient considerably improved during his resi-dence in the Infirmary.

The following case is at present in Dr Balfour's wards. Although it is certainly not a typical exam-ple, I here include it, because the myosis is well marked, presenting similar features to the con-tracted pupils in the other cases, and because there are some slight and obscure nervous symptoms which *may* be indicative of incipient spinal affec-tion.

Robert Clerk, æt. 66, a clerk, was admitted into Dr Balfour's wards on 18th October 1869, com-plaining of general debility. His appearance sufficiently indicates that for a lengthened period he has been in straitened circumstances. He, how-ever, enjoyed good health till three years ago, when he suffered from varicose ulcers on his legs, which, under treatment, disappeared in about six months. Since that time he has never completely regained his strength, although he thinks he has improved of late. For the last two or three years he has been troubled with twitchings and startings of the legs while in bed at night, and for three months he has experienced a great heat in the skin, especially of the legs. He has no incontinence of urine, but states that he cannot expel his water with any force.

On examination no decided impairment of muscular power or of sensation could be anywhere detected. His gait, however, is unsteady, and when he stands with his feet close together and shuts his eyes, his body sways somewhat, but he can stand thus without support for some time.

Both pupils are of the same size, and markedly contracted, measuring barely 1 line in diameter, and only partial dilatation (to 2½ lines) ensues on the application of a strong atropine solution. No alteration in the size of the pupil is observable under the influence of light, but when near ob-jects are looked at contraction at once ensues. Vi-sion is good, though not perfect in both eyes, and there is no colour-blindness.

On ophthalmoscopic examination a slightly atrophic condition of the optic nerves was observa-ble.

(I may mention that in the examination of this patient considerable difficulty was experienced in getting from him an accurate account of his histo-ry and symptoms, as he exhibited a great tendency to modify his statements to what he imagined would please his examiner.)

These four cases serve well to illustrate the con-nexion between certain eye-symptoms and a dis-eased condition of the spinal cord. In all of them there was marked contraction of the pupil, which differed from myosis due to other causes, in that the pupil was insensible to light, but contracted still further during the act of accommodation for near objects, while strong solutions of atropine only induced a medium dilatation of the pupil.[1] In three of the cases a slight degree of atrophy of the optic nerves existed, as was evinced by a shal-low excavation and lighter colour of the optic disc. In one, we observed a symptom which has been noticed occasionally in spinal disease by Brown-Sequard and others—namely, a drooping of the upper lids. In none of the cases was there any appreciable colour-blindness. As regards the nature of the spinal lesion, in one case the charac-ters of locomotor ataxy were well marked; in the other two the form of spinal affection is doubtful; while in the fourth patient, as I have already men-tioned, the symptoms of spinal disease are by no means well marked.

To most of the eye-symptoms found in these cases I alluded at length in a previous communica-tion to this Journal. I will therefore pass them over without remark at this time. But I now de-sire to direct special attention to a very remarkable circumstance which I noticed in the case that formed the subject of my previous paper, and which I again observed in all the above cases, viz., that although the retina is quite sensitive, and the pupil contracts during the act of accommodation for near objects, yet an alteration in the amount of light admitted to the eye does not influence the size of the pupil. This cannot be explained by the supposition that the pupil is already so small as to be incapable of further contraction under light; because (in the healthy eye) a still further degree of contraction of the pupil may be effected by the use of the Calabar bean, and yet the pupil varies in size according to the intensity of the light. The only possible solution of the difficulty is to be found in the theory, that for contraction of the pu-

---

[1] I may mention, that the patients have been frequently carefully examined as to these points with a like result by Mr Walker, Professor Sanders, Dr G. W. Balfour, Dr Barde of Geneva, and many others.

pil under light it is necessary that the cilio-spinal nerves remain intact, and, as in these cases of myosis the cilio-spinal nerves are paralyzed, light does not influence the pupil. But hitherto this contraction of the pupil under light has been invariably referred to reflex stimulation of the ciliary branches of the third pair which supply the circular fibres of the iris. If this latter view were correct, I see no reason why in these cases light did not influence the pupil. In all of them the retina was thoroughly sensitive to light, and in all of them the ciliary branches of the third pair were healthy and active (as was shown by the further contraction of the pupil during the act of accommodation, which can only be referred to these nerves). But in all there were symptoms of spinal disease, and in all myosis due to paralysis of the cilio-spinal nerves. I am therefore inclined to the former view, in which case it is necessary to assume that the contraction of the pupil which naturally occurs when light is admitted to the eye is not as has been hitherto sup-

posed an excellent example of reflex action, but an isolated example of normal, temporary, reflex paralysis.

I am aware that a dilated immobile condition of the pupil has been found to follow division of the third pair in animals, and that in cases of complete paralysis of the third pair, the pupil is dilated usually and insensible to light. This would rather tend to the conclusion that the contraction of the pupil under light is due to the motor oculi; but in division of this nerve, so many tissues are injured at the same time as to render deductions from effects observed open to many fallacies, while in cases of paralysis of the third pair, we not unfrequently observe the pupil to act partially under the influence of light; and where this is not the case, the immobility may be due to degenerative changes in the nervous or muscular tissue. For a thorough solution of this question, further experiments and clinical observation are necessary.

XII   Horner's Syndrome

THE use of eponyms to denote medical syndromes is common among physicians and especially among neurologists. A disadvantage of this practice is that the names themselves are not descriptive. Furthermore, confusion arises when more than one person is credited with a single achievement or when one man's name is attached to several discoveries. Despite these drawbacks, the eponym avoids lengthy descriptive terminology and conveys meaning with brevity. In addition, each eponym is a lesson in the history of medicine and keeps alive the names of those who contributed to medical progress. It seems preferable to retain this human element in nosology rather than to replace it with a series of resounding Latin adjectives, many of which will later seem unimportant as the disease is further elucidated. (For a contrary opinion, see Wartenberg.[1])

The convenience of an eponym is exemplified by the complex syndrome resulting from paralysis of the sympathetic fibers supplying the neck, face, and eyes. A variety of pathologic processes within and without the central nervous system is responsible for this syndrome, which consists of ipsilateral miosis, ptosis, and apparent enophthalmos, with cutaneous vascular dilatation and absence of sweating over the neck and face. It is widely known simply as Horner's syndrome.[2]

Johann Friedrich Horner (1831-1886) was a Swiss ophthalmologist who lived and practiced in Zurich.[3] His classic description of cervical sympathetic paralysis was not without precedent. Lesions of the cervical sympathetic system had been studied previously in animals by several investigators, including Claude Bernard.[3] Also, some features of the syndrome had been mentioned in a brief clinical case report by Edward Selleck Hare, but Hare failed to perceive its etiology.[4] To Horner belongs the credit for the first full description in man of the cause and manifestations of this common syndrome.

Although many investigators have contributed more to the understanding of the anatomy, physiology, and pathology of the autonomic nervous system,[5-8] Horner has become better known than most of the others because of eponymic convenience.

References

1. Wartenberg, R.: On Neurologic Terminology. Eponyms and the Lasègue Sign, *Neurology* 6:853-858, 1956.
2. Cogan, D.G.: *Neurology of the Ocular Muscles*, ed 2, Springfield, Ill: Charles C Thomas, Publisher, 1956, pp 177-179.
3. Fulton, J.F.: Horner and the Syndrome of Paralysis of the Cervical Sympathetic, *Arch Surg* 18:2025-2039, 1929.
4. Hare, E.S.: Tumor Involving Certain Nerves, *London Med Gaz* 23:16-18, 1838.
5. Timme, W.: The Vegetative Nervous System: Historical Retrospect, *Res Publ Assoc Res Nerv Ment Dis* 9:1-11, 1930.
6. Sheehan, D.: Discovery of the Autonomic Nervous System, *Arch Neurol Psychiat* 35:1081-1115, 1936.
7. White, J.C.; Smithwick, R.H.; and Simeone, F.A.: *The Autonomic Nervous System: Anatomy, Physiology, and Surgical Application*, ed 3, New York: Macmillan Co., Publishers, 1952, pp 3-15.
8. Monro, P.A.G.: *Sympathectomy: An Anatomical and Physiological Study With Clinical Applications*, London: Oxford University Press, 1959, pp 3-9, 189-195.

ON A FORM OF PTOSIS*

By F. Horner

Many of my colleagues are familiar with long-standing cases of incomplete ptosis in adults, lacking the usual accompanying signs of oculomotor paralysis but exhibiting the striking symptoms of a myosis of the pupil on the same side. This clinical picture was not new to me when at the end of last November a woman, 40 years of age, presented herself with these symptoms; less than a week later I saw them again in a woman of about the same age, but it was not possible for me to obtain such crucial information for the elucidation of the ptosis in this case as it was in the first. I may be permitted, therefore, to report here on the first case.

Frau Anna Brändli, aged 40, a healthy-looking peasant woman of medium size, seems to have suffered since adolescence from generalized headache which in the course of recent years had rather diminished in frequency and intensity.

Six weeks after her last confinement, which occurred a year ago, she noticed a slight drooping of her right upper eyelid, which increased very gradually and for about three months had remained constant. The upper lid covers the right cornea to the upper edge of the pupil; the lid is not loose or wrinkled but somewhat sunken into the orbit and is still capable of movement; it is neither injected nor swollen. The upper convex furrows on the right side of the forehead indicate that the frontalis muscle is working as a substitute [for the levator palpebrae superioris].

The pupil of the right eye is considerably more constricted than that of the left, but reacts to light; the globe has sunk inward very slightly and repeated determinations showed that it was somewhat less firm than the left. Both eyes are emmetropic, and have normal visual acuity and early presbyopia.

During the clinical discussion of the case, the right side of her face became red and warm, the color and heat increasing in intensity under our observation, while the left side remained pale and cool. The right side seemed turgid and rounded, the left more sunken and angular; the one perfectly dry, the other moist. The boundary of the redness and warmth was exactly in the midline.

The patient thereupon told us that the right side had never perspired, and that the flushed feeling, and also the ptosis, had only developed in the course of the last year. The redness of the right side of the forehead and cheek was said to be present in the evening as a rule but was also brought on more or less markedly at other times by any emotion.

By feeling the cheeks with the hand, one could perceive a marked difference in temperature. We took steps to establish this precisely and to determine its range. Dr. Julius Michel and Wilh. von Muralt made accurate determinations, some of which I record here. Very sensitive thermometers were read after being warmed in water at about 25 C., and then fastened against the cheek with a cotton compress and adhesive. The temperature was also taken in other localities—behind the ear (over the mastoid process), in the axilla and in the groin.

I. Temperature of the Cheek.—EXPERIMENT 1.: Immediately after application, the thermometer on the right recorded 35 C., that on the left, 30 C., the former rising in fifteen minutes to 36.3 C., the latter to 34.1 C. After the temperature on the two sides had become nearly equal and the left cheek had been warmed by the compress so that no difference could be felt with the hand, the thermometers were quickly exchanged, and after five minutes the thermometer on the left rapidly fell to 35.3 C., while that on the right rose to 36.3 C.; after ten minutes the temperatures were equal.

*Translation of: Ueber eine Form von Ptosis, *Klinische Monatsblätter für Augenheilkunde* 7:193-198, 1869 (as translated by J. F. Fulton³).

EXPERIMENT 2:

	R.	L.
After 1½ minutes	35.0	29.5
After 4 minutes	35.8	31.4
After 6 minutes	36.1	32.8
After 10 minutes	36.1	33.6
After 14 minutes	36.2	33.9
After 20 minutes	36.4	34.4
After 26 minutes	36.6	35.0
After 34 minutes	36.7	35.7

II. Temperature Behind the Ear—

Time	R.	L.	Time	R.	L.
3.36	34.0	30.0	3.46	36.2	35.4
3.38	35.0	32.0	3.48	36.4	35.8
3.40	35.4	33.8	3.50	36.6	36.2
3.42	35.8	34.6	3.52	36.8	36.3
3.44	35.9	35.0	3.56	36.8	36.6

III. Temperature in the Axilla.—At first the temperature differed by only three tenths of a degree, and finally (after twenty minutes) by six tenths, the curves being practically parallel, the left lower than the right by a constant interval.

IV. Temperature in the Groin.—During the entire period of observation (twenty minutes), the temperature remained the same, 37.6 C. on both sides. The sensation in both cheeks was exactly the same. This investigation thus proves the integrity of the sensory trigeminal nerves, transitory paralysis of the vasomotor fibers in the right trigeminal area; higher initial temperature on the right side with slowly rising (temperature) curve, a low initial temperature on the side with a rapidly rising curve; equalization of both if the observation is continued long enough with the left cheek adequately covered and protected.

Two points necessitate the conclusion that the vasomotor disturbance involves not only the trigeminal area, but also that of the fibers of the cervical sympathetic: first, the slight but distinct variation in temperature in the axillae, secondly, and more important, the small size of the right pupil.

The latter symptom prompted some investigations concerning the action of atropine and calabar. When equal quantities of atropine were instilled into each conjunctival sac the right pupil enlarged slowly and irregularly; after twenty minutes it had not yet reached the size of the left, but remained more constricted and oval, even though more drops were put into the right eye.

When, twenty-four hours after the atropine, equal quantities of calabar were put into the conjunctival sac of each eye, one noticed after ten minutes a marked constriction on the right, and after half an hour almost maximal myosis, while on the left the action of the atropine still continued, and it was only after a half an hour that an insignificant decrease of the effect of the atropine was apparent.

I have already mentioned that the right globe always appeared somewhat softer, but the difference was slight, even if constant. Measurements were made with a Dor tonometer, which is adequate for such comparisons. This difference in tension suggested comparing also the diameter of the retinal vessels. When observed during the stage of elevation of temperature, the veins of the right retina appeared wider and more tortuous than the left, a difference which did not exist when the whole right side was cool, as it was, for example, when the ophthalmoscopic examination was made in the early morning. However, the differences found were so slight that only through repeated examinations by several investigators can the results be securely established.

It is not too much to assert that this experiment with belladonna and calabar speaks for the dual control of the movements of the iris in man; differences in color and caliber of the vessels of the irides have not been found, and therefore it is most probable that we are dealing with right dilator paralysis.

The explanation of the difference in the tension relations of the globe is as yet a matter of personal opinion, since the various functional components of what the anatomist calls the trigeminus cannot yet be accurately distinguished by experimentation.

Let us now turn to the question of the causation of the ptosis. I believe that nobody who had seen all the foregoing symptoms, would be surprised at my considering this ptosis, which comes on gradually but remains incomplete, to be a paralysis of the musculus palpebrae superioris supplied by the sympathetic nerve (H. Müller, Harling), and the appearance of the upper lid as part and parcel of the whole symptom-complex. It would thus appear to be the opposite of the condition in exophthalmic goiter in which the upper lid is drawn upward, or better, into the orbit, which by von Graefe and Remak*) is described as due to the stimulation of the muscle fibers of the lid.

Finally, I may mention that our patient was treated with the constant current, but only for a short period, and therefore without effect.

---

*) *Deutsche Klinik.* 1864 No. 16.—*Kl. Monatsblätter* 1864. p. 185.

XIII   Duchenne's Muscular Dystrophy

G. B. A. Duchenne's description of pseudohypertrophic muscular paralysis contains not only the first clear account of this disease, but also the first report of a practical instrument of muscle biopsy.

Duchenne (1806-1875) was a French neurologist who was led to a careful study of neuromuscular diseases through his interest in the effects of electrical stimulation on muscle.[1] His painstaking observations, combined with an intuitive grasp of his field, enabled him to make many important contributions to nosology at a time when the distinction between primary muscle disease and neurogenic atrophy of muscle was poorly appreciated.

Duchenne's muscular dystrophy remains a well-defined clinical entity, but other forms of muscular dystrophy have since been described.[2,3] Although Duchenne did not recognize the hereditary character of the disease, the muscular dystrophies have subsequently been shown to have a genetic basis, and techniques are now available to detect genetic carriers.[4]

Duchenne correctly ascribed the pseudohypertrophy of muscle to the interstitial accumulation of fat and connective tissue. However, later authors, in general, have not agreed with Duchenne's insistence that this accumulation is the primary disturbance in the muscle. Current theories of the pathogenesis of muscular dystrophy tend to place the primary lesion in the muscle cell itself although the nature of such a lesion is as yet unknown.

It is noteworthy that Duchenne's original patient was mentally dull. The recent report of cerebral malformations in patients with muscular dystrophy[5] provides a morphologic basis for the mental deficiency often seen in association with muscular dystrophy.

Time has not borne out Duchenne's faith in the therapeutic efficacy of electrical stimulation. Neither this treatment nor any other tried thus far can cure muscular dystrophy. The mild cases cited by Duchenne as recovering after his electrical treatment were probably examples of benign congenital hypotonia rather than muscular dystrophy.

The histological punch introduced by Duchenne provided a new method for the diagnosis of muscle disease and was the forerunner of tissue biopsy as we know it in medicine today.

References

1. Chamberlain, O.B.: "Guillame Benjamin Amand Duchenne (1806-1875)," in Haymaker, W. (ed.): *The Founders of Neurology*, Springfield, Ill.: Charles C Thomas, Publisher, 1953, pp 275-279.

2. Walton, J.N.: "Clinical Aspects of Human Muscular Dystrophy", in Bourne, G.H., and Golarz, N. (eds.): *Muscular Dystrophy in Man and Animals*, New York: Hafner Publishing Co., 1963, chapter 7.

3. Pearson, C.M.: Muscular Dystrophy: Review and Recent Observations, *Amer J Med* **35**:632-645 (Nov) 1963.

4. Walton, J.N.: Muscular Dystrophy: Some Recent Advances in Knowledge, *Brit Med J* 1:1344-1348 (May 23) 1964.

5. Rosman, N.P., and Kakulas, B.A.: Mental Deficiency Associated With Muscular Dystrophy, A Neuropathological Study, *Brain* **89**:769-788 (Dec) 1966.

STUDIES ON PSEUDOHYPERTROPHIC MUSCULAR PARALYSIS OR MYOSCLEROTIC PARALYSIS*

By Dr. [G. B. A.] Duchenne (de Boulogne)

A. Definition and Naming of the Disease

The disease I will describe is characterized principally by: (1) weakness of movements, usually settling at first in the muscles of the lower extremities and the lumbar spine, then spreading to the upper extremities at the terminal stage and worsening at the same time until movement is abolished; (2) increase of volume either (ordinarily) in several of the paralyzed muscles or (exceptionally) in nearly all the paralyzed muscles; (3) hyperplasia of the interstitial connective tissue of the paralyzed muscles, with an abundant production of fibrous tissue or of fatty vesicles in the more advanced stage.

I propose to call this disease *pseudohypertrophic muscular paralysis* after its principal objective clinical signs or *myosclerotic paralysis* after its peripheral anatomic characteristics. These terms will be justified by studying the symptomatology and the pathologic anatomy in the living during the course of the disease. I prefer the first of these terms.

B. History of My Investigations

The discovery of pseudohypertrophic muscular paralysis goes back to the beginning of the year 1858. I owe it to the observation of a child who was afflicted with an unusual paralysis and was sent to my private clinic by my friend M. Bouvier.

Having collected, in 3 years, several similar cases, for which I knew nothing analogous in science, I believed myself justified in regarding this muscular affection as a disease entity not previously described and peculiar to childhood. When I published the principal clinical characteristics in 1861,[1] I wished only to attract the attention of observers to a disease that seemed to be rare. Faithful to the rule of conduct which I imposed on myself in my previous pathologic studies, I intended to offer a more complete description as soon as it was possible to base it on a larger number of cases matured by time.

I am happy today to have followed that step because the new cases that I have collected and those that have been observed in France and Germany have somewhat modified my ideas on this disease,

especially as concerns its progression and its nature. These new cases have, at the same time, confirmed the correctness of the principal clinical characteristics that I had outlined and now give me greater authority to enter it into nosology as a new disease.

C. Description of the Disease

I will trace the picture of pseudohypertrophic paralysis by referring to the observation that I chose in 1861 as an example and typical case. This case will be presented in more complete and precise manner because of the reports and the new information given by the young patient's mother. (The history that I previously gave of the patient had been furnished by the father who had observed the early childhood less accurately than the mother.) Furthermore, this report will be of greater interest because I could follow the progression (in extent and severity) of this pseudohypertrophic paralysis from the time of the previous report (1861) for several years until it became generalized and terminated in death.

First Case: *Pseudohypertrophic paralysis; beginning in infancy with weakness of the lower extremities; considerable enlargement of the muscles of the lower extremities and the extensors of the lumbar vertebral column to the age of 7 years; progressive generalization of the paralysis and complete abolition of all movements at 13½ years; intelligence dull; pulmonary death at 15 years.*

Joseph Serrazin, residing in Paris, no. 7 rue Rousselet, was born well built, of a good constitution, and without any apparent difficulty in the mobility of his limbs. The lower limbs were a bit more developed than the upper. His mother said he was a *beautiful baby*. No one in the family had been afflicted with a disease similar to that which he developed. His brother and sister, today aged 14 and 21, are in good health. It was only when attempts were made to teach him to stand and to walk at the age of 8 to 10 months that weakness in his lower extremities was noted. If one tried to stand him up, he collapsed. He could not sit a little while in a chair without fatigue, and he cried until he was taken up in someone's arms. He commenced to walk much later than his brother and sister, at the age of 2½ years, and still always needed support. He could not walk except with legs spread apart for lateral balance (swinging gait) and somewhat arched. Toward the age of 3

---

*Translation of: Recherches sur la paralysie musculaire pseudo-hypertrophique, ou paralysie myosclérosique, *Archives Générales de Médecine* 11:5-25, 179-209, 305-321, 421-443, 552-588, 1868.

[1] Eléctrisation localisée, 2ᵉ édition, 1861, paraplégie hypertrophique congénitale, p. 364.

years, his mother noted that his lower extremities grew in volume. Her attention was first drawn to this by the difficulty in placing his calves in his stockings, which were large enough a short time before. This excessive development of the lower extremities had progressed during 2 years. Since then, the condition of the boy remained stationary until he was presented to me for the first time in 1858 at the age of 7 years.

Here is what I then observed. The muscles of the lower extremities and the lumbar spine were so developed and made such a contrast with those of the upper extremities, which were slender, that I immediately made a photograph. . . . They were firm and even hard, like hypertrophies, and the gastrocnemius and the lumbar spinal (muscles) seemed to bulge through the thinned and distended skin. Therefore, I was not a little surprised to learn that these athletic appearing muscles had been lacking power since birth and had hardly been exercised. The child disliked moving his lower extremities and consequently was almost always resting, seated or lying down. All the movements of the lower extremities could be performed, but the strength of each measured individually was very feeble except for extension of the foot on the leg, which had retained great power. If he bent forward when seated he could not straighten up even though the lumbar muscles were enormously distended. On standing, he had to hold to a support to prevent falling. Supported, he could walk, but laboriously, spreading his legs and inclining his trunk with each step to the side of the lower extremity that rested on the ground. These efforts (standing and walking) tired him greatly and could not be maintained more than a short time. All the muscles responded perfectly to electrical stimulation. On each side there was an equinovarus of first degree. As soon as the child attempted to flex the foot on the leg, the muscles effecting this movement went into action, but their antagonists, the triceps surae, were already retracted and opposed them. The foot thus appeared extended instead of flexed. The upper extremities, although thin in comparison with the lower extremities, utilized all their mobility and served the child normally. The intellect was dull, and speech was difficult. The temporal regions were extremely projecting as in certain hydrocephalics. Nothing that I prescribed ameliorated this disease state, neither faradization (30 treatments) nor hydrotherapy nor massage, etc.

The pseudohypertrophic paralysis was still localized in the lower extremities in 1863. . . . But toward the end of 1863, the weakness increased rapidly to the point that the child was obliged to remain constantly in bed or chair. In the first months of 1864, the paralysis progressed to involve the upper extremities, where the muscles had not yet increased in volume. Six months later, the paralysis, was generalized, and movements were almost completely abolished.

His general health had been rather good, and the excessive volume of the lower extremities was maintained until June 1865. From that date the digestive functions became deranged. He suffered alternating constipation and diarrhea, and the lower extremities lost their volume little by little. Finally, in January 1866, he succumbed to a phthisis in a state of extreme emaciation, at the Frères Saint-Jean-De-Dieu, rue de Sèvres, where he had been given asylum since 1863. He was 15 years of age. There was no autopsy. . . .

Apparent Muscular Hypertrophy

The pathological phenomenon with which I shall deal invariably surprises the physician the first time he sees it coexisting with weakness of movement. I refer to the increase in the volume of the muscles producing these movements. If this type of apparent muscular hypertrophy is limited to a few muscles, . . . then one may at first, attribute it to a swelling of the structures adjacent to these muscles, to the existence of a tumor, or finally to the hypertrophy of the basic substance of the muscle itself. These were, at least, my first impressions. But, when I noted that the gastrocnemius muscles bulged through a thin skin and that their mass had increased in volume, I abandoned the two first hypotheses. Then, during voluntary contraction, when I saw them harden and form good-looking contours as do athletes' muscles, I must admit that I was led to believe in the existence of either a hypertrophy of the muscle fibers or an increase in their number. Therefore, when I found myself faced with a child all of whose muscles moving his weakened limbs had been affected by this apparent muscular hypertrophy, just as I encountered it in the first case which presented itself to me. . . , I did not at first perceive that the

[Plate I].—Fig 3.—Pseudohypertrophic paralysis in a 10 year old boy seen from the back. The monstrous and widespread development of the muscles gives to the subject an exaggerated athletic build. Fig 4.—The same subject in profile, showing his saddleback while standing and walking. Fig 5.—The Farnese Hercules, ideal of physical strength in antique statuary. The musculature is a perfect imitation of nature and is far from resembling the monstrous musculature of the paralytic child represented in Fig 3 and 4.

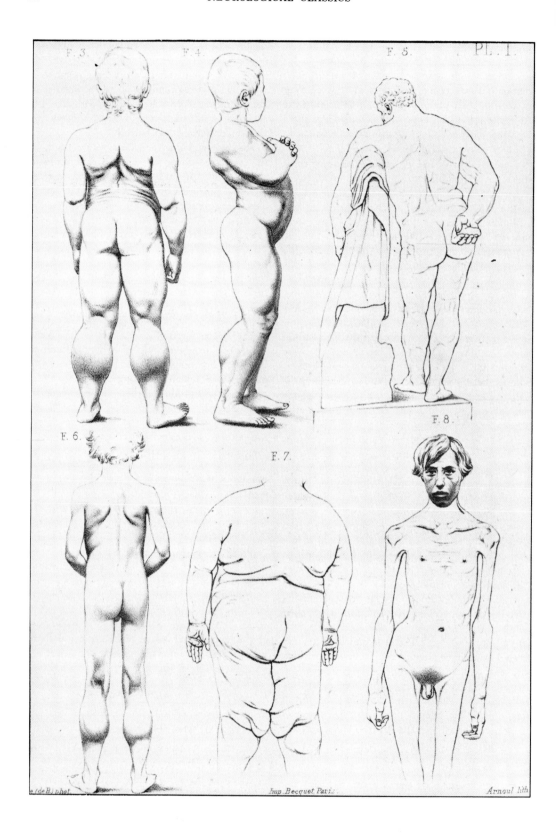

child had a serious disease. I preferred to share the illusions of the mother who exhibited, with a sort of pride, the large limbs of her child. Seeing the other boy, ten years old, whose limbs and body presented an athletic appearance (see fig. 3, 4, pl. I and 11, pl. II, Case XII), who could have guessed that this excessive richness of musculature always accompanies a paralysis which usually progresses fatally? Nevertheless, this is what clinical observation taught me and what I will soon demonstrate.

It is important to determine: at what stage of the disease the apparent muscular hypertrophy appears; in which muscles it usually develops; if it is always located in all the paralyzed muscles; and if the degree of paralysis is directly related to the increase in volume of the muscles.

1. Since I was not present at the onset of the pseudohypertrophic paralysis in almost all cases and did not observe this disease except at an advanced stage when the weakness of the lower limbs coexisted with a more or less marked increase of muscle mass, I have had to turn to the reports of the parents of my little patients for information on this point and on the first manifestations of paralysis. It is evident from the information I have received on the subject that, in most cases observed up to now, the muscular hypertrophy appeared some time after the beginning of weakness of movements. . . .

2. In 1861, when I published the [first] case. . . , the other cases of pseudohypertrophic paralysis that I had collected offered an analogous group of characteristics: the same weakness in the move-

ments of the lower limbs and of the trunk and the same functional disturbances, namely, lordosis on standing erect and walking and lateral swinging of the trunk during ambulation. In addition, the gastrocnemii and the lumbar spinal muscles were, in all cases, of a huge size, and the other muscles of the lower limbs . . . . were somewhat more developed than normal.

But later observation soon showed me that in this disease the large volume of the muscle masses is not always, as I had deduced from my first facts, restricted to the lower extremities and certain muscles of the trunk. . . .

M. Bergeron had the kindness to let me observe, during his service at the Sainte-Eugénie hospital (see Case XII), a case that I photographed from the back, side, and front (see fig. 3, 4, and 11) because of its importance and its rarity. This case shows that apparent muscular hypertrophy can be still more generalized. In fact, we see that with the exception of the pectorals, the latissimus dorsi and the sternomastoids, hypertrophy has involved all the muscles of the limbs, the trunk, and even the face, especially the temporals.

This case is among the most remarkable, not only for the generalization of the muscular hypertrophy, but also for the degree and uniformity of the hypertrophy. Indeed, the volume of the muscle masses is enormous and considerably more than in the other cases. . . .

([Footnote] M. Bergeron notes how the joints of his young patient are small, how the tendons stand out clearly, how free the articulations are, and how the skeleton is in good proportion to the age of the subject. He also notes that his skin is thin and pliable and that nowhere are there fatty pads. I shall add that, if he were not so saddle-backed, his proportions would leave little to desire and that he could serve as a model, in a certain style, for representing an infant Hercules.

We read further in the report of M. Bergeron: "All the muscle masses, with the exception of the pectorals, present a truly monstrous volume for the age of the child, *who brings to mind very exactly the Farnese Hercules and Michelangelo's studies of musculature.*" My honored colleague, with whose perfect taste in art I am well acquainted, said to me on showing me his small patient: *it is the caricature of the Farnese Hercules* (see figure 5, pl. 1, and compare with figures 3 and 4, pl. 1 and 11, pl. II). If this perfectly apt expression is not found in his report, it can be attributed only to an oversight.

The Farnese Hercules is the ideal of physical strength in antique statuary. One can criticize only the smallness of the head (which perhaps represents an intelligence limited in the service of physical strength). The musculature is of admirable proportions and quite natural. (One cannot get an idea of the beauty of this classic from the

line figure in the illustration. I thought it was too well known to require a more finished drawing.) It would be a misunderstanding of its esthetic beauty to compare it with the monstrous musculature of hypertrophic paralysis, represented in figures 3, 4, and 11. This false infant Hercules brings to mind only the school of Michelangelo, who was carried away by the power of his conceptions. His intention was to represent physical strength better than nature by exaggerating the musculature. Such exaggeration can be justified only because of his genius. Current pathological study reveals that this excessive development of the musculature is a sign of weakness. Pathological anatomy will show that these muscular contours, in appearance so formidable, are formed principally by muscles *stuffed* with connective tissue and interstitial fibrosis [End of footnote]).

[Plate II].—Fig 11.—The subject, represented in Fig 3 and 4, seen from the front; showing atrophy of the pectorals. Almost all the other muscles have a hypertrophic appearance. Fig 12, 13, 14.—Primitive fascicles at 45 diameters magnification from subjects affected with pseudohypertrophic paralysis of differing severity; showing the considerable quantity of connective and fibrous interstitial tissue, most marked in the last two. Fig 15, 16, 17, 18.—Same fascicles at 200 diameters showing the thinness of the striations compared with the normal state represented in Fig 19. Fig 20, 21, 22.—Different degrees of fatty degeneration of the muscle fiber. Fig 23.—Necrosis of the muscle fiber in *a* and proliferation of elements of fibrous tissue in *b*.

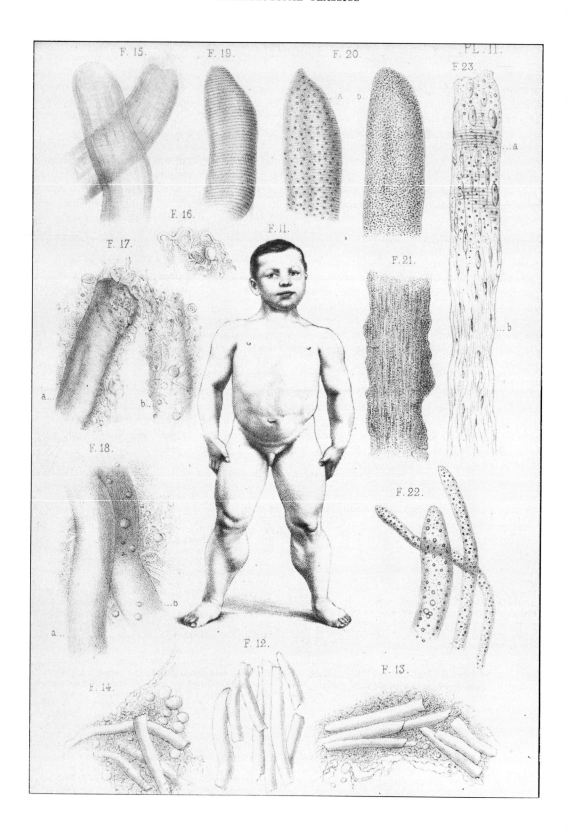

His muscles, regularly developed, make such bulges through the skin, that his limbs present a herculean form. Seen from the front or in profile, as I photographed him in figures 4 and 11, one might call him a wrestler standing proudly, defying an opponent.

In the midst of the apparent richness of his general musculature, this individual, like those I have seen affected by the same disease, presents one of the constant characteristics of pseudohypertrophic paralysis; namely, the atrophy of some muscles, contrasting with the excessive development of others. His pectoralis major and latissimus dorsi muscles are atrophic, as I have already said. We can recognize this easily by electrical exploration, by palpation, and also by the convexity of the transverse diameter of the anterior superior surface of his thorax (see figure 11), which should present, on the contrary, a flat surface in that region if the contours of the pectorales majores were normally developed. In the other small patients, the atrophy of their upper limbs contrasted with the excessive volume of their lower limbs . . . . or of other muscles. . . .

3. Those who have seen only cases similar to [Case I] are right to conclude that in pseudohypertrophic paralysis all weakened muscles become more or less increased in volume. This proposition could be deduced from the observations I had made before 1861. But since then, I have encountered cases in which muscle weakness was more or less generalized almost from the start while the hypertrophy was limited to the muscles of the calf and to the lumbar spinal muscles. . . .

4. There remains to be mentioned one clinical fact showing that in this disease the degree of paralysis is not in direct proportion to the degree of apparent muscular hypertrophy. We have observed without doubt that in all the above cases the muscles of the calf (the gastrocnemii) were the most hypertrophied. If, then, the weakness is in direct ratio to the exaggeration of volume, extension of the foot should have been weaker than flexion, which is controlled by muscles that are much less hypertrophic. However, we observe just the opposite. All my patients could extent the foot strongly, but raised it, on the contrary, with extreme feebleness.

Moreover, the predominance of the tonic force of their gastrocnemii over their antagonists (the flexors of the foot) was such that all these patients had a horselike gait with a resulting claw foot. The equine gaint, as I have shown above, is one of the characteristics of pseudohypertrophic paralysis.

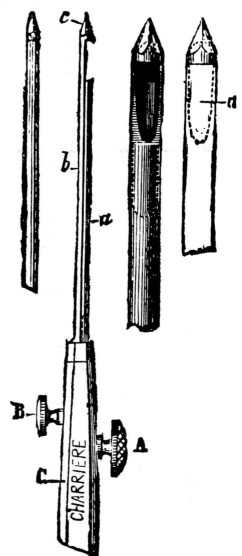

F. 24. F. 25. F. 26. F. 27.

[Plate III].—Fig 24.—Closed shaft of the histological punch. Fig 25.—The closed shaft [Translator's note—This is apparently a typographical error in the original text; the shaft is open] and a portion of its handle. Fig 26, 27.—The shaft enlarged three times to show the cavity that receives the piece of muscle removed by the instrument.

It is evident, in summary, that in this disease not all the paralyzed muscles are affected by apparent hypertrophy and that the degree of paralysis is not in direct proportion to the hypertrophy. . . .

Investigations Made in France

I shall now show that the examination on the

living of the anatomical state of the muscles not only throws great light on the diagnosis of pseudohypertrophic paralysis but is very useful in the prognosis of this disease. . . .

At first I employed the instrument known under the name of *Mideldorff's harpoon,* which was generally used in Germany for investigating trichinous human muscles. However, after one single attempt I had to give it up because it brought back not only the tissue of the muscle into which I inserted it but also foreign tissues, especially subcutaneous adipose tissue. Furthermore, the terminal hook caused intense pain on withdrawal. In addition, it seemed to me to present some dangers.

I preferred a small instrument constructed, under my direction, by the late M. Charriére fils. I called it a *histological punch.*[1] It was improved recently by MM. Robert and Colin (see figs. 24, 25, 26, and 27). Here is its description and the procedure for using it.

It consists of a cylindrical shaft, *a, b, c,* fig. 25, divided into two parts. One of these parts, *b,* is fastened on a handle, C, by the screw B. The other part, *a,* is moved along the first part by pushing the button, A.

The handle, C, of this instrument is held in the right hand, with the three last fingers flexed. The tip of the index finger, more or less extended, is placed on the shaft, *a, b, c,* fig. 25, to limit the depth of penetration. Then the punch, closed as in figure 24, is inserted through the skin. When it has reached the desired depth, it is opened, as in figure 25. The small piece of muscle tissue caught under the hook of the point, *c,* fig. 25, is divided by its sharp edges and by the free end of the other part, *a,* and finds itself closed up in the cavity, *a,* fig. 27. One can then withdraw the punch without catching the tissues which it has crossed. (Figures 26 and 27 represent, enlarged three times, the cavity which receives the tissues one wishes to examine.)

Since 1865 I have used my histological punch in the course of examining the anatomical state of the muscles in the living. It has been a great help in the diagnosis and especially the prognosis of a large number of paralyses and atrophies. With this procedure and with the precautions I shall indicate, it involves only a little pain and has never caused the slightest accident.

To decrease the pain that it can cause, I hold the skin tightly; then I insert and withdraw the instrument rapidly. The subject feels nothing but the

faint sensation of a slight impact. Children scarcely cry if one takes care not to let them see the instrument.

The histological punch should be introduced perpendicular to the direction of the muscle. Its hook should grasp the muscle transversely even at the risk of not bringing anything back.

These small operations have not been followed by a single accident. It is true that I have never neglected to displace the skin laterally as I hold it, so that the external wound and the muscle wound lose their continuity after the operation. Also, the instruments are carefully cleaned. (The dangers of anatomical punctures are too well known for me to insist on this point. Furthermore, if the instrument were not well cleaned, the preparations for microscopy would be contaminated with foreign matter.)

To clean the instrument, it is necessary to separate the different pieces. The parts that have penetrated the tissue are wiped after having been soaked in alcohol, which does not expose them to rusting as does water.

Case VII (continued—*Pseudohypertrophic paralysis; examination, on the living, of the anatomical state of the muscles.* In February 1864, I removed, for the first time, bits of the gemellus muscle with the aid of my histological punch. The patient was a small boy of 8 years, who had suffered, since the age of 5 years, with pseudohypertrophic paralysis in its second stage. I have reported his history earlier. . . . I proceeded to examine on different occasions and at intervals of three to four weeks other pieces of the right deltoid, which was hypertrophied, of the left deltoid, which was comparatively atrophied, and of the gemelli for the second time. . . .

In summary, my personal observations are as follows:

1. Hyperplasia of the interstitial connective tissue, with proliferation of more or less abundant fibrous tissue (see fig. 13, 14, 17, 18, pl. II), is the fundamental anatomical lesion of the muscles in pseudohypertrophic paralysis.

2. It is present in all the paralyzed muscles, whether or not they are increased in volume. This justifies the name *myosclerotic paralysis,* which I propose to give it. Its symptomatological name is *pseudohypertrophic paralysis.*

3. It is this [hyperplasia] that produces the considerable and sometimes monstrous increase in muscle volume, which is in direct proportion to the quantity of hyperplastic interstitial connective and fibrous tissue.

---

[1] This histological punch was presented to the Paris Academy of Medicine at its meeting of August 1, 1865.

4. The hyperplastic interstitial connective and fibrous tissue is associated with a slight (see fig. 13, pl. II) or moderate (see fig. 14, pl. II) number of fatty vesicles. According to the observations in Germany, it is replaced by a considerable quantity of adipose tissue.

This last condition appears to me to be the most advanced degree of alteration of interstitial muscular tissue in pseudohypertrophic paralysis.

5. According to my personal observations, the transverse striation is preserved in the whole length (see a, fig. 17, pl. II) or in a rather large portion of most muscle fibers (see fig. 18, pl. II), but it becomes extremely fine and less apparent. Where the transverse striation has disappeared, we see the longitudinal striations. Sometimes these longitudinal striations themselves are obliterated, and the sarcolemma seems to contain fatty vesicles (see b, fig. 18, pl. II), which, in reality, arise from the surrounding interstitial tissue, and which, moreover, differ essentially in their appearance and their confluence from the fatty granulations that characterize the fatty degeneration of muscle.

6. The hyperplasia of the interstitial connective tissue usually does not appear until the second stage of the disease. It seems to me to be preceded by an inflammatory condition of the muscles, which may give rise to a slight increase in their volume.

In this period, the transverse striation of the muscle fiber is already extremely thin. (see fig. 15 pl. II).

Diagnosis

The basis for the diagnosis of pseudohypertrophic paralysis is of two kinds: one draws on the symptomatology and the other draws on the pathological anatomy of the paralyzed muscles, examined *in vivo* with the aid of my histological punch.

I. *Basis of the diagnosis from clinical observation in pseudohypertrophic paralysis*

The diagnostic signs furnished by clinical observation can be reduced to the six principal ones which follow:

1. Decrease in strength, at the beginning of the disease, usually in the muscles of the lower limbs.

2. Lordosis and spreading of the lower limbs on standing and walking.

3. Excessive development of volume, during a second stage, either of some or of all the weakened muscles.

4. Progressive course of the disease, during a third stage, with worsening of the paralysis and with its generalization if it was limited to the inferior members.

5. Decrease or abolition of electromuscular contractility in an advanced stage of the disease.

6. Absence of fever, sensory disturbance, and impairment in the functions of the bladder and intestine during the entire course of the disease.

II. *Basis of the diagnosis from the anatomical state of the muscles in pseudohypertrophic paralysis*

Formerly the diagnosis of a disease could not be clarified by pathological anatomy until after the death of the subject. This was called the *diagnosis of Morgagni*. Today, we can obtain, in the living, small specimens of muscles with a harmless instrument (my histological punch, described above, p. 203) and clarify the diagnosis of muscular disorders by the examination of the anatomical condition of paralyzed muscles. This new basis of diagnosis, furnished by *living pathological anatomy*, has already rendered me great service. We shall shortly see how it is useful in the diagnosis and likewise in the prognosis of pseudophypertrophic paralysis. . . .

Summary

A. The prognosis of pseudohypertrophic paralysis is grave. When I have been called to examine a case that has reached the stage of hypertrophy or of proliferation of interstitial connective tissue, I have always seen it generalize and terminate by complete abolition of movement and death in adolescence.

However, it may heal in the first period, before the pseudohypertrophic or myosclerotic stage. For this reason I have not called it *progressive paralysis,* that is to say, following Requin (who originated that term), paralysis which, once started, always progresses to a fatal termination.

B. I have obtained healing of pseudohypertrophic paralysis in its first stage of muscular faradization, assisted by hydrotherapy and massage.

This treatment applied when the disease had reached its second stage produced only a temporary improvement and did not prevent its progressive course and fatal termination. A variety of medications (strychnine, ergot of rye, potassium iodide, etc.) have likewise failed in this second period.

At present I am trying, in the second stage of pseudohypertrophic paralysis, the therapeutic effect of continuous currents, along with direct muscular faradization.

XIV   Tay-Sachs' Disease

OUR KNOWLEDGE of the amaurotic family idiocies, and especially of Tay-Sachs' disease, has increased during the years in stepwise fashion.[1,2]

In 1881, Waren Tay, an English ophthalmologist, first described the macular changes that were subsequently associated with this condition.[3] Tay later described similar changes in two siblings of the infant first reported.[4] Then in 1887, Bernard Sachs, a neurologist in New York, published the original clinical and pathological description of the disease.[5] In studying additional cases, he noted the familial nature of the condition, which he called amaurotic family idiocy.[6-8] Other physicians published case reports, and Tay-Sachs' disease was established as an entity. Subsequently, this fatal disorder was found to be an autosomal recessive trait, occurring primarily, but not exclusively, in Jewish families from eastern Europe.[2,9]

Early in the twentieth century, other types of cerebroretinal degeneration were described in older patients by Bielschowsky (late infantile form),[10] Batten, Spielmeyer, Vogt (juvenile forms),[11-13] and Kufs (adult form).[14] The exact relationship of these disorders to Tay-Sachs' disease is still being studied.[15]

Newer investigative techniques have contributed further information on Tay-Sachs' disease. Beginning with the biochemical studies of Klenk in the late 1930's, increased amounts of gangliosides were discovered in the brains of patients with this disease.[16,17] Subsequent research using the electron microscope has disclosed ganglioside-rich membranous bodies within the neuronal cytoplasm.[18] At the present time, investigators are attempting to define the biochemical defect responsible for this abnormal accumulation of gangliosides.[17,19]

Thus, the march of research initiated by Tay and Sachs may be coming nearer the final step of finding an effective treatment for this mysterious disease.

References

1. Thannhauser, S.J.: *Lipidoses. Diseases of the Intracellular Lipid Metabolism*, ed 3, New York: Grune & Stratton, Inc., 1958, pp 573-582.
2. Volk, B.W.: "Historical Review," in Volk, B.W. (ed.): *Tay-Sachs' Disease* New York: Grune & Stratton, Inc., 1964, pp 1-15.
3. Tay, W.: Symmetrical Changes in the Region of the Yellow Spot in Each Eye of an Infant, *Trans Ophthal Soc UK* 1:55-57, 1881.
4. Tay, W.: A Third Instance in the Same Family of Symmetrical Changes in the Region of the Yellow Spot in Each Eye of an Infant, Closely Resembling Those of Embolism, *Trans Ophthal Soc UK* 4:158-159, 1884.
5. Sachs, B.: On Arrested Cerebral Development, With Special Reference to its Cortical Pathology, *J Nerv Ment Dis* 14:541-553 (Sept-Oct) 1887.
6. Sachs, B.: A Further Contribution to the Pathology of Arrested Cerebral Development, *J Nerv Ment Dis* 19:603-607 (Aug) 1892.
7. Sachs, B.: A Family Form of Idiocy, Generally Fatal, Associated With Early Blindness (Amaurotic Family Idiocy), *J Nerv Ment Dis* 23:475-479 (July) 1896.
8. Sachs, B.: On Amaurotic Family Idiocy: A Disease Chiefly of the Gray Matter of the Central Nervous System, *J Nerv Ment Dis* 30:1-13 (Jan) 1903.
9. Pratt, R.T.C.: *The Genetics of Neurological Disorders*, London: Oxford University Press, Inc., 1967, pp 7-10.
10. Bielschowsky, M.: Über spätinfantile familiäre amaurotische Idiotie mit Kleinhirnsymptonen, *Deutsch Z Nervenheilk* 50:7-29, 1914.
11. Batten, F.E.: Cerebral Degeneration with

Symmetrical Changes in the Maculae in Two Members of a Family, *Trans Ophthal Soc UK* 23:386-389, 1903.

12. Spielmeyer, W.: Ueber familiäre amaurotische Idiotien, *Neurol Centralbl* 24:620-621 (July) 1905.

13. Vogt, H.: Über familiäre amaurotische Idiotie und verwandte Krankheitsbilder, *Mschr Psychiat Neurol* 18:161-171, 310-357, 1905.

14. Kufs, H.: Über eine Spätform der amaurotischen Idiotie und ihre heredofamiliären Grundlagen, *Z Ges Neurol Psychiat* 95:169-188, 1925.

15. Cumings, J.N.: Some Lipid Diseases of the Brain, *Proc Roy Soc Med* 58:21-28 (Jan) 1965.

16. Klenk, E.: On Gangliosides, *Amer J Dis Child* 97:711-714 (May) 1959.

17. Saifer, A.: "The Biochemistry of Tay-Sachs' Disease," in Volk. B.W. (ed.): *Tay-Sachs Disease*, New York: Grune & Stratton, Inc., 1964, pp 68-117.

18. Samuels, S.; et al: Studies in Tay-Sachs Disease: IV, Membranous Cytoplasmic Bodies; 1. Biochemistry, 2, Ultrastructure, *J Neuropath Exp Neurol* 22:81-97 (Jan-March) 1963.

19. Brady, R.O.: The Sphingolipidoses, *New Eng J Med* 275:312-318 (Aug 11) 1966.

SYMMETRICAL CHANGES IN THE REGION OF THE YELLOW SPOT IN EACH EYE OF AN INFANT.*

By Waren Tay

(With Plate III.)

Mrs. L—brought her infant, aet. 12 months, to the London Hospital, March 7th, 1881. When the baby was a fortnight or three weeks old, it was noticed to have very little power of holding its head up or of moving its limbs. Since that time the weakness had become more and more pronounced. The mother brought the child to the hospital in the hope that something might be done to strengthen it. I could find nothing more than weakness, no absolute paralysis of any part. It seemed to me that its cerebral development was probably deficient, and I was induced to examine the eyes with the ophthalmoscope to ascertain whether there was any affection of the optic nerves. The mother had not suspected there was anything the matter with the sight, though, when questioned closely, she admitted she did not think the baby took as much notice as other babies. I found the optic discs apparently quite healthy, but in the region of the yellow spot in each eye there was a conspicuous, tolerably defined, large white patch, more or less circular in outline, and showing at its centre a brownish-red, fairly circular spot, contrasting strongly with the white patch surrounding it. This central spot did not look at all like a hæmorrhage, nor as if due to pigment, but seemed a gap in the white patch, through which one saw healthy structure. In fact, the appearances may most suitably be compared with those we are familiar with in cases of embolism of the central artery of the retina.

I am quite unable to arrive at any conclusion as to the exact nature of the disease. I believe the changes to be situated in the retina, at any rate chiefly so. They may possibly be congenital. The family history throws no light on the possibilities of the case. This is the first child. There have been no miscarriages. There is no evidence of syphilis whatever to be obtained. There is no history of phthisis in the family. The parents have been married two years, and were not related before marriage.

Dr. Hughlings Jackson kindly saw the child with me, and said there seemed no evidence of any definite cerebral affection. He could only say the baby seemed very weak. He agreed as to the local conditions present, so also did Mr. Hutchinson and others who have examined the child.

The drawing from which Plate III has been made was taken for me by Burgess, and was exhibited to the Society. It shows the conditions well.

Living specimen. April 7th, 1881.

P.S.—July 30th, 1881.—The baby has remained in much the same state as when first seen. There is still no definite sign of localised mischief, but the child lies almost helpless in its mother's arms. It is generally cheerful or else asleep; it is rarely cross. There is an important alteration in one respect, however; the discs are now *undoubtedly becoming atrophic*. The changes in the region of the macula are apparently precisely the same as before.—W.T.

*Reprinted from *Transactions of the Ophthalmological Society of the United Kingdom* 1:55-57, 1881.

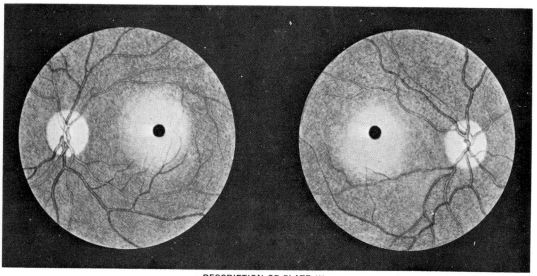

DESCRIPTION OF PLATE III.

Illustrating Mr. Waren Tay's Case of Symmetrical Changes in the Region of the Yellow-spot in each Eye in an Infant.

ON ARRESTED CEREBRAL DEVELOPMENT,
WITH SPECIAL REFERENCE TO
ITS CORTICAL PATHOLOGY.[1]*

By B. Sachs, M. D.

New York

. . . . The following is the history of the case: The little girl S., who was but two years old at the time of death, was the first-born of young and healthy parents. In the families of both parents insanity is not unknown; on the mother's side there is a strong hereditary predisposition to mental disease, and several near relatives of the father have developed various forms of insanity within recent years. During the fifth month of pregnancy, the mother was thrown out of her carriage, but did not sustain any serious injuries; the child was born at full term, and appeared to be a healthy child in every respect; its body and head were well proportioned, its features beautifully regular. Nothing abnormal was noticed until the age of two to three months, when the parents observed that the child was much more listless than children of that age are apt to be; that it took no notice of anything, and that its eyes rolled about curiously (there was evident nystagmus). Allowing for some very slight vacillations, the child remained in practically the same condition up to time of death. The condition was characterized as follows: The child would ordinarily lie upon its back, and was never able to change its position; muscles of head, neck, and back so weak that it was not able either to hold its head straight or to sit upright. It never attempted any voluntary movements; movements that were made were in obedience to peripheral stimulation. All the muscles were extremely flaccid; all reacted perfectly to both forms of current. The child would close its hand upon the finger of the examining person, but objects placed in its hands were quickly dropped. The child as it grew older gave no signs of increasing mental vigor. It could not be made to play with any toy, did not recognize people's voices, and showed no preference for any person around it. During the first year of its life, the child was attracted by the light, and would move its eyes, following objects drawn across its field of vision; but later on absolute blindness set in.

[1]Read before the American Neurol. Assoc., July, 1887.
*Reprinted from *The Journal of Nervous and Mental Disease* 14:541-553 (Sept-Oct) 1887.

Dr. Knapp, who made several ophthalmoscopic examinations of this case, reported the following unusual condition, at the seventeenth meeting of the Heidelberg Ophthalmological Society. The report may be found in the Proceedings of this meeting. Dr. Knapp there says: "Child two to three months; nystagmus vibratorius; pupils contracted as is usual with children at this age. Media clear, optic nerve discs pale. Fovea centralis, of a cherry red color, was surrounded by an intense grayish-white opacity. This opacity was most distinct in the vicinity of the fovea centralis, and for some little distance around it, but faded away gradually into normal retinal field."—Dr. Knapp at first gave a favorable prognosis, except as regards central vision, more particularly as there appeared to be for some time a slight improvement in vision. He could not then, and is not now ready, to give an explanation of this condition.

But two cases of this sort of retinal changes had thus far been reported, by Magnus and Goldzieher, and neither of these authors has any explanation to offer. Dr. Knapp, in private conversation, hinted at a development defect. Unfortunately, the eyes could not be removed after death. Dr. Knapp empowers me to add that "a further examination in May and June, 1886, revealed great changes. Child totally blind, optic nerves completely atrophied (discs as white as paper, with scarcely a trace of blood-vessels). Macula lutea essentially as before."

By way of anticipation, it may be remarked that numerous longitudinal and vertical sections of both optic nerves were variously stained and examined, but that no morbid changes could be made out. Blindness must, therefore, have been due either to the retinal changes, or to the deficient cortical condition, or to both.

Hearing seemed to be very acute; there was unusual hyperexcitability to auditory and tactile impressions; the slightest touch and every sound were apt to startle the child. The child never had convulsions, not even while teething; no marked rigidities at any time. The child never learned to utter a single sound; if left to itself it would occasionally make a low gurgling noise. Bodily functions normal, excepting the frequent recurrence of bronchial troubles and feebleness of its digestive powers. At the age of one it had a severe attack of diphtheria from which it rallied in the course of a few weeks. The child developed unusually high fever with every disturbance, however slight, of its bodily functions. In the way of treatment nothing was recommended but careful nursing and feeding, tonic treatment with malt and the like; phosphorus was given in small doses for a time, and the peripheral muscles and nerves were alternately galvanized and faradized, more in the hope of exciting cerebral activity in a reflex way than of benefiting the nutrition of the flaccid parts.

There were no distinct evidences of inherited or acquired syphilis and none of rachitis.

During last summer (1886), the child grew steadily weaker; it ceased to take its food properly, its bronchial troubles increased, and finally, pneumonia setting in, it died August, 1886.

Immediately after its death, the child was brought to the city, and yet twenty-nine hours had elapsed before the autopsy could be made.

Autopsy.—The autopsy was confined to an examination of skull, brain, and abdominal viscera. The body was in a state of extreme emaciation; all muscles relaxed. The skull was thick, and skull cap unusually heavy. Outer and inner surfaces smooth and showed no unusual appearances or impressions. Skull symmetrical; left frontal fossa a trifle deeper than right; large fontanelle very nearly ossified. A large organized clot was found in the superior longitudinal sinus; there was some thickening of the dura to either side of the sinus, some slight adhesion over the upper portion of the precentral and over the left temporal convolution, but even here and over the entire surface of the brain the pia could be easily removed without injuring the parts below. There was an œdema of the entire convexity; unusual pallor of the convolutions; no marked increase of the fluid in the lateral ventricles. Freed of its dura, the brain weighed exactly two pounds (one thousand grams). Blood-vessels appeared normal and had normal distribution. I may state at once that the cortex was hard to the touch, and that the knife

grated in removing a small portion of the cortex for immediate examination. This grating was due to small calcified plates. On superficial inspection, the great breadth of the fissures, the corresponding narrowness of the convolutions, and the unusual exposure on the left island of Reil were very apparent. A detailed examination of the larger ganglia, of the pons, medulla, etc., will be made and will be reported upon later on.

The spleen was enlarged and the liver hard, but no evidences of hereditary syphilis.

EXAMINATION OF BRAIN.

The brain was immersed at once into Müller's fluid, and as soon as hardened the brain surfaces were photographed.[1] By comparison with the paper[2] which our retiring president read last year, you will recognize certain departures from normal fissuration which are indicative of inferior brain development.

Examination of Brain Surfaces.

Left hemisphere, outer surface. (Plate I.)

The most striking features are the great depth of all fissures, and the comparative simplicity of fissuration, particularly in the frontal lobes; the great exposure of the island of Reil due to the retraction and narrowness of the surrounding convolutions. The central fissure (c) is bifurcated and is clearly confluent with the Sylvian fissure which is broad and long. The first temporal fissure (t. I) —supertemporal, Wilder—would be continuous high up into the parietal region, but for a slight bridging convolution. The parieto-occipital fissure is unusually distinct and in the occipital lobe the three fissures are easily traced. In the frontal lobe, the first and second frontal fissures are well marked, while the second forms the long branch of a zygal formation according to Wilder. The convolutions appear alternately narrowed and broadened; this is particularly true of the first temporal and precentral convolutions. The gyrus angularis is scantily developed.

The mesial surface of left hemisphere exhibits the confluence of the parieto-occipital, the calcarine and hippocampal fissures. The collateral fissure of Wilder well marked. The calloso-marginal fissure well defined though shallow. The præcuneus massive, the cuneus of normal size.

Right hemisphere—*outer surface.*

Here the conditions approach much more nearly to the normal. The island of Reil is scarcely

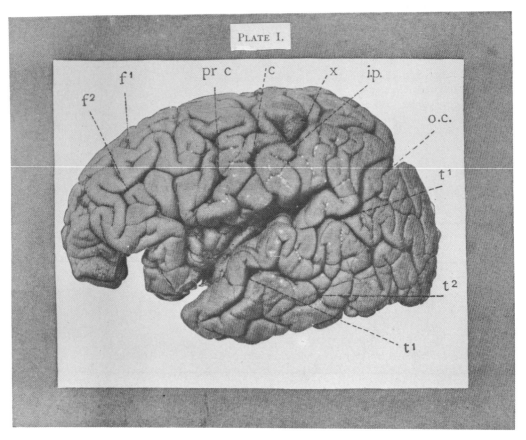

Plate I. Outer aspect of surface of left hemisphere showing the exposure of the island of Reil, and great breadth of fissure of Sylvius.

X denotes region from which first block of cortical tissue had been removed for histological examination; C, central fissure or fissure of Rolando; *pr c,* precentral fissure; *i.p,* interparietal fissure; *oc,* occipital: parieto-occipital fissure; t^1, t^2, first and second temporal fissures; f^1, f^2, first and second frontal fissures; Other explanations in text.

exposed; the fissure of Sylvius of normal breadth and length; the central fissure is confluent with the fissure of Sylvius. The first temporal convolution is *continuous* into the parietal region, and there is a distinct though very narrow angular gyrus. Wilder's interparietal fissure is distinct; in both the occipital and frontal lobes, three typical fissures can be made out; there is an undoubted medifrontal (Wilder) fissure which could not be traced on the left side. The parieto-occipital does not form as distinct an indentation as on left outer surface.

Median surface.—The parieto-occipital, calcarine, and hippocampal fissures are confluent; the collateral fissures well defined; the entire mesial surface is divided into small blocks by numerous secondary fissures. Cuneus and precuneus of normal development.

Microscopical Examination of the Cortex.

The brain surfaces, after they had been thoroughly hardened in Müller's fluid, were cut up into small blocks for histological examination. Sections from the frontal lobes, the motor zones, the base of the third frontal convolution, from the first temporal convolution, and from the occipital apex of both hemispheres have been examined. The cuneus was unfortunately too brittle to permit of section cutting. From the portions thus far examined, it is fair to infer that the changes to be described affect equally every part of the brain surface. The plates herein given represent the changes as seen in sections from the first temporal convolution of the left side. These specimens were stained according to the acid fuchsin method,

PLATE III.

PLATE II.

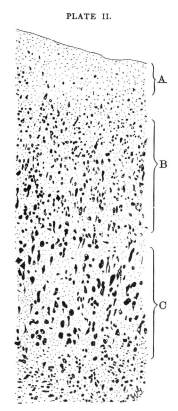

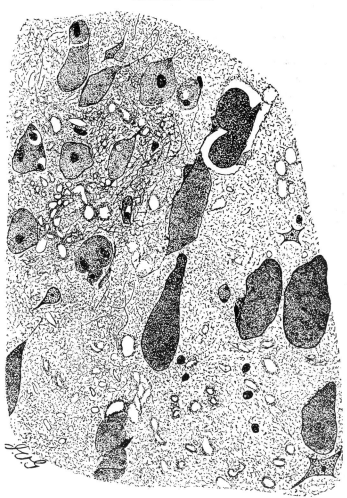

Plate II. X 70 diameters. Section from first temporal convolution; specimen stained with acid fuchsin; drawing made with especial reference to changes in the cells.

Divisions A, B, C, correspond about to layers of superficial neuroglia, of small pyramid cells and of large pyramid cells. Below C is fourth granular layer (Meynert).

It will be noted that with this low magnifying power, the changed appearance of the pyramid cells can be made out. The contours of the cell are altered, the pyramidal shape is often widely departed from; the cell body is altered, and occasionally shows distinct lacunae.

Plate III. X 500 diameters. Section of first temporal convolution, representing a portion of division C under much higher magnifying power. Pyramidal cells have lost their normal shape. The cell body has a homogeneous but altered appearance; nuclei either absent or distorted; smaller cells and neuroglia cells with distinct nuclei; section of capillary vessels normal; in the upper right hand corner a distorted cell mass with pericellular space around.

others were stained with Weigert's two hæmatoxylin methods, and with ammoniacal carmine. You will note that the cellular elements exhibit the same changes, whatever staining method we employed. On the drawing, most carefully made by Dr. Van Gieson, and in these specimens[1] the following conditions may be noted.

We are able to distinguish the external barren

---

[1]Demonstrated at the meeting.

layer, the layer of small pyramidal cells, the layer of the large pyramids, and perhaps a trace of Meynert's fourth granular layer. Examining these sections, very marked changes will be observed in the structure of the small and large pyramid cells. In my search through the entire brain I have not come across more than half a dozen, if as many, pyramid cells of anything like normal appearance. The fewest large and small pyramid cells show well-defined processes. The contours are rounded, and the cell substance exhibits every possible change of its protoplasmatic substance. In some there are a distinct nucleus and nucleolus, surrounded by a detritus-like mass; in many the nucleus and nucleolus are entirely wanting. All these varied changes can be studied best with the acid fuchsin method; in Weigert preparations, the whole pathological cell mass takes up the stain deeply, and it is not always easy to distinguish the nucleus and cell-body. Glancing through the sections, you will also observe that a few of the cells turn their apices downward instead of upward, thus exhibiting a change to which Brückner refers as occurring in his case of tuberous sclerosis and to which no pathological significance is to be attached.

Plate III. exhibits these changes under a very much higher power. In some cells a partly normal and a partly pathological character of the cell-body is visible. In the neuroglia, I have not been able to prove any changes; there is certainly no sclerosis visible in any part I have examined. The white fibres have not undergone morbid changes, but on Weigert specimens they cannot be traced as far towards the periphery as in the normal cortex; the transverse fibers in the outer barren layer could not be made out. There is no evidence whatever of any previous encephalitic process. No infiltration around the blood-vessels; in fact no changes in any of the blood-vessels of the cortex. At the meeting, doubts were expressed whether there was not a paucity of blood-vessels. I have paid special attention to this point, and am now convinced, after examining a very large number of sections from every part of the cortex, that these capillary vessels are of normal calibre and as numerous as in corresponding sections of the normal brain. Nor is there any proliferation of the nuclei of these cells in the walls of the blood-vessels. We have then a simple change affecting the cells and possibly the white fibres only, and the question remains to be decided whether there is mere arrest of development, or an arrest of development the result of a previous inflammatory process. There is nothing in support of the latter proposition, and everything in favor of the former.

I cannot find any evidence of distinct degenerative changes in the cells, and it would seem to me that, if the process were one that had set in after the cells had already matured, we should find some, and many more cells than we actually do, exhibiting a more complete formation than any to be found on the specimens before you. You will note also that there were no gross changes such as are frequently held responsible for insufficient development; there is no evidence of hydrocephalus internus, of a general or a multiple tuberous sclerosis; no traces of a preceding encephalitis.

We have here an agenetic condition pure and simple, affecting the highest nerve elements. As to the cause of this agenetic condition, I am not willing to speculate. I repeat that syphilis is excluded, at least not proved, that there is strong hereditary predisposition to mental troubles, and that there is the etiological factor of traumatism in the case. As the fœtal circulation is easily affected by the slightest disturbances, and the proper nutrition of the most highly differentiated organ of the body may in this way have become impaired, we cannot afford to overlook the factor of traumatism.

XV Little's Disease

PRESENT concepts of infantile cerebral palsy are based largely on the ideas of the English physician, William John Little (1810-1894), and the form of cerebral palsy manifested by bilateral spasticity has become known as Little's disease.[1-6] Afflicted with an equinus deformity of his own left foot, Little made significant contributions to the understanding of clubfoot and other orthopedic disorders.[7,8] In 1861, he presented to the Obstetrical Society of London his classic monograph on cerebral palsy.

The pyramidal and extrapyramidal forms of cerebral palsy had been noted by physicians in random fashion for centuries.[2,3] Little organized this information and related cerebral palsy to trauma, and especially to anoxia, occurring at the time of birth. His astute conclusions profoundly influenced subsequent thought about the nature of cerebral palsy. However, other etiologic factors have more recently been recognized, such as prenatal developmental malformations and kernicterus. Little erred in overemphasizing a single cause, but perinatal anoxia is still considered a major etiologic factor in the development of cerebral palsy.[5]

References

1. Collier, J.: The Pathogenesis of Cerebral Diplegia, *Brain* 47:1-21 (Feb) 1924.

2. Bick, E.M.: *Source Book of Orthopaedics*, ed 2, Baltimore: The Williams & Wilkins Co., 1948.

3. Courville, C.B.: *Cerebral Palsy: A Brief Introduction to Its History, Etiology, and Pathology, With Some Notes on the Resultant Clinical Syndromes and Their Treatment*, Los Angeles: San Lucas Press, 1954.

4. Collis, E., et al: *The Infantile Cerebral Palsies*, Springfield, Ill: Charles C Thomas, Publisher, 1957.

5. Crothers, B., and Paine, R.S.: *The Natural History of Cerebral Palsy*, Cambridge, Mass: Harvard University Press, 1959.

6. Rang, M.: *Anthology of Orthopaedics*, Edinburgh: E. & S. Livingstone, Ltd., 1966.

7. Little, W.J.: Course of Lectures on the Deformities of the Human Frame, *Lancet* 1:5-8, 38-44, 78-82, 141-144, 174-177, 238-241, 285-288, 318-322, 350-354, 382-386, 534-538, 564-568, 598-602, 679-683, 705-712, 745-750, 777-781, 809-815, 1843-1844.

8. Little, W.J.: *On the Nature and Treatment of the Deformities of the Human Frame: Being a Course of Lectures Delivered at the Royal Orthopaedic Hospital in 1843: With Numerous Notes and Additions to the Present Time*, London: Longman, Brown, Green & Longmans, 1853.

ON THE INFLUENCE OF ABNORMAL PARTURITION, DIFFICULT LABOURS, PREMATURE BIRTH, AND ASPHYXIA NEONATORUM, ON THE MENTAL AND PHYSICAL CONDITION OF THE CHILD, ESPECIALLY IN RELATION TO DEFORMITIES.*

By W. J. Little, MD

Senior-Physician to The London Hospital; Founder of The Royal
Orthopaedic Hospital; Visiting-Physician to Asylum
for Idiots, Earlswood; Etc.

(Communicated by Dr. Tyler Smith)

. . . . The object of this communication is to show that the act of birth does occasionally imprint upon the nervous and muscular systems of the nascent infantile organism very serious and peculiar evils. When we investigate the evils in question, and their causative influences, we find that the same laws of pathology apply to diseases incidental to the act of birth as to those which originate before and after birth. We are, in fact, afforded another illustration that there exists no such thing as exceptional or special pathology.

Thirty-five years ago the pathology of deformities, if not invested with fable, was wrapped in obscurity; it was then scarcely perceived that the materials for extensive inductive observation existed.

Nearly twenty years ago, in a course of lectures published in the 'Lancet,' and more fully in a 'Treatise on Deformities,' published in 1853, I showed that premature birth, difficult labours, mechanical injuries during parturition to head and neck, where life had been saved, convulsions following the act of birth, were apt to be succeeded by a determinate affection of the limbs of the child, which I designated spastic rigidity of the limbs of new-born children, spastic rigidity from asphyxia neonatorum, and assimilated it to the trismus nascentium and the universal spastic rigidity sometimes produced at later periods of existence.

Dugès, Cruveilhier, Smellie, Davis, Evory, Kennedy, Doherty, Weber and Hecker, who have described the condition of stillborn children, suspended animation, asphyxia neonatorum and apoplexy of new-born children, are almost entirely silent respecting the after consequences to the infant, when not fatal. The first named is the only one who distinctly enunciates that hemiplegia and idiocy may follow injury received at birth. The others seem quite unaware that abnormal parturi-

tion, besides ending in death or recovery, not unfrequently has another termination, i.e. in the language of medical writers, has a third termination "in other diseases." My friends, Drs. West, Tyler Smith, and Barnes, have informed me that instances of such a termination of abnormal labour have not fallen under their notice. Dr. Ramsbotham says he can remember two instances. It is obvious that the great majority of apparently stillborn infants, whose lives are saved by the attendant accoucheur, recover unharmed from that condition. I have, however, witnessed so many cases of deformity, mental and physical, traceable to causes operative at birth, that I consider the subject worthy the notice of the Obstetrical Society. In orthopaedic practice alone, during about twenty years, I have met with probably two hundred cases of spastic rigidity from this cause. I omit reckoning the subjects of idiot and other asylums, in which probably such cases abound, but of which I have been able to obtain no history. I revert to the subject at the present moment because I believe I am now enabled to form an opinion of the nature of the anatomical lesions and the particular abnormal event at birth on which the symptoms depend. Moreover, as the study of the proximate cause of the affections which I shall describe requires the light of such facts as the members of this Society have peculiar opportunities of supplying, I make no further apology for occupying the Society's time.

Before I describe the mental and physical derangements of the infant which can be referred to the effects of abnormal parturition and asphyxia at birth, I may be permitted to dwell upon the principal phenomena which occur in the fœtal organism immediately before, during, and immediately after, the act of normal parturition.

. . . . The fœtus, during the uterine contractions, especially after evacuation of liquor amnii, is subjected, together with the placenta and umbilical

---

*Reprinted from *Transactions of the Obstetrical Society of London* 3:293-344, 1861.

cord, to a gradually increasing amount of pressure, through which it may reasonably be conjectured that the circulatory system, and consequently the capillary system, as of the lungs and nervous centres, are gradually prepared for the altered offices which are about to devolve upon them. This pressure is at first intermittent, the duration of the period of repose at first greatly exceeding the period of disturbance; as the final exit approaches, the pressure simply remits, until at length it is so considerable that prompt escape from the mother alone prevents mischievous results to the nascent organism. During the uterine contractions a certain amount of impediment to placental respiration or to placental interchange of material is unavoidable, so much of undecarbonized or deteriorated blood is contained in the fœtal tissues—amongst other tissues, in those of the excitor of respiratory acts, the medulla oblongata—as suffices to give notice to the medulla oblongata of the need of inspiratory movements and of the admission of air into the lungs. Hence is explained the first-observed phenomenon of normal, independent, extra-uterine existence, the effectual act of inspiration, accompanied with the welcomed, characteristic, expressive cry of the new-born child. The normal impediment to placental interchange reaches its maximum at the moment of birth. Should any departure from the normal act of birth take place, should the act of normal respiration not be established at the moment of birth, the child presents itself in a state either of manifest death (stillborn), apparently stillborn, or in a state of more or less completely suspended animation, and does not utter the characteristic expressive cry of the new-born child.

The new-born child that has not yet attained to thorough independent existence tolerates a longer duration of suspended animation than the child in which pulmonary respiration has been thoroughly established or than the adult; yet reflection on the nature of a delay of only a few moments in the substitution of pulmonary for the ceased placental respiration would lead to the apprehension that even the want of a few breathings, if not fatal to the economy, may imprint a lasting injury upon it. The observations I have recorded of the direct connection between suspended animation at birth and mental and physical impairment of the individual, prove that the proportion of entire recoveries from the effects of asphyxia neonatorum is smaller than has hitherto been supposed.

It will be acknowledged that the state of things in the fœtus at the moment of birth, at the moment of entire withdrawal of placental or maternal circulatory influence, is one of imminent failure in decarbonization of the blood. If pulmonary respiration be not immediately established, the state of suspended animation—asphyxia neonatorum—takes place. From analogy with other forms of suffocation in later life, as from drowning, when the air-passages are suddenly and forcibly obstructed, suffocation also from inhalation of certain gases which exclude oxygen from the lungs, we may infer that the want of respiration in the new-born child is followed by stagnation of blood in all the large venous channels. We may direct our thoughts to the necessary consequences of blood stagnation in the sinuses of the brain, the venous plexuses surrounding the spinal cord, the venae cavae, the right side of heart, and the pulmonary system. We can apprehend the inevitable congestions of the capillary system of the brain and spinal cord, and a prompt result in death, if the mischievous circle of affairs is not relieved by suitable respiration.

The forms of abnormal parturition which I have observed to precede certain mental and physical derangements of the infant consisted of difficult labours, i.e. unnatural presentations, tedious labours from rigidity of maternal passages or apertures, instrumental labours, labours in which turning was had recourse to, breech presentations, premature labours, and cases in which the umbilical cord had been entangled around the infant's neck or had fallen down before the head. To these abnormal forms of labour I believe Cases LII and LIII justify me in adding labours in which, from want of due attention immediately after birth or after expulsion from the mother, the child has been partially suffocated in the maternal secretions or under her clothes.

Doubtless in some of the instances I have recorded sufficient mechanical injury to head and neck was inflicted to account for whatever unfavorable consequences, whether these were fatal or not, may have ensued, but the more the facts I shall adduce are studied the more apparent, in my opinion, it will be that a larger proportion of infants, either dead, stillborn, apoplectic, or asphyxiated at birth, have been rendered so by interruption of the proper placental relation of the fœtus to the mother, and non-substitution of pulmonary respiration, than from direct mechanical injury to the brain and spinal cord.

. . . . The detailed autopsies of Hecker and Weber, with the carefully appended histories of the nature of the fatal impediment at birth, have

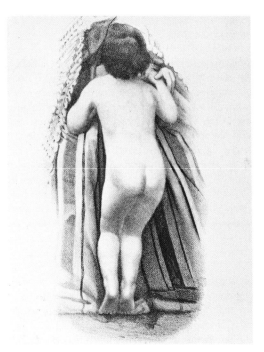

Plate VI.—General spastic contraction of the lower extremities. Premature birth. Asphyxia neonatorum of thirty-six hours' duration. Hands unaffected. See Case XLVII.

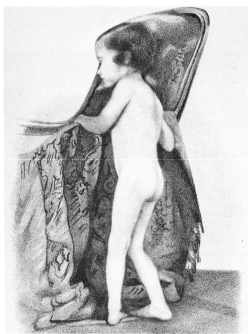

Plate VII.—Contraction of adductors and flexors of lower extremities. Left hand weak. Both hands awkward. More paralytic than spastic. Born with navel-string around neck. Asphyxia neonatorum one hour. See Case XLIII.

greatly facilitated an explanation of the spastic rigidity and paralysis of limbs, which appeared from my observations to be produced by so many different forms of unnatural parturition. The dissections of these obstetricians show the important fact that mechanical injury of the fœtal head, neck, or trunk, is not necessary for the production of intense congestion and blood extravasation of serous surfaces of chest, brain, and spinal cord. The other phenomenon commonly observed in difficult and abnormal parturition is that of interruption of placental respiration and circulation with nonsubstitution of pulmonary breathing and circulation. To this phenomenon alone, when mechanical injury or impediment has not existed, can we attribute the internal congestions, capillary extravasations, serous effusions which correspond with, or produce the symptoms of asphyxia, suspended animation, apoplexy, torpidity, tetanic spasms, convulsions of new-born children, and the spastic rigidity, paralysis, and idiocy subsequently witnessed. I am justified in regarding the dissections of Hecker and Weber as confirmatory of the opinion emitted by me, that asphyxia neonatorum, through resulting injury to nervous centres, is the cause of the commonest contractions which origi-

nate at the moment of birth, namely, more or less general spastic rigidity, and sometimes of paralytic contraction.

The former class of affections may be described as impairment of volition, with tonic rigidity and ultimately structural shortening in varying degrees, of a few or many of the muscles of the body. Both lower extremities are more or less generally involved. (See plate) Sometimes the affection of one limb only is observed by the parent, but examination usually shows a smaller degree of affection in the limb supposed to be sound. The contraction in the hips, knees, and ankles, is often considerable. The flexors and abductors of thighs, the flexors of knees, and the gastrocnemii, preponderate. In most cases, after a time, owing to structural shortening of the muscles and of the articular ligaments, and perhaps to some change of form of articular surfaces, the thighs cannot be completely abducted or extended, the knees cannot be straightened, nor can the heels be properly applied to the ground. The upper extremities are sometimes held down by preponderating action of pectorals, teres major and teres minor, and latissimus dorsi; the elbows are semi-flexed, the wrists partially flexed, pronated, and the fingers incapable of perfect voluntary direction. Sometimes the upper extremities appear unaffected with spasm or want of volition, sometimes a mere awkwardness in using them exists. Not unfrequently the parent reports that the hands were formerly affected. Participation of the muscles of trunk is sometimes shown by the shortened, flattened aspect of pectoral and abdominal surfaces, as compared with the more elongated and rounded form of the back. The prominence of back partially disappears on recumbency, but the greater weakness of muscles on dorsal aspect of trunk is obvious when the individual again attempts to sit upright. The muscles feel harder than natural to the age. Micturition is sometimes observed to be rare, and the bowels usually confined, either from deficient exercise of voluntary expulsive power or from implication of the sphincters. The muscles of speech are commonly involved, varying in degree from inability to utter correctly particular letters up to entire loss of articulating power. Sometimes articulation is only slow and difficult, like other acts of volition, the child or adult reminding us of a tardigrade animal. Sometimes the speech is nervous, impulsive, or stuttering. Often during the earliest months of life deglutition is impaired, and the power of carrying saliva into the fauces is not acquired until late. The intellectual functions are sometimes quite unaffected, but in the majority of cases the intellect suffers—from the slightest impairment which the parent unwillingly acknowledges or fails to perceive up to entire imbecility. The functions of organic life are unexceptionably performed, except, perhaps, that of development of caloric, although the depression of temperature in later life is more probably dependent upon the want of proper exercise. The frame is often lean and wiry, but not wasted. On the contrary, it is generally well nourished. The appetite is good, the child is often described as the healthiest of the family. These subjects often lead a more precarious existence during the first weeks after birth, at first even vegetative existence languishes, sometimes, perhaps, because premature birth or difficult labour, by impairing the maternal supply of nutriment, renders more difficult the infant's recovery from the shock its system received at birth. However, in the majority of instances, after restoration of the vegetative functions, a gradual but slow amelioration of all the functions of animal life is perceived. Some cases present distinct convulsive twitchings of face or limbs during first days after birth, open or suppressed convulsions, opisthotonos, or laryngismus. In some instances the persist-

ent rigidity of muscles commences or is observed shortly after birth, in others it escapes observation until the lapse of some weeks or months. The child's limbs are sometimes reported to have been simply weaker, to have shared in the general debility, the question of viability having alone occupied the attention of the attendants during the first month. Occasionally the weakness of the limbs has been recognised as a genuine paralysis in the first instance, of which the rigidity of muscles has been the sequel. Before the age of three or four months, though sometimes in slight cases not until ordinary time for walking arrives, the nurse perceives that the infant never thoroughly straightens the knees, that these cannot be properly depressed or separated, that she is unable to wash and dress the infant with the ordinary facility, that the hands are not properly used. The upper extremities recover before the lower limbs. Sometimes the trunk is habitually stiffened, so that the infant is turned over in the lap "all of a piece," as the nurse expresses it. Occasionally the head is habitually retracted. Where the symptoms of convulsions or "inward convulsions" exists, the rigidity is attributed to the convulsions. In many cases convulsions have been absent. As the child approaches the period at which the first attempts at standing and progression should be made, it is observed to make no use of the limbs, or he is incapable of standing except on the toes, or the feet are disposed to cross each other. Even children slightly affected rarely "go alone" before three or four years of age, many are unable to raise themselves from the ground at that age, and others do not walk, even indifferently, at puberty. On examination, the surgeon finds that the soles of the feet are not properly applied to the ground, that the knees always incline inwardly, and continue bent. When locomotion is accomplished, the movements are characterised by inability to stand still and balance the body in erect attitude. In the best recoveries from *general* spastic rigidity, even in the adult, the gait is shuffling, stiff; each knee, by forcible spastic rubbing against its fellow, obstructs progression.

The external form of cranium occasionally exhibits departure from the normal or average type, such as general smallness of skull, depression of frontal or occipital region only, sometimes one lateral half of skull, sometimes of one half of occiput, or forehead only. In slight cases the head has been well developed.

In cases even with great inertia as to exercise of volition in any part of the body, common sensibility appears little, if at all, deficient. The child often, indeed, manifests uncommon sensitiveness to external impressions, even when approaching adolescence he is alarmed at trifling noises. The sleep after the first weeks of life is light, easily disturbed. Often there is extreme sensibility to touch, the whole condition reminding the observer of tetanus. In a few cases a distinct resemblance to severe chorea is perceptible. It is probable that some of the cases designated by authors congenital chorea have been cases of the affection I have described.

Amongst the more uncommon consequences of difficult or premature labour and asphyxia, I may refer to Cases XLVIII and XLIX, in which wry-neck apparently resulted from one or other of these causes, and Cases VII, X, XX, and others, in which a distinct hemiplegic contraction resulted. I have occasionally met with the slightest amount of single spastic talipes equinus referable to this cause. Such a case has commonly been attributed to dentition, a fit or illness during infancy, the first link in the pathological chain of nervous suscepti-bility caused by the asphyxia having been disre-garded or overlooked.

A survey of the history of forty-seven cases, appended, shows that one fact is common to all the cases of persistent spastic rigidity of new-born children, namely, that some abnormal circumstance attended the act of parturition, or rather, the several processes concerned in separating the fœ-tus from the parent and its establishment in the world as an independent being. I cannot recall positively to mind, or find recorded in my jour-nals, more than a single case in which this persist-ent *spastic* rigidity affected a numerous series of muscles of the trunk and extremities which could be unequivocally referred to any illness subsequent to the establishment of proper pulmonary respira-tion as its starting-point. Often it has been found that convulsions in infancy had occurred, to which the disease had been attributed. Spastic contraction of a single set of muscles, as the gastrocnemii of one or both limbs, commonly of one limb only, or of the muscles of the forearm and calf on one side, is certainly an everyday occurrence after infantile convulsions, convulsions *during* dentition, and during early childhood without convulsions or other marked illness. But general spastic rigidity I have, with one exception, found to have been preceded by some abnormal act connected with mode of birth. Occasionally several causes, either of which may be competent to produce cerebro-spinal disorder and deformity, may coexist. Thus,

in Case XLIII uterine hæmorrhage occurred two months before labour; labour was tedious, accou-cheur was absent at birth, the child was born with navel-string around neck and legs, and did not cry for an hour afterwards, and a large, hard sub-stance, as large as another child—possibly a blasted twin conception—was discharged with the after-birth. I may remark that asphyxia neonatorum, from whatever amount of disturbance in separa-tion of fœtus from the uterus it may have resulted, is, as might be surmised, very apt to be accompa-nied with, and to be succeeded by, convulsions at variable periods after birth. It will be borne in mind that convulsions at birth, or subsequently to it, are but a symptom of lesion of nervous centre, and that we cannot refer one symptom of disorder of the nervous system to another symptom of the kind. The convulsions may doubtless react upon the nervous centres, upon the lungs and heart, and probably aggravate the disorder.

. . . . It is impossible not to connect the persist-ent affections of the intellect, of volition, and of organic life, with the injury the several nervous centres suffered in some instances before the fœtus had reached the maternal pelvis, in others whilst in transit through it; and in a third set of cases, where the fœtus was exposed to neither of these kinds of injury, it suffered from asphyxia neo-natorum, suspended animation, and its concomitant congestions, effusions, capillary apoplexies of brain, medulla oblongata, and spinal cord. Hither-to I have been afforded only one opportunity of learning the post-mortem condition of any of the cases of spastic rigidity which I have referred to asphyxia at birth, viz., Case LX, kindly furnished by my colleague, Dr. Down. It is certain that if, examined after death, after living many years, and such cases I find may live at least past the meridian of life, an anatomical condition very different from that present at or soon after birth would be found. Without going so far as Weber, as to assert that capillary apoplexies are necessarily absorbed when immediate death does not result from them, we may conclude that although the effused blood-particles may be absorbed, perma-nent lesion—atrophy of the nervous tissue—re-sults (see Case LX). Possibly a state of chronic meningitis, with effusion, or of chronic meningeal hyperæmia or congestion, or a certain amount of chronic myelitis, may maintain the spastic excita-ble tetanoid, sometimes choreal contractions, with rigidity of the trunk and extremities. My experi-ence as Physician to the London Hospital has afforded me some facts which support the idea that spinal meningitic and myelitic affections may play a considerable part in the phenomena of spastic rigidity. Thus the only case of persistent general spastic rigidity of upper and lower extremities, commencing after adult age, which I had the opportunity of seeing at intervals during twenty years, and the general appearance of which appeared to me similar in many respects to spastic rigidity from asphyxia neonatorum, was found by me after death to have depended upon chronic spinal meningitis and myelitis. A case related by Cruveilhier, of pus found in medulla spinalis, in a case of death of infant on the fifth day, after difficult labour, supports this view.

The greater or smaller impairment of intellect may safely be attributed to the greater or less mischief inflicted upon the cerebrum. As already observed, the considerable extravasations of blood on the surface of the brain are usually fatal. The autopsy, Case LX, showing cicatrized apoplexies on surface and interior of brain, is an exception. The only fatal instance of partially stillborn infant, which I have had the opportunity of postmortem examination, was one which came rapidly into the world, preceded by uterine hæmorrhage, nearly at full time, owing to fright to which the mother was exposed. Death of child ensued seventy hours after birth. In this case considerable effusion of blood was discovered in both ventricles of brain—a true apoplexy in the new-born child without mechanical injury. The autopsy, Case XLI, illustrates congestive apoplexy, no pelvic obstruction having existed.

I formerly found much difficulty in the analysis of various symptoms met with in different cases of spastic rigidity traceable to something abnormal in the act of birth. It soon became apparent that the symptoms, *of the living* at least, attributable to mechanical injury of head were a minority of the whole. This is consistent with the remark of Ollivier ('Traité sur les Maladies de la Moelle Epinière,' vol. i, p. 152), that whilst at natural birth the spinal cord is perfectly developed, the brain is still in a very rudimentary state, and consequently able to bear considerable disturbance without ultimate injury to its functions. In fact, in the new-born child brain-life is entirely absent; any injury it may have received at birth is at that period unaccompanied with special brain-symptoms, and, if not too severe, the child may entirely recover. Ollivier says (p. 244) "the brain of the new-born child is often found softened and destroyed without any external sign having permitted the practitioner to suspect it during life." In

the present day, with the experience we now possess of the causes of death at or shortly after birth, the accoucheur will suspect the existence of some form of apoplexy in every case.

The severe lesions caused by mechanical compression and laceration, and extensive hæmorrhages within the skull, when they do not destroy life, give rise to permanent deformity of cranium, to atrophy of injured portions of brain, and are the cause of many cases erroneously described as *congenital* idiocy. Dr. J. Crichton Browne ("Psychical Diseases of Early Life," 'Journal of Mental Science,' April, 1860) is one of the few observers who have traced idiocy to difficult labours (see also Dr. Howe, 'Causes of Idiocy,' Edinburgh, 1858). But in addition to the undoubted instances in which cranial injury and some imperfect development of intellect stand in the relation of cause and effect, the Appendix shows impaired intellect in Cases IV and VIII, in which no mechanical injury had taken place, but in which suspended animation, asphyxia neonatorum, and probably its consequent general and capillary congestion and ecchymoses—capillary apoplexies of the brain as well as of the spinal cord—perhaps even a moderate amount of larger apoplectic extravasation, had taken place, and had been imperfectly recovered from. I have observed that in impaired intellect from abnormal birth the degree of impairment met with in private practice often does not exceed feebleness of intellect; it varies much in degree, a elsewhere mentioned; it is often not sufficient to exclude the individual from family society. The individual may acquire a fair knowledge of music, the memory is good, the constructive tendency may exist, a fair capacity for arithmetic and languages may be displayed, but there commonly exists a great want of application, a slowness of intellect similar to the slowness of volition. In other cases, where intellectual powers are good, a preternatural impulsive nervous condition of mind exists, combined with an agitated, eager, anxious mode of performing acts of volition. Making every allowance for family peculiarities, there undoubtedly exists a considerable pathological resemblance, even in intellectual character and physiognomical expression, in these subjects of more or less general spastic rigidity. The occurrence of this feeble intellect in those who have not been exposed to mechanical injury of head, but in whom premature birth or pressure on umbilical cord has been recorded, appears explicable only on the supposition that the asphyxia and feebleness at birth had been followed by the usual capillary or larger hæmorrhage or effusions in brain, and their transformations and consequences to the nervous tissue; and the degree and variety of impaired function of brain may be due to the degree and variety of situation of these hæmorrhages.

. . . . Reference to more than fifty cases of injury of mind or body from abnormal parturition which are appended, will show that whilst in many cases the subsequent symptoms indicated that the brain and medulla oblongata had permanently suffered, the only one of the nervous centres which invariably presented symptoms of lesion was the medulla spinalis.

If—from analogy with the contractions of limbs observed to follow well-known diseases of spinal cord in later life, and from the fact of capillary apoplexy, larger blood-extravasations, and serous effusions being met with after death in spinal cord of infants who have died still-born from premature birth, descent of funis before head, &c., without mechanical injury to head and neck—I am justified in referring the spastic rigidity which follows asphyxia at birth to lesion of spinal cord, and not to lesion of brain or medulla oblongata, it is obvious, from the greater frequency of this evidence of lesion of spinal cord than of lesion of brain and medulla oblongata, that from some cause this nervous centre suffers most often from the asphyxia, or least frequently recovers its integrity. It seems almost superfluous to add, as

further proof of non-dependence of spastic rigidity of limbs upon mechanical injury at birth, that the lower extremities are oftenest affected and are the slowest to recover, although they derive their nerve-power from the lower part of the spinal column, which is assuredly the part of the cerebro-spinal axis least obnoxious to mechanical injury.

. . . . I trust the views of the pathology of the lesions of mind and body referable to the influence of the act of birth upon the child, which I hope to have somewhat unravelled, will promote the beneficial treatment of the disorders when detected in the early stages. In the later stages, the general principles of orthopaedy, and mental training when the intellect is affected, are successfully applicable in the inverse proportion to the extent of the permanent disorganization of the nervous centres and of peripheral structures. The length to which this paper has already extended prevents my dwelling upon the subject of treatment. I have had many of these cases under observation from one to twenty years, and may mention as an encouragement to other practitioners that treatment based upon physiology and rational therapeutics effects an amelioration surprising to those who have not watched such cases. Many of the most helpless have been restored to considerable activity and enjoyment of life. Even cases which exhibit impaired intellect may be benefited in mind and body to an unexpected extent.

XVI   Sydenham's Chorea

R HEUMATIC chorea is named for Thomas Sydenham, who first described this disorder and mistakenly called it St. Vitus's dance.

St. Vitus's dance was actually an entirely separate phenomenon. During the Middle Ages, in a setting of widespread religious mysticism, ignorance, and superstition, mass outbreaks of wild emotional dancing occurred throughout Europe. The victims were frequently brought to the chapels of St. Vitus, a Sicilian boy who had been martyred in the year 303 during the persecution of the Christians by Diocletian. St. Vitus thus became the patron saint of those afflicted with the dancing mania.[1]

.... So early as the year 1374, assemblages of men and women were seen at Aix-la-Chapelle who had come out of Germany, and who, united by one common delusion, exhibited to the public both in the streets and in the churches the following strange spectacle. . . . They formed circles hand in hand, and appearing to have lost all control over their senses, continued dancing, regardless of the bystanders, for hours together, in wild delirium, until at length they fell to the ground in a state of exhaustion. They then complained of extreme oppression, and groaned as if in the agonies of death, until they were swathed in cloths bound tightly round their waists, upon which they again recovered, and remained free from complaint until the next attack. . . . While dancing they neither saw nor heard, being insensible to external impressions through the senses, but were haunted by visions, their fancies conjuring up spirits whose names. . . they shrieked out; and some of them afterwards asserted that they felt as if they had been immersed in a stream of blood, which obliged them to leap so high. . . .[1]

In 1686, the famous English physician,

Thomas Sydenham (1624-1689), described a different disorder. Sydenham, who has been called the English Hippocrates, made important contributions to medicine by accurately recording the natural history of a variety of diseases.[2-5] He relied upon his powers of observation at the bedside and had little interest in theorizing. Rheumatic fever and chorea were two of the entities that he described. However, he did not relate them, and his account of chorea was brief and incomplete.

The relationship between Sydenham's chorea and rheumatic arthritis and carditis was emphasized by Sée in 1850.[6] Many, but not all, cases of Sydenham's chorea are now considered to be part of the clinical picture of rheumatic fever.[7-9] The disease is rare in adulthood except during pregnancy when it may be especially severe. In addition to the adventitious movements and weakness noted by Sydenham, psychic disturbances also occur in acute chorea. Since most of the victims of Sydenham's chorea recover completely, there have been few pathologic studies, and these have shown no striking or consistent abnormalities.[7]

Although Thomas Sydenham's account of this disease was limited and his treatment preposterous, nevertheless his priority has caused it to become known as Sydenham's chorea.

References

1. Hecker, J.F.C.: *The Epidemics of the Middle Ages*, B.G. Babington (trans.), London: Sydenham Society, 1844, pp 87-93.
2. Payne, J.F.: *Thomas Sydenham*, New York: Longmans, Green & Co., 1900, pp 1-264.
3. Bett, W.R.: Some Paediatric Eponyms: IV. Sydenham's Chorea, *Brit J Child Dis* 29:283-288 (Oct-Dec) 1932.
4. Kelly, E.C.: Thomas Sydenham, *Med Classics* 4:287-301 (Dec) 1939.
5. Dewhurst, K.: *Dr. Thomas Sydenham (1624-1689), His Life and Original Writings,* London: Wellcome Historical Medical Library, 1966, pp 1-191.
6. Sée, G.: De la Chorée: Rapports du rhuma-

tisme et des maladies du coeur avec les affections nerveuses et convulsives, *Mem Acad Nat Med* **15**:373-525, 1850.

7. Lessof, M.: Sydenham's Chorea, *Guy's Hosp Rep* **107**:185-206 (July-Sept) 1958.

8. Paradise, J.L.: Sydenham's Chorea Without Evidence of Rheumatic Fever: Report of Its Association With the Henoch-Schönlein Syndrome, and With Systemic Lupus Erythematosus, and Review of the Literature, *New Eng J Med* **263**:625-629 (Sept 29) 1960.

9. Copeman, W.S.C.: *Textbook of the Rheumatic Diseases,* Edinburgh: E. & S. Livingstone, Ltd., 1964, pp 1-8, 156-159.

ON THE APPEARANCE OF A NEW FEVER*

. . . . Saint Vitus's dance is a sort of convulsion which attacks boys and girls from the tenth year until they have done growing. At first it shows itself by a halting, or rather an unsteady movement of one of the legs, which the patient *drags.* Then it is seen in the hand of the same side. The patient cannot keep it a moment in its place, whether he lay it upon his breast or any other part of his body. Do what he may, it will be jerked elsewhere convulsively. If any vessel filled with drink be put into his hand, before it reaches his mouth he will exhibit a thousand gesticulations like a mountebank. He holds the cup out straight, as if to move it to his mouth, but has his hand carried elsewhere by sudden jerks. Then, perhaps, he contrives to bring it to his mouth. If so, he will drink the liquid off at a gulp; just as if he were trying to amuse the spectators by his antics.

Now this affection arises from some humour falling on the nerves; and such irritation causes the spasm. Hence the treatment is first to bleed and purge, and then to restore the strength. To this end I act thus: I bleed from the arms to seven ounces, more or less according to the patient's age. Next day I order half (or more) of the previous purgative of tamarinds, senna-leaves, &c.; the quantity being regulated by the age, habit, and aptitude for purgative medicines of the patient.

In the evening I order as follow:

    Rx Water of black cherries, ʒ j;
        Aqua epileptica Langii, ʒ iij;
        Venice treacle (old), Ə j;
        Liquid laudanum, viij.

    Make into a draught.

This cathartic draught I repeat three times on alternate days, with a paregoric the same three nights. Then I bleed afresh; then purge. So I bleed and purge, in turns, until a vein has been breathed three or four times, with purges proportionate— this being regulated by the strength of the patient. All the while, however, I look carefully, lest, between the alternate evacuations, any bad symptoms should arise.

The days when there is no purging I order—

    Rx Conserve of Roman wormwood,
        Conserve of orange-peel, āā ʒ j;
        Conserve of rosemary, ʒ ss;
        Venice treacle (old),
        Candied nutmeg, āā ʒ iij;
        Candied ginger, ʒ j;
        Syrup of lemon-juice, q. s.

Make into an electuary; of which take a part the size of a nutmeg, every morning at five p.m. Wash this down with—

    Pœony-root,
    Elecampane,
    Masterwort,
    Angelica, āā ʒ j;
    Rue-leaves,
    Sage,
    Betony,
    Germander,
    White horehound,
    Tops of lesser centaury, of each a handful;
    Juniper-berries, ʒ vj;
    The rind of two oranges.

Slice and steep in six pints of Canary wine. Strain and set by for use.

    Rx Rue-water, ʒ iv;
        Aqua epileptica Langii,
        Compound bryony-water, āā, ʒ j
        Syrup of pœonies, ʒ vj,

Mix, and make into a julep. Take four spoonfuls, every night at bedtime, with eight drops of spirits of hartshorn.

Apply to the feet the *emplastrum a caranna.*

Just in proportion as the patient improves, he drags his leg less, keeps his hand steadier, and lifts a cup more readily to his mouth. These are the surest signs of recovery. To accomplish this I do not recommend bleeding beyond the third or fourth time. Cathartics and alteratives, however, may be kept on until the cure is complete. Since, too, the disease is liable to return again, I think it well for the patient to be bled and purged about the same time, or a little earlier, the following year. . . .

---

*Sydenham, T.: "Schedula monitoria de novae febris ingressu," in R. G. Latham (trans.-ed.): *The Works of Thomas Sydenham, M.D.: Translated from the Latin Edition of Dr. Greenhill with a Life of the Author,* London: Sydenham Society, 1848-1850, vol 2, pp 198-200.

XVII   Parkinson's Syndrome

JAMES Parkinson (1755-1824), a general practitioner in London, was a man of many talents.[1,2] He made major scientific contributions in paleontology and geology, and he was a prominent political reformer. Likewise, in the field of medicine he wrote on a variety of subjects, the best remembered of which is the syndrome that now bears his name.[3-6]

Parkinson's graphic description established paralysis agitans as a recognizable entity. However, additional clinical features have since been described, including a distinction between the rigidity and the akinesia occurring in this syndrome.[7] In some cases there is an initiating cause such as encephalitis lethargica,[8,9] but in the majority the etiology remains unknown.

Parkinson had no autopsy material, and predicted erroneously that the lesions of paralysis agitans would be found in the cervical spinal cord. Later pathological studies of idiopathic parkinsonism have shown characteristic abnormalities in the brain, consisting of widespread neuronal degeneration, especially in the substantia nigra, and Lewy intracellular inclusion bodies.[10-12]

Parkinson's skeptical attitude toward the medicinal treatment of the disease could also apply to the anticholinergic compounds,[7,13] which later became the mainstay of medical management. These compounds have only limited value, but current research gives hope of providing more effective drug therapy.[14] Meanwhile, a fruitful approach has been the treatment of parkinsonism by stereotactic surgery.[15-19] In many cases, stereoencephalotomy has resulted in striking amelioration of tremor and rigidity. Moreover the development of these techniques has prompted a resurgence of interest in the pathophysiology of the basal ganglia.[20]

The recent work in stereotactic surgery and in the biochemistry of the basal ganglia[14,20] is bringing a better understanding of the disorder first described in 1817 by James Parkinson.

References

1. McMenemey, W.H.: "James Parkinson, 1755-1824: A Biographical Essay" in Critchley, M. (ed.): *James Parkinson (1755-1824): A Bicentenary Volume of Papers Dealing with Parkinson's Disease, Incorporating the Original 'Essay on the Shaking Palsy'*, London: Macmillan & Co., Ltd., 1955, pp 1-143.
2. Brain, R.: The Neurological Tradition of the London Hospital: Or The Importance of Being Thirty, *Lancet* 2:575-581 (Oct 17) 1959.
3. Parkinson, J.: *An Essay on the Shaking Palsy*, London: Sherwood, Neely, and Jones, 1817.
4. Ostheimer, A.J.: An Essay on the Shaking Palsy, by James Parkinson, M.D., Member of the Royal College of Surgeons, With a Bibliographic Note Thereon, *Arch Neurol Psychiat* 7:681-710 (June) 1922.
5. Parkinson, J.: An Essay on the Shaking Palsy, *Med Classics* 2:964-997 (June) 1938.
6. Parkinson, J.: "An Essay on the Shaking Palsy" in Critchley, M. (ed.): *James Parkinson (1755-1824): A Bicentenary Volume of Papers Dealing with Parkinson's Disease, Incorporating the*

Original 'Essay on the Shaking Palsy,' London: Macmillan & Co., Ltd., 1955, pp 145-218.

7. Onuaguluchi, G.: *Parkinsonism*, London: Butterworth & Co., 1964.

8. Duvoisin, R.C., and Yahr, M.D.: Encephalitis and Parkinsonism, *Arch Neurol* 12:227-239 (March) 1965.

9. Wilkins, R.H., and Brody, I.A.: Neurological Classics IV: Encephalitis Lethargica, *Arch Neurol* 18:324-328 (March) 1968.

10. Greenfield, J.G.: "The Pathology of Parkinson's Disease" in Critchley, M. (ed.): *James Parkinson (1755-1824): A Bicentenary Volume of Papers Dealing with Parkinson's Disease, Incorporating the Original 'Essay on the Shaking Palsy'*, London: Macmillan & Co., Ltd., 1955, pp 219-243.

11. Earle, K.: Pathology of Extrapyramidal Diseases: Introduction to the Panel, *J Neurosurg* 24:247-249 (Jan) 1966.

12. Lewy, F.H.: Zur pathologischen Anatomie der Paralysis Agitans, *Deutsch Z Nervenheilk* 50:50-55, 1914.

13. England, A.C., Jr., and Schwab, R.S.: Parkinson's Syndrome, *New Eng J Med* 265:785-791 (Oct 19), 837-844 (Oct 26) 1961.

14. Cotzias, G.C.; Van Woert, M.H.; and Schiffer, L.M.: Aromatic Amino Acids and Modification of Parkinsonism, *New Eng J Med* 276:374-379 (Feb 16) 1967.

15. Cooper, I.S.: *Parkinsonism: Its Medical and Surgical Therapy*, Springfield, Ill: Charles C Thomas Publisher, 1961.

16. Wilkins, R.H.: Neurosurgical Classic XXVII: *J Neurosurg* 22:102-125 (Jan) 1965.

17. Gillingham, F.J.: Stereotactic Surgery—Past, Present, and Future, *Clin Neurosurg* 13:189-203, 1965.

18. Spiegel, E.S.: Development of Stereoencephalotomy for Extrapyramidal Diseases, *J Neurosurg* 24:433-439 (Jan) 1966.

19. Meyers, R.: "Historical Background and Personal Experiences in the Surgical Relief of Hyperkinesia and Hypertonus" in Fields, W.S. (ed.): *Pathogenesis and Treatment of Parkinsonism*, Springfield, Ill: Charles C Thomas, Publisher, 1958, pp 229-270.

20. Martin, J.P.: Remarks on the Functions of the Basal Ganglia, *Lancet* 1:999-1005 (Dec 5) 1959.

21. Barbeau, A.: Some Biochemical Disorders in Parkinson's Disease: A Review, *J Neurosurg* 24:162-164 (Jan) 1966.

AN ESSAY ON THE SHAKING PALSY*

By

JAMES PARKINSON

Member of the Royal College of Surgeons

London: Printed by Whittingham and Rowland, Goswell Street, for Sherwood, Neely, and Jones, Paternoster Row, 1817

Preface

. . . . The disease, respecting which the present inquiry is made, is of a nature highly afflictive. Notwithstanding which, it has not yet obtained a place in the classification of nosologists; some have regarded its characteristic symptoms as distinct and different diseases, and others have given its name to disease differing essentially from it; whilst the unhappy sufferer has considered it as an evil, from the domination of which he had no prospect of escape.

The disease is of long duration: to connect, therefore, the symptoms which occur in its later stages with those which mark its commencement, requires a continuance of observation of the same case, or at least a correct history of its symptoms, even for several years. Of both these advantages the writer has had the opportunities of availing himself; and has hence been led particularly to observe several other cases in which the disease existed in different stages of its progress. By these repeated observations, he hoped that he had been led to a probable conjecture as to the nature of the malady, and that analogy had suggested such means as might be productive of relief, and perhaps even of cure, if employed before the disease had been too long established. He therefore considered it to be a duty to submit his opinions to the examination of others, even in their present state of immaturity and imperfection. . . .

Chapter I. Definition-History-Illustrative Cases
Shaking Palsy (Paralysis Agitans)

(Involuntary tremulous motion, with lessened muscular power, in parts not in action and even when supported; with a propensity to bend the trunk forwards, and to pass from a walking to a running pace: the senses and intellects being uninjured)

The term Shaking Palsy has been vaguely employed by medical writers in general. By some it has been used to designate ordinary cases of Palsy, in which some slight tremblings have occurred; whilst by others it has been applied to certain anomalous affections, not belonging to Palsy. . . .

Tremor has been adopted, as a genus, by almost every nosologist; but always unmarked, in their several definitions, by such characters as would embrace this disease. . . .

*Reprinted from *Medical Classics* 2:964-997 (June) 1938.

History

So slight and nearly imperceptible are the first inroads of this malady, and so extremely slow is its progress, that it rarely happens, that the patient can form any recollection of the precise period of its commencement. The first symptoms perceived are, a slight sense of weakness, with a proneness to trembling in some particular part; sometimes in the head, but most commonly in one of the hands and arms. These symptoms gradually increase in the part first affected; and at an uncertain period, but seldom in less than twelve months or more, the morbid influence is felt in some other part. Thus assuming one of the hands and arms to be first attacked, the other, at this period becomes similarly affected. After a few more months the patient is found to be less strict than usual in preserving an upright posture: this being most observable whilst walking, but sometimes whilst sitting or standing. Sometime after the appearance of this symptom, and during its slow increase, one of the legs is discovered slightly to tremble, and is also found to suffer fatigue sooner than the leg of the other side: and in a few months this limb becomes agitated by similar tremblings, and suffers a similar loss of power.

Hitherto the patient will have experienced but little inconvenience; and befriended by the strong influence of habitual endurance, would perhaps seldom think of his being the subject of disease, except when reminded of it by the unsteadiness of his hand, whilst writing or employing himself in any nicer kind of manipulation. But as the disease proceeds, similar employments are accomplished with considerable difficulty, the hand failing to answer with exactness to the dictates of the will. Walking becomes a task which cannot be performed without considerable attention. The legs are not raised to that height, or with that promptitude which the will directs, so that the utmost care is necessary to prevent frequent falls.

At this period the patient experiences much inconvenience, which unhappily is found daily to increase. The submission of the limbs to the directions of the will can hardly ever be obtained in the performance of the most ordinary offices of life. The fingers cannot be disposed of in the proposed directions, and applied with certainty to any proposed point. As time and the disease proceed, difficulties increase: writing can now be hardly at all accomplished; and reading, from the tremulous motion, is accomplished with some difficulty. Whilst at meals the fork not being duly directed frequently fails to raise the morsel from the plate: which, when seized, is with much difficulty conveyed to the mouth. At this period the patient seldom experiences a suspension of the agitation of his limbs. Commencing, for instance in one arm, the wearisome agitation is borne until beyond sufferance, when by suddenly changing the posture it is for a time stopped in that limb, to commence, generally, in less than a minute in one of the legs, or in the arm of the other side. Harassed by this tormenting round, the patient has recourse to walking, a mode of exercise to which the sufferers from this malady are in general partial; owing to their attention being thereby somewhat diverted from their unpleasant feelings, by the care and exertion required to ensure its safe performance.

But as the malady proceeds, even this temporary mitigation of suffering from the agitation of the limbs is denied. The propensity to lean forward becomes invincible, and the patient is thereby forced to step on the toes and fore part of the feet, whilst the upper part of the body is thrown so far forward as to render it difficult to avoid falling on the face. In some cases, when this state of the malady is attained, the patient can no longer exercise himself by walking in his usual manner, but is thrown on the toes and forepart of the feet; being, at the same time, irresistibly impelled to take much quicker and shorter steps, and thereby to adopt unwillingly a running pace. In some cases it is found necessary entirely to substitute running for walking; since otherwise the patient, on proceeding only a very few paces, would inevitably fall.

In this stage, the sleep becomes much disturbed The tremulous motion of the limbs occur during sleep, and augment until they awaken the patient, and frequently with much agitation and alarm. The power of conveying the food to the mouth is at length so much impeded that he is obliged to consent to be fed by others. The bowels, which had been all along torpid, now, in most cases, demand stimulating medicines of very considerable power: the expulsion of the faeces from the rectum sometimes requiring mechanical aid. As the disease proceeds towards its last stage, the trunk is almost permanently bowed, the muscular power is more decidedly diminished, and the tremulous agitation becomes violent. The patient walks now with great difficulty, and unable any longer to support himself with his stick, he dares not venture on this exercise, unless assisted by an attendant, who walking backwards before him, prevents his falling forwards, by the pressure of his hands against the fore part of his shoulders. His words are now scarcely intelligible; and he is not only no longer able to feed himself, but when the food is conveyed to the mouth, so much are the actions of the muscles of the tongue, pharynx, etc. impeded by impaired action and perpetual agitation, that the food is with difficulty retained in the mouth until masticated; and then as difficultly swallowed. Now also, from the same cause, another very unpleasant circumstance occurs: the saliva fails of being directed to the back part of the fauces, and hence is continually draining from the mouth, mixed with the particles of food, which he is no longer able to clear from the inside of the mouth.

As the debility increased and the influence of the will over the muscles fades away, the tremulous agitation becomes more vehement. It now seldom leaves him for a moment; but even when exhausted nature seizes a small portion of sleep, the motion becomes so violent as not only to shake the bed-hangings, but even the floor and sashes of the room. The chin is now almost immovably bent down upon the sternum. The slops with which he is attempted to be fed, with the saliva, are continually trickling from the mouth. The power of articulation is lost. The urine and faeces are passed involuntarily; and at the last, constant sleepiness, with slight delirium, and other marks of extreme exhaustion, announce the wished-for release.

[Six case reports follow. Three of these subjects were casually met or seen in the street, and were not Parkinson's patients]

Chapter II. Pathognomonic Symptoms Examined—Tremor Coactus— Scelotyrbe Festinans

It has been seen in the preceding history of the disease, and in the accompanying cases, that certain affections, the tremulous agitation, and the almost invincible propensity to run, when wishing only to walk, each of which has been considered by nosologists as distinct diseases, appear to be pathognomonic symptoms of this malady. To determine in which of these points of view these affections ought to be regarded, an examination into their nature, and an inquiry into the opinions of preceding writers respecting them, seem necessary to be attempted.
I. *Involuntary tremulous motion, with lessened voluntary muscular power, in parts, not in action, and even supported*

. . . . It is. . . necessary to bear in mind, that this affection is distinguishable from tremor, by the agitation, in the former, occurring whilst the affected part is supported and unemployed, and being even checked by the adoption of voluntary motion: whilst in the latter, the tremor is induced immediately on bringing the parts into action. Thus an artist, afflicted with the malady here treated of, whilst his hand and arm is palpitating strongly, will seize his pencil, and the motions will be suspended, allowing him to use it for a short period; but in tremor, if the hand be quite free from the affection, should the pen or pencil be taken up, the trembling immediately commences.
II. *A propensity to bend the trunk forwards, and to pass from a walking to a running pace*

This affection, which observation seems to authorise the being considered as a symptom peculiar to this disease, has been mentioned by few nosologists: it appears to have been first noticed by Gaubius, who says, "Cases occur in which the muscles duly excited into the action by the impulse of the will, do then, with an unbidden agility, and with an impetus not to be repressed, accelerate their motion, and run before the unwilling mind. It is a frequent fault of the muscles belonging to speech, nor yet of these alone: I have seen one, who was able to run, but not to walk. . . ." . . . .

Mons. de Sauvages attributes this complaint to a want of flexibility in the muscular fibres. Hence, he supposes, that the patients make shorter steps, and strive with a more than common exertion or impetus to overcome the resistance; walking with a quick and hastened step, as if hurried along against their will. . . .

Chapter III. Shaking Palsy Distinguished From Other Diseases With Which It May be Confounded

Treating of a disease resulting from an assemblage of symptoms, some of which do not appear to have yet engaged the general notice of the profession, particular care is required whilst endeavoring to mark its diagnostic characters. . . .

Palsy, either consequent to compression of the brain, or dependent on partial exhaustion of the energy of that organ, may, when the palsied limbs become affected with tremulous motions, be confounded with this disease. In those cases the abolition or diminution of voluntary muscular action takes place suddenly, the sense of feeling being sometimes also impaired. But in this disease, the diminution of the influence of the will on the muscles comes on with extreme slowness, is always accompanied, and even preceded, by agitations of the affected parts, and never by a lessened sense of feeling. The dictates of the will are even, in the last stages of the disease, conveyed to the muscles; and the muscles act on this impulse, but their actions are perverted.

Anomalous cases of convulsive affections have been designated by the term Shaking Palsy: a term which appears to be improperly applied to these cases, independent of the want of accordance between them and that disease which has been here denominated Shaking Palsy. . . .

Unless attention is paid to one circumstance, this disease will be confounded with those species of passive tremblings to which the term Shaking Palsies has frequently been applied. These are, tremor tremulentus, the trembling consequent to indulgence in the drinking of spirituous liquors; that which proceeds from the immoderate employment of tea and coffee; that which appears to be dependent on advanced age; and all those tremblings which proceed from the various circumstances which induce a diminution of power in the nervous system. But by attending to that circumstance alone, which has been already noted as characteristic of mere tremor, the distinction will readily be made. If the trembling limb be supported, and none of its muscles be called into action, the trembling will cease. In the real Shaking Palsy the reverse of this takes place, the agitation continues in full force whilst the limb is at rest and unemployed; and even is sometimes diminished by calling the muscles into employment.

Chapter IV. Proximate Cause—Remote Causes—Illustrative Cases

Before making the attempt to point out the nature and cause of this disease, it is necessary to plead, that it is made under very unfavourable circumstances. Unaided by previous inquiries immediately directed to this disease, and not having had the advantage, in a single case, of that light which anatomical examination yields, opinions and not facts can only be offered. Conjecture founded on analogy, and an attentive consideration of the peculiar symptoms of the disease, have been the only guides that could be obtained for this research, the result of which is, as it ought to be, offered with hesitation.

Supposed Proximate Cause

. . . . By the nature of the symptoms we are taught, that the disease depends on some irregularity in the direction of the nervous influence; by the wide range of parts which are affected, that the injury is rather in the source of this influence than merely in the nerves of the parts; by the situation of the parts whose actions are impaired, and the order in which they become affected, that the proximate cause of the disease is in the superior part of the medulla spinalis; and by the absence of any injury to the senses and to the intellect, that the morbid state does not extend to the encephalon.

Uncertainty existing as to the nature of the proximate cause of this disease, is remote causes must necessarily be referred to with indecision. Assuming however the state just mentioned as the proximate cause, it may be concluded that this may be the result of injuries of the medulla itself, or of the theca helping to form the canal in which it is inclosed. . . .

Chapter V. Considerations Respecting The Means of Cure

The inquiries made in the preceding pages yield, it is to be much regretted, but little more than evidence of inference; nothing direct and satisfactory has been obtained. All that has been ventured to assume here, has been that the disease depends on a disordered state of that part of the medulla which is contained in the cervical vertebrae. But of what nature that morbid change is; and whether originating in the medulla itself, in its membranes, or in the containing theca, is, at present, the subject of doubt and conjecture. But although, at present, uninformed as to the precise nature of the disease, still it ought not be considered as one against which there exists no countervailing remedy. . . .

From this review. . . the chance of relief from the proposed mode of treatment may appear to be sufficient to warrant its trial.

In such a case then, at whatever period of the disease it might be proposed to attempt the cure, blood should be first taken from the upper part of the neck, unless contra-indicated by any particular circumstance. After which vesicatories should be applied to the same part, and a purulent discharge obtained by appropriate use of the Sabine Liniment; having recourse to the application of a fresh blister, when from the diminution of the discharging surface, pus is not secreted in a sufficient quantity. Should the blisters be found too inconvenient, or a sufficient quantity of discharge not be obtained thereby, an issue of at least an inch and a half in length might be established on each side of the vertebral column, in its superior part. These, it is presumed, would be best formed with caustic, and kept open with any proper substance. . . .

Until we are better informed respecting the nature of this disease, the employment of internal medicines is scarcely warrantable; unless analogy should point out some remedy the trial of which rational hope might authorize. Particular circumstances indeed must arise in different cases, in which the aid of medicine may be demanded: and the intelligent will never fail to avail themselves of any opportunity of making trial of the influence of mercury, which has in so many instances, manifested its power in correcting derangement of structure.

The weakened powers of the muscles in the affected parts is so prominent a symptom, as to be very liable to mislead the inattentive, who may regard the disease as a mere consequence of constitutional debility. If this notion be pursued, and tonic medicines, and highly nutritious diet be directed, no benefit is likely to be thus obtained since the disease depends not on general weakness, but merely on the interruption of the flow of the nervous influence to the affected parts.

It is indeed much to be regretted that this malady is generally regarded by the sufferers in this point of view, so discouraging to the employment of remedial means. Seldom occurring before the age of fifty, and frequently yielding but little inconvenience for several months, it is generally considered as the irremediable diminution of the nervous influence, naturally resulting from declining life; and remedies therefore are seldom sought for. . . .

Before concluding these pages, it may be proper to observe once more, that an important object proposed to be obtained by them is, the leading of the attention of those who humanely employ anatomical examination in detecting the causes and nature of disease, particularly to this malady. By their benevolent labours its real nature may be ascertained, and appropriate modes, of relief, or even of cure, pointed out.

To such researches the healing art is already much indebted for the enlargement of its powers of lessening the evils of suffering humanity. Little is the public aware of the obligations it owes to those who, led by professional ardour, and the dictates of duty, have devoted themselves to these pursuits, under circumstances most unpleasant and forbidding. Every person of consideration and feeling, may judge of the advantages yielded by the philanthropic exertions of a HOWARD; but how few can estimate the benefits bestowed on mankind by the labours of a MORGAGNI, HUNTER, or BAILLIE.

Finis

XVIII   The Thalamic Syndrome

may be related to release of the thalamus from cortical inhibition.[10] As Dejerine and Roussy noted, the pain is resistant to analgesic medications. However, recent experience with stereotactic thalamotomy and mesencephalotomy give hope that this pain may eventually be controlled.[11,12]

References

1. Zabriskie, E.G.: "Joseph Jules Dejerine (1849-1917)," in Haymaker, W. (ed.): *The Founders of Neurology*, Springfield, Ill: Charles C Thomas, Publisher, 1953, pp 271-275.

2. Heuyer, G.: "Jules Joseph Dejerine (1849-1917)," in Kolle, K. (ed.): *Grosse Nervenärzte*, Stuttgart: Georg Thieme, 1963, Vol 3, pp 133-142.

3. Miller, H.: Three Great Neurologists, *Proc Roy Soc Med* 60:399-405 (April) 1967.

4. Klumpke, A.: Contribution a l'étude des paralysies radiculaires du plexus brachial, *Rev Med* 5:519-616 and 739-790, 1885.

5. Dejerine, J., and Egger, M.: Contribution a l'étude de la physiologie pathologique de l'incoordination motrice, *Rev Neurol* 11:397-405 (April 30) 1903.

6. Dejerine, J., and Roussy, G.: Le syndrome thalamique, *Rev Neurol* 14:521-532 (June 30) 1906.

7. Roussy, G.: *La couche optique. Le syndrome thalamique*, Paris: G. Steinheil, 1907.

8. Foix, C., and Masson, A.: Le syndrome de l'artère cérébrale postérieure, *Presse Med* 31:361-365 (April 21) 1923.

9. Foix, C., and Hillemand, P.: Les syndromes de la region thalamique, *Presse Med* 33:113-117 (Jan 28) 1925.

10. Langworthy, O.R., and Fox, H.M.: Thalamic Syndrome: Syndrome of the Posterior Cerebral Artery: A Review, *Arch Intern Med* 60:203-224 (Aug) 1937.

11. Davis, R.A., and Stokes, J.W.: Neurosurgical Attempts to Relieve Thalamic Pain, *Surg Gynec Obstet* 123:371-384 (Aug) 1966.

12. Nashold, B.S., Jr.; Wilson, W.P.; and Slaughter, D.G.: Stereotaxic Midbrain Lesions for Central Dysesthesia and Phantom Pain: Preliminary Report, *J Neurosurg* 30:116-126 (Feb) 1969.

FEW physicians have been more honored by eponyms than Jules Dejerine (1849 to 1917), the French neurologist.[1-3] Among the diseases that bear his name are facioscapulohumeral muscular dystrophy (Landouzy-Dejerine), hypertrophic interstitial neuritis (Dejerine-Sottas), olivopontocerebellar atrophy (Dejerine-Thomas), and the thalamic syndrome (Dejerine-Roussy). His American wife, Augusta Klumpke, was also a talented neurologist whose name is now associated with lower brachial plexus palsy.[4]

Beginning in 1903, Dejerine and his associates discovered and studied the clinical and pathological features of the thalamic syndrome.[5-7] Little has been added to their thorough presentations. Twenty years after Dejerine's initial paper on the subject, Foix, Masson, and Hillemand demonstrated the most common cause of the syndrome—occlusion of the thalamogeniculate branches of the posterior cerebral artery.[8-10]

The most distressing feature of the thalamic syndrome is the intense pain, which

The Thalamic Syndrome*

by J. Dejerine and G. Roussy

. . . . *Definition.*—The term *thalamic syndrome,* as it appears from our personal observations and those of the authors cited above, must now be understood as a syndrome characterized by:

1. *A slight hemiplegia, usually without contracture and rapidly regressive.*

2. *A persistent superficial hemianesthesia of an organic character, which can in some cases be replaced by cutaneous hyperesthesia, but is always accompanied by marked and persistent disturbances of deep sensation.*

3. *Mild hemiataxia and more or less complete astereognosis.*

To these three principal and constant symptoms are ordinarily added:

4. *Severe, persistent, paroxysmal, often intolerable, pains on the hemiplegic side, not yielding to any analgesic treatment.*

5. *Choreoathetoid movements in the limbs on the paralyzed side.*

Such are the various symptoms which, by their occurrence together, allow us to affirm the existence of a lesion involving the thalamus and localized at a particular point in this ganglion that we will indicate later. Besides these cardinal symptoms, there occur signs of a second order: sphincteric disturbances (rectal and vesical tenesmus) and hemianopsia. We shall neglect these signs since they are more rarely observed and are not really part of the syndrome. . . .

Clinical Study

A patient presenting the various symptoms of the thalamic syndrome is a hemiplegic whose illness began without great disturbance, as is the rule with small areas of softening. Most often, at the onset there is no true ictus and the patient perceives the paralysis coming on after a dizzy spell or a very slight impairment of consciousness for a few hours. With the motor hemiplegia, there appear sensory disturbances that follow a different course from the motor disturbances. While the motor phenomena will continue to improve and diminish considerably, the sensory phenomena will usually persist until death, which may occur some years after the beginning of the illness.

At the onset, difficulties with micturition may

appear (retention with tenesmus or incontinence), which the patients complain of a great deal. However, this symptom is not found in every case.

In our analytical study of the symptoms of the thalamic syndrome, we shall examine the signs as they appear a few months, or even better a year, after the onset of the hemiplegia.

It is, in fact, in this period that the syndrome appears in all its purity, and then it is easiest to affirm its existence.

A. Disturbances of motility.

These consist of a slight hemiplegia or hemiparesis. . . .

More important are the phenomena of posthemiplegic motor excitation, such as *hemichorea* and *hemiathetosis,* which we find noted in several cases. They are, in fact, frequent. . . .

It is not a major hemichorea that we observe here, but small movements in the distal portions of the limbs, localized especially in the fingers and hand. Sometimes they have the disturbed character of chorea, sometimes they take on the slow and worm-like aspect of athetosis.

We noted no case of *unilateral tremor.*

Finally, among the motor disturbances, *hemiataxia* is one of the most interesting signs of the thalamic syndrome.

The ataxia of hemiplegics differs in intensity from one case to another, but it retains some characteristics of its own, which distinguish it from ataxias of peripheral or medullary origin. One of us, in an earlier work, has already drawn attention to this fact.[1] The hemiataxia from a cerebral lesion is slight, limited and restricted, and is never as severe as the marked ataxia of tabetics. In the patient's movements, there is a certain uneasiness, a certain hesitation attributable to the ataxia. But the patient can coordinate a succession of movements, such as opening the fingers one after the other, which a tabetic cannot do. When the patient is asked to put his index finger on the tip of his nose with his eyes closed, he makes errors of localization, hesitates very often, but, in these various acts, the movement slows before reaching the end. Although the patient cannot direct his fingers exactly to a given point, at least he can regulate the amplitude and

*Translation of: Le Syndrome Thalamique, *Revue Neurologique* 14:521-532 (June 30) 1906.

1. *Revue de Neurologie,* no. 8, 1903.

speed of movement. Thus, he does not make gross errors such as moving his index finger to his head or shoulders as a tabetic will do.

To sum up, this is a slight ataxia, apparently not connected with the intensity of superficial and deep sensory disturbances, as we shall see. . . .

B. Reflexes.

The state of the tendon reflexes is that found in long-standing mild hemiplegia. Sometimes they are slightly exaggerated; sometimes almost normal.

The cutaneous reflexes (cremasteric, abdominal, epigastric) and the plantar reflex are normal or absent. *The absence of the Babinski response in all our cases,* despite the pyramidal degeneration noted on our sections, deserves mention. In fact, one may ask if this indicates only slight motor involvement in the thalamic syndrome, or if—and this is the opinion that seems most likely—the injured optic thalamus does not participate in the production of this phenomenon. . . .

C. Sensory disorders.

The disorders of sensation take on major importance in the clinical picture we are studying by virtue of their intensity, their constancy, their character, and their modality. They dominate the symptomatology of the thalamic syndrome.

It is not only a matter here of disorders of objective sensation but also of disorders of subjective sensation, of pain on the hemiplegic side, which we shall comment on later.

a. *Objective sensation.*

Superficial sensation is affected by the thalamic lesions in its three modalities: touch, pain, and temperature. There is not a complete abolition of peripheral sensations but modification of sensory impressions as they occur in the cerebral anesthesias with all their classical characteristics. We will only enumerate them rapidly: The anesthesia is never absolute as in hysterical hemianesthesia; it predominates in the distal portion of the limb and diminishes from the periphery proximally; and finally, on the trunk and the face this anesthesia goes slightly over the midline of the body, 1 to 2 cm. on the healthy side. . . .

Deep sensation is affected much more, and in its various components: articular, muscular, tendinous, osseous. In fact, one notices in many cases the diminution or reduction of osseous sensitivity, tested with the tuning fork, and the complete loss of muscle sense.

In our patients, the awareness of active or passive movements is diminished, and sometimes lost; likewise, the awareness of resistance and

strength. The sensation of weight is completely lost on the injured side. Finally, position sense, or the awareness of the attitudes of body parts, is strongly affected (akinesia).

There is more or less complete loss of "stereognosis," which is always affected, but to different degrees. . . .

b. *Subjective sensation.*

The presence of pain on the hemiplegic side is important to note. . . . These pains should be grouped with the pains thought to be "of central origin" by Anton, Edinger, Golscheider, etc. They appear early, dating from the onset of the hemiplegia, or a few months later. They reside not only in the paralyzed limbs, but also in the face and trunk. . . . It is very hard to obtain from the patients an exact idea of the localization of these pains concerning whether they are superficial or deep. Most of the patients, though, insist that they are rather superficial and that it is the skin and the subjacent adipose tissue which are painful.

In any case, these pains are continuous with paroxysmal exacerbations, sometimes bringing cries from the patients and keeping them from sleep or awakening them rudely.

One of our patients keeps telling us that what prevents her from moving her left hand, or walking, are the intense pains in her arm and leg. Here is a true *painful impotence.*

Moreover, the pain is not exclusively spontaneous. In some cases it may be provoked by simply touching the skin with the finger. Pinprick, contact with cold and heat, and pressure are very painful. The patients are sometimes very hyperesthesic.

The patients sometime compare their pains to superficial or deep burns, sometime to twinges, to violent and painful pressure placed on the skin, sometimes to the stabbing of a dagger. These phenomena have a paroxysmal character. Between crises, there are formications, numbness in the tips of the limbs and sometimes around the face.

Finally we note another important characteristic. These pains are not suppressed by any internal or external analgesic treatment. Nothing gives relief to the patient, whose suffering is sometimes intolerable. . . .

Pathologic Anatomy

. . . The anatomical ideas we offer today are the result of the study of *three specimens* examined in rigorously serialized microscopic sections. . . .

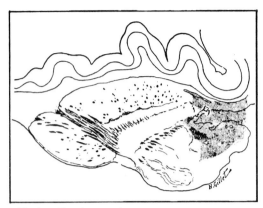

Fig 1.—(Cas Joss . . .)

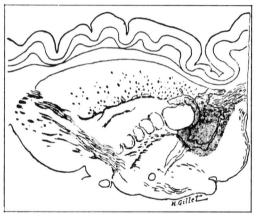

Fig 2.—(Cas Hud . . .)

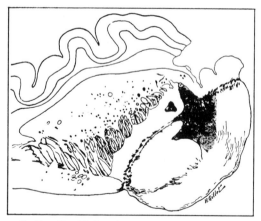

Fig 3.—(Cas Thal . . .)

In the first case (Joss . . .), the original lesion occupies the posterior part of the optic thalamus through almost its entire height. In the superior part of the thalamus the focus of destruction involves, in its posterior third, a large part of the external and internal nuclei (fig. 1). Lower, the lesion diminishes in extent but still involves mostly the external nucleus, continuing medially through the internal nucleus and the median nucleus, and, posteriorly, through the pulvinar. In the inferior part of the optic thalamus, the lesion is represented only by a line crossing directly through the external nucleus. At its highest point the lesion laterally cuts the posterior part of the posterior limb of the internal capsule. Finally, there exists, as a small secondary focus, a lacuna of cerebral disintegration in the posterior part of the putamen.

In the second case (Hud . . .), there is an equally large focus of destruction occupying principally the optic thalamus in its two inferior layers (fig. 2). It terminates at the upper limit of the subthalamic region. This focus is located in the external nucleus, which it largely destroys. Furthermore, it injures the internal, median and pulvinar nuclei. From the thalamus the lesion passes through the posterior and retrolenticular segments of the internal capsule, which it destroys, and divides the posterior part of the putamen.

Finally, in the third case (Thal . . .), study of the series of sections reveals a lesion much less extensive than in the previous cases, but involving exactly the same regions. It should be noted that the clinical signs, although evident, were much less prominent than in the first two cases. The lesion occupies the middle part of the optic thalamus and involves principally the posterior part of the external nucleus. (See fig. 3). From there, it passes medially to damage the internal and median nuclei (in relation to the pulvinar), and laterally to cut the posterior segment of the internal capsule and also a very small portion of the posterior part of the lenticular nucleus. The capsular lesion is only visible in the superior sections. Below, the thalamic lesion does not go beyond the optic thalamus. . . .

The cases we studied and present here allow us to add that *when the lesion occupies the external nucleus (external and posterior part) extending through the internal and median nuclei of the thalamus, involving only a part of the fibers of the posterior limb of the internal capsule, the clinical picture of the thalamic syndrome results.*

XIX   Raynaud's Phenomenon

EPISODIC vasospasm with discoloration of the digits was first described in 1862 by the French physician Maurice Raynaud (1834 to 1881).[1,2] A typical attack, as noted by Raynaud, consists of a cyclic discoloration of the skin, proceeding from white to blue to red.[3] At present, these attacks are usually referred to as "Raynaud's disease" if they occur in isolation; if they accompany another disorder, such as cryoglobulinemia, the term "Raynaud's phenomenon" is used.

Raynaud postulated that the transient discoloration of the digits is due to a disturbance in the sympathetic nervous system, and sympathectomy was later introduced as a treatment for the condition. The success of this operation has led to a better understanding of the autonomic nervous system and has promoted the use of sympathectomy in the management of a variety of vascular disorders.[4-8]

References

1. Raynaud, M.: *De l'asphyxie locale et de la gangrène symétrique des extrémitiés*, Paris: Rignoux, 1862.

2. Raynaud, M.: *On Local Asphyxia and Symmetrical Gangrene of the Extremities*, T. Barlow (trans), London: The New Sydenham Society, 1888.

3. Allen, E.V.; Barker, N.W.; and Hines, E.A., Jr.: *Peripheral Vascular Diseases*, Philadelphia: W. B. Saunders Co., ed 3, 1962, pp 124-171.

4. Sheehan, D.: Discovery of the Autonomic Nervous System, *Arch Neurol Psychiat* 35:1081-1115 (May) 1936.

5. White, J.C., and Smithwick, R.H.: *The Autonomic Nervous System: Anatomy, Physiology and Surgical Application*, New York: Macmillan Co., ed 2, 1941, pp 7-21.

6. Atkinson, W.J.: "Surgery of the Autonomic Nervous System," in Walker, A.E. (ed.): *A History of Neurological Surgery*, Baltimore: The Williams & Wilkins Co., 1951, pp 428-450.

7. Monro, P.A.G.: *Sympathectomy: An Anatomical and Physiological Study With Clinical Applications*, London: Oxford University Press, 1959, pp 3-9, 189-195.

8. Greenwood, B.: The Origins of Sympathectomy, *Med Hist* 11:165-169 (April-June) 1967.

ON LOCAL ASPHYXIA
and
SYMMETRICAL GANGRENE OF THE
EXTREMITIES*
by
Maurice Raynaud

Symptoms

. . . In its simplest form, local syncope is a condition perfectly compatible with health. Persons who are attacked with it, and who are ordinarily females, see under the least stimulus, sometimes without appreciable cause, one or many fingers become pale and cold all at once; in many cases it is the same finger which is always first attacked; the others become dead successively and in the same order. It is the phenomenon known under the name of the "dead finger." The attack is indolent, the duration varies from a few minutes to many hours. The determining cause is often the impression of cold; but that which is only commonly produced under the influence of the most severe cold, appears in the subjects of whom I speak on the occasion of the least lowering of temperature; sometimes even a simple mental emotion is enough. It would appear that the same cause which acts upon the capillaries of the face, and brings the red colour to the face, may in other circumstances act specially on the capillaries of the extremities; the skin of the affected parts assumes a dead white or sometimes a yellow colour; it appears completely exsanguine. The cutaneous sensibility becomes blunted, then annihilated; the fingers become like foreign bodies to the subject. They can be pinched and pricked with impunity; they may entirely lose the sense of contact and yet be able to distinguish heat and cold. Their temperature is notably lowered; this can be easily ascertained by touching them. It was established in one case that the temperature remained constantly one degree R. above that of the surrounding air. Ought the loss of movement in these cases to be attributed to a momentary paralysis of the flexor and extensor muscles? This is hardly possible if one considers that this syncopal state is often limited to a single digit, whilst a single muscle gives rise to many tendinous insertions. It is more reasonable to admit that the diseased part no longer transmitting sensation to the brain, the

brain itself loses temporarily, for want of excitant, the power of determining movements. In rare cases the secretions are affected and the dead finger becomes covered with a cold sweat. The slight importance of this local abolition of the circulation is probably due to the fact that it is so transient. The fingers are not the sole subjects of the affection, and if they appear to be more frequently attacked it is solely because they are of more immediate need for the usages of life than the toes. The attack is followed by a period of reaction, which is often very painful, and which gives place to a sensation quite analogous to that of being benumbed by cold.

We must not confound this condition with the numbness which succeeds the concussion or compression of a nerve. In the latter case it is the sensibility and motility which are primarily attacked, the circulation remaining intact; it is precisely the reverse which occurs in local syncope. When this, in place of affecting one or many digits, occupies the whole of a limb, then the circulatory troubles which one was forced to admit in some sort by induction become very evident.

In Case III. there was noted an excessive feebleness of the pulse at the moment of the commencement of the attack, which might have suggested some arterial obstruction if the increase of the pulsations during the intermissions had not appeared to negative this supposition.

In the more pronounced cases, those in which the asphyxial phenomena predominate, the pallor of the extremities is replaced by a cyanotic colour. This colour offers many different shades. Sometimes it is of a bluish white; it seems as though the skin had acquired a greater transparence than natural, so as to allow the subjacent tissues to be perceived; sometimes it is violet or slate-coloured, even becoming black, quite comparable to that which a slight blot of ink produces on the skin. When one presses on the parts thus altered in colour, the patch of dead white produced by pressure, in place of disappearing instantly, as happens to a healthy extremity, takes a considerable time before recovering the colour of the neighbouring parts, which denotes an excessive slowness of the capillary circulation.

*Reprinted from Raynaud, M.: *On Local Asphyxia and Symmetrical Gangrene of the Extremities*, T. Barlow (trans), London: The New Sydenham Society, 1888, pp 99-101, 110-111, 138-140, 143-145, and 147-150.

Habitually to this is added a little swelling in the neighbourhood. Very frequently also we see marked out up to a variable height livid venous marblings and which are very like those produced along the legs and thighs of persons who make use of foot-warmers. Pain is almost a constant phenomenon, it may be sufficiently sharp to draw forth cries from the patients; to a painful numbness there succeeds a sensation of burning and shooting which increases on pressure. Meanwhile the cutaneous anaesthesia is complete, and interferes with the prehension of small objects. The period of reaction is accompanied by irritating tingling sensations, which the patients compare to tingling from cold, or to the stinging of nettles.

Then less livid patches appear on the cyanosed parts; they extend and join one another, at the same time a vermilion colour shows itself at the margin; little by little it gains ground, chasing before it the bronzed colour which persists longest in the parts where it commenced, that is, in the most peripheral portions. Finally, a patch of deep red is formed on the extremities of the fingers. This patch gives place to the normal pink colour, and then the skin is found to have entirely returned to the primitive condition. . . .

Diagnosis

The diagnosis of the affection is generally easy. Nevertheless, especially at the outset, it is well to take precaution against several causes of error.

The phenomenon of "dead finger" is too well known by everybody for it to be necessary for me to delay in discussing it. The affection might be confounded with the state of habitual pallor which the extremities so often present in chlorotic females. But the preservation of movement and of sensibility in the latter case, and especially the persistence of the anaemic state, joined to the general trouble, of which it is only the expression, would suffice to remove all difficulties. Is it possible to establish a diagnosis between local asphyxia and frost bite? The phenomena are so similar that in truth it is not a simple analogy that they present to us, it is a perfect identity. But there is this important difference, that frost bite has a constant and perfectly known cause—the impression from excessive cold—whilst syncope and local asphyxia occur under the influence of an insignificant lowering of temperature, or even in the absence of this adjuvant circumstance. . . .

Diagnosis may offer more difficulties when pain precedes by a longer or shorter interval the appearance of a livid colour of the extremities. We have seen in one case of this kind (X) the malady taken for rheumatism by a distinguished surgeon, and treated for that disease; in this case the pain was situated not in the extremities, which subsequently mortified, but in the tibiotarsal joint and in that of the wrist. It will suffice to recall that in acute articular rheumatism the pain of the joints is almost always accompanied by redness, tumefaction, synovial effusion, and fever, and that in the disease in question nothing of this kind occurs. Sometimes in place of this pseudo-rheumatic appearance the malady assumes a neuralgic form. In this case, and before the appearance of the morbid colour of the skin, the error would be an easy one to commit, especially if there were well-marked periodicity. . . .

Nature of the Disease

. . . It appears then to be proved that lesions of nerves may lead in certain circumstances to alterations of nutrition, which are somewhat profound. But let it be noted that in all these cases there is a traumatic antecedent, which is wanting in our observations; that generally, if not always, there is the coincidence of a true paralysis; finally, and above all, that it is not true gangrene which is produced, and that the anatomical form of the lesion differs essentially from that which we have described. . . . Moreover, when we reflect on the numerous anastomoses which the nerves of the cerebro-spinal system have with the great sympathetic more or less near their origin, we cannot affirm that the lesion of nutrition, when it occurs, is not dependent on a lesion of the ganglionary system. This appears to result from M. Claude Bernard's experiments, and this leads us naturally to consider the bearing of his experiments on our subject.

The physiology of the circulation has been enriched in late years by one of the most beautiful discoveries of the century, with which is coupled the name of the illustrious professor whom I have just quoted. In repeating the experiments of Pourfour du Petit on the section of the great sympathetic of the neck, M. Bernard recognised that this lesion is accompanied always by a very notable elevation of temperature in the corresponding parts of the head. The same fact, studied subsequently by M. Brown-Séquard, and by M. Schiff, of Berne, has been not only verified but generalised. Since then the doctrine of vaso-motor nerves has passed from the domain of hypothesis to that of fact. On the one hand anatomy demonstrated the existence of smooth muscular fibres in the middle coat of the arteries, on the other physiology established the subordination of these fibres to nervous influence. Thus Valentin's phrase was realised, "The vascular contractility is the moderator of the course of the blood."

It was reserved to M. Bernard to add another discovery to the preceding. He demonstrated that the branches of the lingual nerve which go to the submaxillary gland have a property which is precisely inverse to that of the great sympathetic; when cut they provoke an acceleration of the blood current in that vascular region; galvanised at their peripheral end they cause slowing of the circulation; these vessels are thus subjected to two opposite local influences, of which the equilibrium is necessary for the maintenance of the normal circulation. Whence arises this conclusion: the pressure of the arterial system and the cardiac impulse are common mechanical conditions which the general circulation dispenses to all the organs. But the special nervous arrangment which has to do with each capillary system and each organic tissue regulates in each part the course of the blood in relation with the chemical functional conditions of the organs; these nervous modifications of the capillary circulation take place on the spot, and without any disturbance of the circulation of the neighbouring organs, or still less of the general circulation. Each part is united to the whole by the common conditions of the general circulation, and at the same time by means of the nervous system each part can have a circulation of its own and become physiologically individualised. Now whether this takes place only in the fine arterioles, the capillaries properly so called remaining foreign to it, in consequence of the constitution of their walls; or whether, on the contrary, according to Hastings and Milne Edwards, the capillary vessels themselves may take part, is of little importance from the physiological and pathological point of view; that which is certain is that on the confines of the arterial and venous systems important phenomena take place having to do with the volume, the temperature, and the colour of the parts, and of which the vascular contractility can and ought to render an account. . . .

(Local syncope and asphyxia) . . . commences by a spasm of the capillary vessels, and let us remark that this spasm occurs in subjects who are characterised by a nervous predominance, young women, hysterical people, children, etc. In the simplest cases those in which the malady remains,

if I may so say, in a rough state, the exaggerated peristaltic contraction of the capillaries drives the blood before it, the extremities become pale, withered looking, and insensible. This is the "dead finger." But this phenomenon does not persist long enough for gangrene to follow. To contraction succeeds relaxation, the circulation is re-established, and everything returns to the normal state after a period of reaction more or less painful. Such is *local syncope,* in which the venules participate in the contraction of the arterioles.

Local asphyxia is only a more advanced condition. After an initial period of capillary spasm there occurs a period of reaction, but it is incomplete reaction. The vessels which return first to their primary calibre, or even beyond, are naturally those which present in their structure the fewest contractile elements, viz, the venules. At the moment when these are opened, the arterioles being still closed, the venous blood, which had been at first driven back into the great trunks of the dark blood system, flows again into the finest vascular divisions, and then the extremities will take on that tint varying from blue to black which is a certain index of the presence of venous blood in the capillary network. This explains two phenomena to which I have called attention in speaking of the symptoms. The first is that the cyanotic tint of the extremities succeeds in general to an extreme pallor, or in other terms that syncope precedes asphyxia.

The second is that at the outset at least the asphyxiated parts have not that very deep tint which one observes following on a violent constriction of a limb; in this last case, in fact, there is venous blood extending into arteries of a calibre which is relatively considerable. In local asphyxia the venous reflux does not go beyond the capillary network properly so-called; it results therefrom that the colour which is observed has a certain transparence; it is a mixture of cyanosis and pallor. During the convulsions or painful crises, effort determines a more abundant reflux still of venous blood, and the extremities become warm at the same time that they become black (Case VII.).

In the meantime the vis a tergo having ceased its action on the venous side, the return circulation is no longer favoured except by the causes which in the physiological state are limited to the part of accessory conditions; such are the muscular contraction of the limbs, the play of the valves, the aspiration exercised by the thoracic cavity, etc. Consequently the blood stagnates even in the great venous trunks, and then are produced along with a very slight oedematous suffusion those subcutaneous livid venous markings which have been rightly compared to those which the prolonged use of warming pans produces.*

This state may be chronic, and the spasm of vessels may only have a limited duration so as to return in irregular or intermittent attacks. This case is itself susceptible of many degrees: at one time everything is comprised in local asphyxia pure and simple; at another, each attack having a longer duration, the tendency to gangrene is more pronounced; bullae form with very small sloughs, then at the moment when gangrene is on the point of becoming confirmed the parts revive momentarily, to be soon afterwards attacked in the same way; and this may go on for years. Finally it may happen, although much more rarely (but we have collected several examples of it), that the capillary spasm comes on all at once with an intensity and a duration altogether extraordinary. Syncope and local asphyxia succeed one another rapidly; the venous blood becomes insufficient to nourish the parts; the colour becomes deeper and deeper; small blood-stained infiltrations take place through the walls of the venules; these walls may themselves become granular; in one word, there is confirmed gangrene, and gangrene which may go on to the fall of many ends of fingers or toes. . . .

Treatment

It will, I trust, be readily understood that for a malady of which so many points are still obscure, I am not quite prepared to formulate a complete treatment. It is desirable, nevertheless, to state the principal indications which are to be fulfilled, and especially some gross errors which are to be avoided.

We have seen that in one case (XV.), dominated by the desire of irritating and stimulating the torpid parts, I advised the patient at the beginning of the affection to use local mustard baths. I have reported the disastrous results which immediately followed the employment of these means. This is what I think takes place in such a case: the application to the extremities of a powerful modifying agency, whilst locally combating the vascular spasm, causes the vascular spasm in some sort to retrograde to the larger arteries;

hence the sudden eruption of venous blood into parts which it did not previously occupy, and consequently blackness of the extremities rising much higher towards the root of the limbs. Whether this be the explanation or not, we must avoid the use of a therapeutic measure which is as treacherous as it is dangerous, and in general terms we must forbid the employment of energetic rubefacients. . . .

It is hardly necessary to add, that to all these methods of treatment it will always be opportune to add the envelopment of the affected limb in close fitting material, and especially in cotton wool. If radiation has upon the progress of the symptoms the dangerous influence which I have attributed to it, it is evident that it must be useful to try to neutralise this cause of chilling. . . .

Finally, all these local means are only secondary, since manifestly we have to do with a malady of general origin. If I am not deceived as to the mechanism which produces it, the desideratum is to find a medicament which would have a constant resolving action on the smooth muscular fibres of the arterial coats.

Is opium such a medicament? We know the unbounded confidence which Pott accorded to it as curative of gangrene. Since his time we have been compelled to abate some of the enthusiasm roused by the early cases in which this drug was employed. Nevertheless in every causal condition, and quite apart from all theory, we must acknowledge that opium, being the first of the narcotics, at least responds to this primary indication—viz, to calm the atrocious pains of mortification of the extremities. In this respect it will always find its use, which, moreover, is free from any inconvenience. . . .

Moreover, in conclusion, I repeat that this malady, so strange, so formidable in appearance, is far from having in reality all the gravity which at first one would be tempted to attribute to it. To moderate the pains, to prevent the use of unsuitable measures and doubtful remedies, such ought to be in the majority of cases the part played by the physician. Nature will do the rest. We shall be sufficiently satisfied, although we cannot immediately relieve our patients, if we can still encourage them with the hope of a probable and approaching recovery, and should this point be the only one which clearly results from the work just completed, I should not regret the pains which I have bestowed upon it.

---

*Are the spontaneous pains of syncope and of local asphyxia in relation to the vascular contraction a sort of painful cramps of arteries?

XX   Alzheimer's Disease

ALZHEIMER'S original description of presenile dementia in 1907 showed the value of clinical-pathological correlation in psychiatry. With his close associate Franz Nissl, the German neuropathologist Alois Alzheimer (1864 to 1915) devoted his career to investigating the anatomical changes underlying dementia.[1-3] In the course of these studies, he discovered the disorder now known as Alzheimer's disease, which is characterized clinically by presenile dementia and pathologically by cerebral atrophy, senile plaques, and neurofibrillary degeneration.

Alzheimer was not the first to describe senile plaques.[4] These microscopic foci are often found in the brains of the elderly, and some degree of plaque formation seems to accompany normal aging. However, Alzheimer correctly recognized that the presence of senile plaques in large numbers was abnormal. The neurofibrillary changes, consisting of tangles of thick argentophilic fibrils within the cytoplasm of neurons, were new to Alzheimer. Although he considered them specific for presenile dementia, subsequent investigations have also demonstrated these neurofibrillary tangles in cases of senile dementia as well as in elderly individuals without dementia.[4-7]

The occurrence of similar pathological changes in presenile and senile dementia makes their characterization as separate nosologic entities somewhat artificial. However, it was Kraepelin who began the tradition of applying Alzheimer's name to the presenile form of the disease, and the tradition continues.[1]

References

1. Young, A.W.: "Franz Nissl, 1860-1918, Alois Alzheimer, 1864-1915," in *Neurological Biographies and Addresses, Foundation Volume, Published for the Staff, to Commemorate the Opening of the Montreal Neurological Institute, of McGill University*, London: Oxford University Press, 1936, pp 107-113.

2. Lewey, F.H.: "Alois Alzheimer (1864-1915)," in Haymaker, W. (ed.): *The Founders of Neurology*, Springfield, Ill: Charles C Thomas, Publishers, 1953, pp 165-168.

3. Meyer, J.E.: "Alois Alzheimer (1864-1915)," in Kolle, K. (ed.): *Grosse Nervenärzte*, Stuttgart Georg Thieme, 1959, vol 2, pp 32-38.

4. McMenemey, W.H.: "The Dementias and Progressive Diseases of the Basal Ganglia," in Blackwood, W., et al (eds.): *Greenfield's Neuropathology*, ed 2, Baltimore: Williams & Wilkins Co., 1963, pp 520-576.

5. Margolis, G.: Senile Cerebral Disease: A Critical Survey of Traditional Concepts Based Upon Observations With Newer Technics, *Lab Invest* 8:335-370 (March-April) 1959.

6. Hirano, A., and Zimmerman, H.M.: Alzheimer's Neurofibrillary Changes: A Topographic Study, *Arch Neurol* 7:227-242 (Sept) 1962.

7. Tomlinson, B.F.; Blessed, G.; and Roth, M.: Observations on the Brains of Non-Demented Old People, *J Neurol Sci* 7:331-356 (Sept-Oct) 1968.

On a Peculiar Disease of the

Cerebral Cortex*

Alzheimer—Munich

A. reports a patient observed in the insane asylum in Frankfurt am Main, whose central nervous system had been given to him for investigation by Director Sioli.

Clinically the patient presented such an unusual picture that the case could not be categorized under any of the known diseases. Anatomically the findings were different from all other known disease processes.

*Translation of: Über eine eigenartige Erkrankung der Hirnrinde. *Allgemeine Zeitschrift für Psychiatrie und Psychisch-Gerichtlich Medicin* 64:146-148, 1907. (Also *Zentralblatt für Nervenheilkunde und Psychiatrie* 30:177-179, 1907.)

A woman, 51 years old, showed jealousy toward her husband as the first noticeable sign of the disease. Soon a rapidly increasing loss of memory could be noticed. She could not find her way around in her own apartment. She carried objects back and forth and hid them. At times she would think that someone wanted to kill her and would begin shrieking loudly.

In the institution her entire behavior bore the stamp of utter perplexity. She was totally disoriented to time and place. Occasionally she stated that she could not understand and did not know her way around. At times she greeted the doctor like a visitor, and excused herself for not having finished her work; at times she shrieked loudly that he wanted to cut her, or she repulsed him with indignation, saying that she feared from him something against her chastity. Periodically she was totally delirious, dragged her bedding around, called her husband and her daughter, and seemed to have auditory hallucinations. Frequently, she shrieked with a dreadful voice for many hours.

Because of her inability to comprehend the situation, she always cried out loudly as soon as someone tried to examine her. Only through repeated attempts was it possible finally to ascertain anything.

Her ability to remember was severely disturbed. If one pointed to objects, she named most of them correctly, but immediately afterwards she would forget everything again. When reading, she went from one line into another, reading the letters or reading with a senseless emphasis. When writing, she repeated individual syllables several times, left out others, and quickly became stranded. When talking, she frequently used perplexing phrases and some paraphrastic expressions (milk-pourer instead of cup). Sometimes one noticed her getting stuck. Some questions she obviously did not comprehend. She seemed no longer to understand the use of some objects. Her gait was not impaired. She could use both hands equally well. Her pateller reflexes were present. Her pupils reacted. Somewhat rigid radial arteries; no enlargement of cardiac dullness; no albumin.

During her subsequent course, the phenomena that were interpreted as focal symptoms were at times more noticeable and at times less noticeable. But always they were only slight. The generalized dementia progressed however. After 4½ years of the disease, death occurred. At the end, the patient was completely stuporous; she lay in her bed with her legs drawn up under her, and in spite of all precautions she acquired decubitus ulcers.

The autopsy revealed a generally atrophic brain without macroscopic lesions. The large cerebral vessels were altered by arteriosclerosis.

In sections prepared with the Bielschowsky silver method, remarkable changes in the neurofibrils appeared. In the interior of a cell that otherwise appeared normal, one or several fibrils stood out due to their extraordinary thickness and impregnability. At a later stage, many fibrils appeared, situated side by side and altered in the same way. Then they merged into dense bundles and gradually reached the surface of the cell. Finally, the nucleus and the cell disintegrated, and only a dense bundle of fibrils indicated the site where a ganglion cell had been.

Since these fibrils could be stained with different dyes than normal, a chemical alteration of the fibrillar substance must have taken place. This then could be the reason why the fibrils survived the death of the cell. The alteration of the fibrils seemed to go hand in hand with the deposition in the ganglion cell of a pathological metabolic product not yet investigated further. About ¼ to ⅓ of all ganglion cells in the cerebral cortex showed such changes. Numerous ganglion cells, particularly in the upper cell layers, had disappeared entirely.

Scattered through the entire cortex, especially in the upper layers, one found miliary foci that were caused by the deposition of a peculiar substance in the cerebral cortex. It could be recognized without staining, but was very refractory to dyes.

The glia had formed abundant fibers. Furthermore, many glial cells exhibited large fat vesicles.

Infiltration of the vessels was entirely absent. However, one saw evidence of endothelial proliferation and also neovascularization in some places.

In summary, we are apparently confronted with a distinctive disease process. An increasing number of unusual diseases have been discovered during the past few years. These observations show that we should not be satisfied to take a clinically unclear case and, by making great efforts, fit it into one of the known disease categories. Undoubtedly there are many more psychiatric diseases than are included in our textbooks. Often a subsequent histological examination would show the peculiarity of the case. Then gradually we would be able to separate individual diseases clinically from the large classes of diseases in our textbooks and define their clinical characteristics more precisely.

(From our own correspondent)

XXI   The Signs of Kernig and Brudzinski

A NEW clinical sign, like a new treatment, often seems to have its greatest value in the hands of its promulgator. Josef Brudzinski (1874-1917), a Polish pediatrician,[1] claimed that his neck sign for meningitis was present in a higher percentage of cases than Kernig's sign, which had been described earlier for the same condition.[2,3] The usefulness of Brudzinski's test has been well documented by later observers, but its superiority to Kernig's sign has not been established.[4]

In 1884, Vladimir Kernig (1840-1917), a Russian physician,[1] described a sign consisting of limitation in passive extension at the knee because of spasm of the hamstring muscles.[3] Kernig preferred to elicit his sign with the patient in the sitting position, though the test is rarely done this way now. It is more convenient to allow the patient to remain in the supine position and attempt to extend the knee after the thigh has been brought perpendicular to the trunk. Kernig's description, though detailed, failed to include a striking aspect of a positive test: the intense pain inflicted on the patient by the maneuver. The basis for Kernig's sign was later interpreted as a protective reaction to prevent the pain induced by stretch of the inflamed and hypersensitive sciatic nerve roots.[4]

In 1909, Brudzinski described his neck sign, consisting of flexion at the knees and hips in response to passive flexion of the neck.[2] He explained the sign in terms of unmasking latent patterns of muscle tone, and this view has since been developed into the theory that the sign represents release of a primitive tonic neck reflex.[5,6] However, this idea is disputed by those who look upon the sign as a protective reaction preventing stretch of inflamed sciatic nerve roots in a manner similar to Kernig's sign.[4,6] Forward flexion of the head has been found to put traction on the intradural roots, which attain maximal relaxation when both hip and knee are placed in intermediate degrees of flexion.[4]

In his original paper, Brudzinski also reviews another "Brudzinski sign" of meningitis: the contralateral leg phenomenon.[7] However, Brudzinski's leg sign was not destined to attain the popularity of his neck sign.

The tests of Kernig and of Brudzinski are often performed together. These signs may be present not only in infectious meningitis but also when the meninges are affected by bleeding, chemical agents, or carcinomatosis.[6] As bedside indicators of meningeal irritation, the two signs are now considered to have equal value.

References

1. Hall, G.W.: Neurologic Signs and Their Discoverers, *JAMA* **95**:703-707 (Sept 6) 1930.
2. Brudzinski, J.: Un signe nouveau sur les

membres inferieurs dans les meningites chez les enfants (signe de la nuque), *Arch Med* 12:745-752, 1909.

3. Kernig, W.: Ueber ein Wenig Bemerktes Meningitis-Symptom, *Berlin Klin Wschr* 21:829-832, 1884.

4. O'Connell, J.E.A: The Clinical Signs of Meningeal Irritation, *Brain* 69:9-21, 1946.

5. Brock, S., and Krieger, H.P.: *The Basis of Clinical Neurology,* ed 4, Baltimore: Williams & Wilkins Co., 1963, p 455.

6. Wartenberg, R.: The Signs of Brudzinski and of Kernig, *J Pediat* 37:679-684 (Oct) 1950.

7. Brudzinski, J.: Ueber die Kontralateralen Reflexe an den Unteren Extremitaeten bei Kindern, *Wien Klin Wschr* 21:255-261, 1908.

Concerning a Little Noted Sign of Meningitis*

By Dr. W. Kernig, Ordinator at Obuchow Hospital in St. Petersburg

For a number of years I have noted in cases of meningitis a sign that appears to be little known although its practical value is, in my opinion, not insignificant. I refer to the occurrence of flexion in the legs, and sometimes in the arms as well, when the patient sits up.

It is well known that the great majority of patients with tuberculous and epidemic cerebrospinal meningitis have the classical rather intense stiffness of the neck and back (although a few patients with acute meningitis have no muscle spasm at all, particularly with purulent secondary meningitis). As long as the patient is lying, there exists, in some of the cases, spasm of the extremities. In other cases—and these appear, in our observations up to now, to constitute the great majority—we find the recumbent patient to have stiffness of neck and back but no spasm in the extremities. Neither an extension nor a flexion spasm is present in the arms or legs, and if the patient by chance holds his extremities flexed, they can be passively extended without notable resistence. If we now place the patient upright on the edge of the bed so that the legs hang down (in cases with very intense stiffness of the neck and back, this maneuver is not easily accomplished), the spasm of the neck and back usually becomes much more marked. There then appears a flexion at the knees and occasionally also at the elbows. If we attempt to extend the legs of the sitting patient at the knee, we can succeed only to an obtuse angle of about 135°. When the phenomenon is very marked, the leg remains at a right angle. This striking phenomenon is the difference between nothing and something: between the complete lack of spasm in the patient lying down and the presence of it in the patient sitting up. It is so clear-cut that special attention should be directed

to this sign and it should be looked for in every case. In view of the ease with which the test is performed, it is very useful in the midst of pressing hospital activities, especially as a quick orientation sign, if I may so express myself. Nuchal rigidity is sometimes barely noticeable in the recumbent position and does not always become more conspicuous upon sitting up. The sensorium in any given moment may seem so clear that, as is known, the first examination may not arouse the suspicion of meningitis. Then it is valuable to be able to elicit, by simply sitting the patient up, such a pregnant sign as a distinct flexion spasm at the knee joints. When suspicion is already present, the diagnosis will be established further. When there is no suspicion, the sign points to meningitis, or rather, as I will discuss, to affections of the pia specifically. . . .

The great constancy of the sign under discussion must be strongly emphasized. During the entire illness, from the development of the meningitis till far into convalescence and long after the disappearance of the fever, it is possible to evoke spasm in the legs through sitting the patient up. It corresponds with the appearance of spasm in the back and neck, which also, as is known, grows in intensity and is present continuously. On the other hand, the spasms in the extremities of recumbent patients are, as far as I have seen, present only intermittently.

Closer observation has further taught us that as soon as we bring the patient from the sitting to the standing position, the spasm at the knee disappears. This came to my attention strikingly and indeed for the first time, when I saw a person convalescing from meningitis who had slight neck spasm and spasm in the knees on sitting, but who walked freely about the room. As soon as she stood, the contractions disappeared. Thereafter I made the same observation on several other patients and have convinced myself that when one tries to bring the extended lower limb to a right

*Translation of: Ueber ein wenig bemerktes Meningitis-Symptom, *Berliner Klinische Wochenschrift* 21:829-832, 1884.

angle with the trunk of the recumbent patient, spasm begins with the flexion of the thigh on the trunk. In patients with other illnesses there is no tendency to bring the leg in flexion up to the thigh. . . .

In general, I can assert the following: the spasm at the knee joint, which is under discussion, occurs when the meningitis patient has the thigh in some degree of flexion in relation to the trunk (about at a right angle). Here lies the explanation why this phenomen has not been noticed up to now. One ordinarily straightens the thighs in relation to the trunk when looking for spasm in the recumbent patient. Consequently, the form of spasm under discussion disappears. . . .

[Six case reports follow in which clinical meningitis was not present.]

If we review these six cases with reference to the anatomical findings in the cerebral and spinal meninges, we have in the first case, edema of the pia; in the third, hemorrhagic meningitis of the dura and intermeningeal bleeding; in the fourth, circumscribed pachy- and lepto-meningitis and thrombosis of the petrosal sinus; in the fifth, adhesion of the dura with the cranium and chronic lepto-meningitis; in the sixth, again extensive intermeningeal bleeding of the brain and spinal cord, with slight, very fresh meningitis of the convexity. Only in the second case is the involvement of the pia insignificant, consisting of moderate hyperemia. However, we have seen that the possibility of a very early stage of tuberculous meningitis has not been excluded.

Except for this one case out of 21, we find that when the classic anatomical picture of one of the usual forms of meningitis did not exist, the pia nevertheless participated in some way in the pathological process which during life caused the symptom I have been emphasizing. Edema, intermeningeal bleeding, circumscribed meningitis, and chronic inflammation were the changes found.

Nowhere in the literature do I find the symptom described by me brought into focus and explicity emphasized. . . .

A NEW SIGN OF THE LOWER EXTREMITIES IN MENINGITIS OF CHILDREN (Neck Sign)*

By Dr. J. Brudzinski, Chief Physician of the Anne-Marie Hospital, Lodz, Poland

In my work entitled *Contralateral Reflexes in the Lower Limbs of Children,* I have drawn attention to a sign that appears in tuberculous and epidemic meningitis, among other conditions. It concerns the corresponding reflex movement of a lower limb when one passively flexes the opposite lower limb (the identical contralateral reflex). Sometimes a lower limb first placed in flexion makes a reflex movement of extension after the passive flexion of the other limb (the reciprocal contralateral reflex). In the eight cases of tuberculous meningitis observed at that time, I noted the identical contralateral reflex six times and the reciprocal contralateral reflex once. In one case, I could find neither of these reflexes. In the two cases of epidemic cerebrospinal meningitis seen at that time, the identical contralateral reflex appeared very clearly in both lower limbs. In that work I stated that the sign described by me can be useful for differential diagnosis of meningitis along with the signs already known.

Subsequent investigations have confirmed my conviction. I have found this sign in both lower limbs, although sometimes only in one, in 17 cases of tuberculous meningitis, and it has greatly facilitated diagnosis since the signs of Babinski and of Kernig were sometimes lacking. I have also observed it in six cases of epidemic cerebrospinal meningitis.

Recently, Mlle. Zaimovsky, in her thesis *On the State of Reflexes in Children,* inspired by M. Hutinel, has mentioned the contralateral reflex and has expressed herself thus on its value for the diagnosis of meningitis: "We can say that the reflex of Brudzinski is almost constant in children with disease of the meninges."

In the course of these investigations, I have observed a new sign in cases of meningitis: *passive flexion of the neck forward causes the lower limbs to flex at the knees and the hips, and the limbs sometimes make a very marked flexion on the pelvis.*

Comparative studies on a series of children of all ages, both healthy and suffering from various diseases other than affections of the meninges, have demonstrated to me the complete absence of

*Translation of: Un Signe Nouveau sur les Membres Inférieurs dans les Méningites chez les Enfants (Signe de la Nuque), *Archives de medécine des enfants* 12:745-752, 1909.

this sign. Since a careful search of the literature has been negative with regard to this phenomenon, I can publish it as a new sign of meningitis in children.

In the case reports, I shall mention only information relating to the reflexes. The diagnosis of meningitis was confirmed in our cases by lumbar puncture and examination of cerebrospinal fluid, and in some cases by autopsy.

I shall designate this sign: *the neck sign.*

I observed this sign for the first time in a little girl of five years, Marianne F . . . , offspring of a tuberculous family. She had been sick ten days. The illness began with headache and vomiting. The child, semi-conscious, restless. Dermatographia very distinct. Patellar reflex very active. Positive Babinski sign. Positive Kernig sign. Contralateral reflex (Brudzinski) positive—reflex flexion of a lower extremity after passive flexion of the opposite extremity. Equal pupils, a little dilated; pupillary reaction very sluggish. Stiffness of the neck not marked; the sensitivity of the neck is not increased.

When I flexed the neck passively to convince myself of its stiffness, I noticed flexion of the lower extremities in the two joints and flexion of the lower extremities on the pelvis.

I have observed this sign in 21 cases of tuberculous meningitis, 11 cases of cerebrospinal meningitis, eight cases of serous meningitis in the course of various infectious diseases, and two cases of pneumococcal meningitis following pneumonia with slow resolution. In one of these cases, the discovery of the sign in the course of the pneumonia raised doubts about the value of the sign for the diagnosis of meningitis. However, the pneumonia did not resolve, and the child assumed a more and more meningitic appearance. It was brought to the hospital, and lumbar puncture yielded purulent fluid containing pneumococci. The value of this sign was thus confirmed.

For these four kinds of meningitis, comprising 42 cases, the frequency of these four signs per 100 was as follows:

Kernig's sign............57%
Babinski's sign 50%
Contralateral reflex 66%
Neck sign 97%

It appears from our investigations and from the data in the literature that the signs known up to now sometimes do not suffice for the diagnosis of meningitis. Therefore, it is hoped that the signs described by us, the contralateral reflex and above all the neck sign, will make the diagnosis of meningitis easier.

The neck sign, as we have shown above, was present in all the cases of meningitis of diverse type, except for a case of tuberculous meningitis in an agonal state. The contralateral reflex can occupy at least the same rank as the other known signs.

The technique of examining for the neck sign is very simple. One takes the head of the supine child in his left hand and flexes the head and the neck while resting his right hand on the chest of the child to prevent its being raised.

The examination is, in general, without inconvenience. With the very young, one sometimes does not accomplish it quickly because the restlessness of the child keeps the lower extremities from remaining extended. In such a case, one holds them gently at the knee joints. To avoid errors, it is necessary to make repeated examinations. The examination is so convenient that one cannot forget it since one always tests the stiffness of the neck in suspicious cases, and it is then that the sign appears.

I cannot give an adequate explanation of the cause of this sign. Increased pressure in the cerebral canal does not play the preponderant role since we have not found the sign in cases of hydrocephalus with very increased pressure. The spastic state of the lower extremities appears to play an important role in cerebrospinal meningitis, but the flexion of the limbs on the pelvis is also marked in cases of tuberculous meningitis, where the spasticity is barely present. This sign was not found in several cases of Little's disease examined for it. The pain caused by the forced flexion is not decisive even momentarily since one finds this sign in cases of meningitis where stiffness is minimal. Furthermore, in hydrocephalic children flexion is very painful, and this sign is not forthcoming. Furthermore, in normal children, especially in nursing infants, flexion was at times rather painful and the children struggled with their feet, but these movements were completely disorderly and were movements of defense.

It is probable that, in accordance with Chaufards hypothesis concerning Kernig's sign, the most important factor is a muscular hypertonia of the lower limbs and a physiological predominance of the extensor muscles of the neck and back over the flexor muscles of the lower extremities. We can only hope that later investigations will give us a more precise explanation.

XXII   Lasègue's Sign

T HE Lasègue test, used in the evaluation of patients with sciatica, is sometimes confused with the Kernig test, which it closely resembles.[1-4]

Sciatica, which is now defined as pain along the course of the sciatic nerve, was first described by the early Greek and Roman physicians.[5] However, it was not related to dysfunction of the sciatic nerve until 1764, when Domenico Cotugno of Naples published his *De Ischiade Nervosa Commentarius*.[6] Irritation of the sciatic nerve and its component nerve roots was subsequently found to result from different underlying conditions, such as spinal arthritis, intraspinal and extraspinal neoplasms, and spondylolisthesis.[7] Recently, it has become apparent that sciatica is often caused by nerve root compression from a herniated nucleus pulposus of a lumbar intervertebral disk.[8] The common awareness of lumbar disk disease at the present time has led to widespread use of the Lasègue test.

Charles Ernest Lasègue (1816 to 1883), a French clinician and pathologist, never published a description of his test. The description was given by his pupil, J. -J. Forst, in his doctoral thesis in 1881.[9-14] The Lasègue test consists of two maneuvers. First, the involved lower extremity of a supine patient is raised with the knee extended. Then the maneuver is repeated, but the leg is flexed on the thigh as the thigh is flexed on the pelvis. The Lasègue sign is present if the first maneuver produces sciatic pain but the second maneuver does not.

Forst and Lasègue concluded that the pain produced by raising the involved lower extremity with the knee extended was due to muscular compression of the sciatic nerve. The current view, implicating stretch of the sciatic nerve and its component nerve roots, is attributed to De Beurmann,[15] who wrote on the subject in 1884. However, Laza Lazarević, a Yugoslavian physician writing in the *Archivum serbicum pro universa scientia et arte medica recipienda* in 1880, was actually the first to describe the straight-leg-raising test in sciatica and to identify the stretching of the sciatic nerve as the cause of the pain.[16,17]

The Kernig test, first described in 1884, is usually performed by attempting to extend the flexed knee of the supine patient after the thigh has been flexed on the pelvis.[4] It is therefore not exactly the same as the Lasègue test. However, its underlying mechanism, the stretching of the sciatic nerve and its roots, is identical, and a positive test produces similar sciatic and low-back pain.[1] Both the Lasègue sign and the Kernig sign may be present bilaterally in patients with meningeal irritation and unilaterally in those with unilateral sciatica.

In view of their similarity, it seems arbitrary that medical tradition insists upon maintaining the minor differences between the two tests. The Kernig test is used primarily in the diagnosis of meningitis, whereas the Lasègue test is now applied almost solely to the diagnosis of the herniated lumbar disk.

References

1. Wartenberg, R.: The Signs of Brudzinski and of Kernig, *J Pediat* 37:679-684 (Oct) 1950.

2. Spurling, R.G.: *Lesions of the Lumbar Intervertebral Disc: With Special Reference to Rupture of the Annulus Fibrosus with Herniation of the Nucleus Pulposus,* Springfield, Ill: Charles C Thomas, Publisher, 1953, pp 53-54.

3. Borden, J.N.: The Lasègue Test, *JAMA* 201:641 (Aug 21) 1967.

4. Brody, I.A., and Wilkins, R.H.: Neurological Classics XXI: The Signs of Kernig and Brudzinski, *Arch Neurol* 21:215-218 (Aug) 1969.

5. Mettler, C.C.: *History of Medicine: A Correlative Text, Arranged According to Subjects,* F.A. Mettler (ed.) Philadelphia: Blakiston Co., 1947, pp 493,813-814.

6. Viets, H.R.: Domenico Cotugno: His Description of the Cerebrospinal Fluid, With a Translation of Part of His *De Ischiade Nervosa Commentarius*

(1764) and a Bibliography of His Important Works, *Bull Inst Hist Med* 3:701-738 (Nov) 1935.

7. Gray, C.: The Causes and Treatment of Sciatic Pain, *Int Abstr Surg* 85:417-441 (Nov) 1947.

8. Wilkins, R.H.: Neurosurgical Classic-XV, *J Neurosurg* 21:73-81 (Jan) 1964.

9. Hall, G.W.: Neurologic Signs and Their Discoverers, *JAMA* 95:703-707 (Sept 6) 1930.

10. Sjöqvist, O.: The Mechanism of Origin of Lasègue's Sign, *Acta Psychiat Neurol,* 461 (suppl 46): 290-297, 1947.

11. Woodhall, B., and Hayes, G.J.: The Well-Leg-Raising Test of Fajersztajn in the Diagnosis of Ruptured Lumbar Intervertebral Disc, *J Bone Joint Surg* 32A:786-792 (Oct) 1950.

12. Wartenberg, R.: Lasègue Sign and Kernig Sign: Historical Notes, *Arch Neurol Psychiat* 66:58-60 (July) 1951.

13. Wartenberg, R.: On Neurologic Terminology, Eponyms and the Lasègue Sign, *Neurology* 6:853-858 (Dec) 1956.

14. Bazzi, F., and Donadi, G.: Storia di un Sintoma: Il Lasèguè, *Riv Stor Med* 8:159-171 (July-Dec) 1964.

15. De Beurmann, (L): Note Sur Un Signe Peu Connu de la Sciatique: Recherches Expérimentales, *Arch Physiol Norm Path* 16:375-380, 1884.

16. Lazarević, L.K.: Ischias postica Cotunnii: Ein Beitrag zu deren Differential-Diagnose, *Allg Wien Med Ztg* 29:425-426, 1884.

17. Dimitrijevic, D.T.: Lasègue Sign, *Neurology* 2:453-454 (Sept-Oct) 1952.

Contribution to the Clinical Study of Sciatica*

J. -J. Forst

We do not intend to make a complete study of sciatica. We will limit ourselves to a clinical sign of very great diagnostic value. In spite of all that has been written on sciatica, we have found no mention of the symptom that we are about to bring to light.

It was our master, Professor Lasègue, who called our attention to this clinical sign. . . .

The patient is placed on the bed in the supine position, and we take the foot of the affected limb in one hand, as in figure 1. We place the other hand on the knee of the same limb, and, holding the leg in extension, we flex the thigh on the pelvis. Raising the limb only a few centimeters produces a sharp pain at the level of the sciatic

*Translation of: *Contribution a l'Étude Clinique de la Sciatique. Thèse pour le Doctorat en Médecine,* Paris: Faculté de Médecine de Paris, 1881.

notch, just at the emergence of the nerve. We replace the limb on the bed and proceed to another maneuver, which is only a confirmatory test. We have just seen that the patient experiences pain when the thigh is flexed on the pelvis with the limb in extension. If we now flex the leg on the thigh, as in figure 2, we can flex the thigh on the pelvis without producing any painful sensation. For this second maneuver to succeed, it is necessary to take certain precautions. One must flex the leg on the thigh slowly, sliding the heel on the bed so as to avoid any movement in the joint other than that caused by the flexion of the leg on the thigh.

This precaution is understandable, for if we flex the leg on the thigh in a rough manner, there is a good chance of producing some pain. Thus, it is necessary to flex the leg on the thigh and the

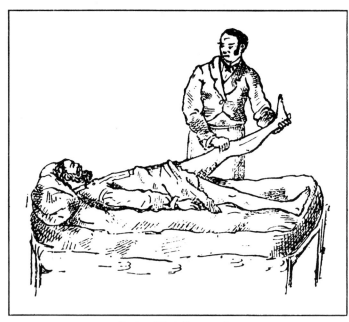

Fig 1.—[First Maneuver].

Fig 2.—[Second Maneuver].

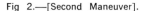

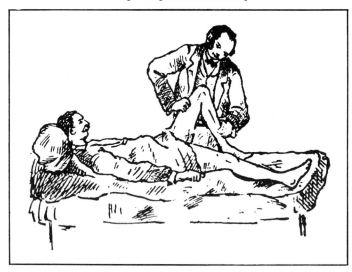

level. . . . If, however, we flex the leg on the thigh, we can then flex the thigh on the pelvis further and we do not encounter this vague sensation of pulling.

What is happening?

The explanation of the difficulty in flexing the thigh on the pelvis with the leg in extension is evidently that the flexor muscles are counterbalanced by their antagonists, the extensors of the thigh, which are very powerful. In the action of raising the limb, all the muscles contract; hence, the sensation of pulling is very probably due to compression of the sciatic nerve by muscular contraction. On the other hand, if we flex the leg on the thigh, we paralyse the extensors of the thigh on the pelvis. They are in complete relaxation. The action of the flexors of the thigh is thus more effective and there is greater ease in raising the limb with less compression of the sciatic nerve. Consequently, the sensation of numbness at the gluteal level is absent.

Let us return to the patient's bedside. . . . It appears to us— and it is the opinion of our master, Professor Lasègue— that the sharp pain experienced by the patient may be attributed to compression of the sciatic nerve by the muscle mass. . . .

The sciatic nerve is in relationship at the level of the buttocks, with the inferior border of the piriformis, under

thigh on the pelvis at the same time. It is also necessary for the patient to cooperate in the test, and he must relax his limb completely. . . .

The pain that we have just produced by raising the patient's extended leg is, in our opinion, only the exaggeration of a physiological phenomenon. In the physiological state we find a certain difficulty in raising the extended limb. There is a pulling and a certain constraint at the gluteal

which it emerges, with the gluteus maximus, which covers it, and with the gemelli, obturator internus and the quadratus femoris, located under it. The sign that we have just described. . . appears as a result of compression by muscular contraction, or by tension of the same muscles. . . .

We consider this sign to be pathognomonic of sciatica, for we have not found it in any other affection of that region.

XXIII   Lhermitte's Sign

"LHERMITTE'S sign" is not a sign, nor was it first described by Lhermitte. As a phenomenon perceived only by the patient, it is more properly called a symptom, and the first description was given by Josef Babinski,[1] who also gave neurology the extensor toe sign[2,3] and the inverted radial reflex.[4] The contribution of Jean Lhermitte, the French neurologist, was to point out the value of this symptom as an indicator of early multiple sclerosis.[5,6]

Unlike many of the other symptoms of early multiple sclerosis, the electrical sensation is rarely encountered in hysterical subjects, and, therefore, it may provide the only evidence of organic disease in an otherwise perplexing case.

Lhermitte correctly surmised that the lesion responsible for the electrical sensation is located in the cervical cord. However, he overemphasized the specificity of this symptom for demyelinating disease. Cervical spondylosis, cervical-cord tumor, and subacute combined degeneration of the cord, in addition to multiple sclerosis and cervical-cord trauma, may each give rise to the same electrical sensation.[7,8] Alajouanine and coworkers[7] claim that the phenomenon is the result of irritation of the posterior columns of the cervical cord, and they were able to evoke the electrical sensation by mechanical stimulation of the exposed posterior columns of a human subject during the course of a surgical operation.

Although "Lhermitte's sign" may be a misnomer, it has proved to be of great value for neurologic diagnosis, and both its name and its clinical importance are likely to persist.

References

1. Babinski, J., and Dubois, A.: Douleurs à forme de décharge électrique, consécutives aux traumatismes de la nuque, *Presse Med* **26**:64, 1918.

2. Babinski, J.: Du phénomène des orteils et de sa valeur sémiologique, *Sem Méd* **18**:321-322, 1898.

3. Wilkins, R.H., and Brody, I.A.: Babinski's Sign, *Arch Neurol* **17**:441-446 (Oct) 1967.

4. Babinski, J.: Inversion du réflexe du radius, *Bull et Mem de la Soc Méd des Hôp de Paris* **30**:185-186 (Oct 14) 1910.

5. Lhermitte, J.; Bollak; and Nicholas, M.: Les douleurs à type de décharge électrique consécutives à la flexion céphalique daus la sclérose en plaques. Un cas de forme sensitive de la sclérose multiple, *Rev Neurol* **2**:56-62, 1924.

6. Lhermitte, J.: Multiple Sclerosis: the Sensation of an Electrical Discharge as an Early Symptom, *Arch Neurol Psych* **22**:5-8 (July) 1929.

7. Alajouanine, T.; Thurel, R.; and Papaioanou, C.: La douleur a type de décharge électrique, provoquée par la flexion de la tête et parcourant le corps de haut en bas, *Rev Neurol* **81**:89-97, 1949.

8. McAlpine, D.; Compston, N.D.; and Lumsden, C.E.: Multiple Sclerosis, London: E. & S. Livingston Ltd., 1955, pp 81-83.

PAIN RESEMBLING AN ELECTRICAL DISCHARGE FOLLOWING CEPHALIC FLEXION IN FOCAL SCLEROSIS. A CASE OF THE SENSITIVE FORM OF MULTIPLE SCLEROSIS,

by J. Lhermitte, Bollak, and M. Nicholas.*

Neurologists agree that sensory disturbances frequently occur in the initial phase of multiple sclerosis. This was brought out at the last Paris neurological meeting. Professor G. Guillain's paper quite rightly emphasized the special characteristics of these subjective disturbances and showed that it is proper to rely upon them in establishing an early diagnosis of multiple sclerosis.

The patient we present now seems to be a fine example of the "sensitive form" of multiple sclerosis. We think her clinical history deserves attention because of the number and diversity of her disordered sensations.

Case. Mrs. D., cashier, 43 years old, without significant personal or hereditary background, married, and mother of a healthy child, became ill in July 1923 with an acute intestinal attack accompanied by abdominal pains and diarrhea. A few days after the end of this episode, she suffered a rather violent headache accompanied by tingling in the feet and knees. At this time, walking became difficult. . . .

*Translation of: Les douleurs à type de décharge électrique consécutives à la flexion céphalique dans la sclérose en plaques. Un cas de forme sensitive de la sclérose multiple, *Revue Neurologique* 2:56-62, 1924.

In August 1923, the patient first noticed a phenomenon that she described thus: When I try to lower my head, I feel a violent shock in the nape of my neck, and a pain like an electric current runs through my whole body, from my neck to my feet, down my vertebral column.

During the same month, these phenomena became more marked and each flexion movement of the head or the trunk brought about this sensation of electrical discharge radiating from the nape of the neck to the tips of the toes and also of the fingers. The patient could not dress herself, put on her shoes, or pick up an object from the ground without carefully keeping her head in line with her trunk.

Until May 1924, the condition of the patient did not change appreciably despite the treatments employed. At this period a new and disturbing symptom appeared: marked impairment of vision of the right eye. . . . On June 11, 1924, the patient consulted us for the first time. . . .

We would like to direct our attention to a particular manifestation that we believe has never before been pointed out in the symptomatology of multiple sclerosis: *the pains resembling an electric shock.* This phenomenon was described to us spontaneously by the patient, for we never suspected its existence in a case of this kind. The sensations are uncomfortable but not really painful, and they closely resemble those produced by a faradic current. They never appear spontaneously when the subject is at rest but occur exclusively with movements that are accompanied by forward flexion of the head. Thus, they occur in many acts of daily life, such as bending over to pick up an object or to lace the shoes, or arranging the hair, or saying an energetic yes. These sensations usually radiate from the head to the upper limbs and to the legs. For months our patient could not bend over without a shudder running down her spinal column to the tips of her toes.

These sensations are always rapid and brief because, by an instinctive reflex, the patient corrects the position of her head by straightening her neck. Moreover, since these electric-like pains appear exclusively on bending the head, the patient carefully avoids any such movement, and she succeeds quite well.

We investigated whether passive flexion would produce the same phenomenon and noted that even a slight movement sufficed to evoke it. It is also interesting to note that the intensity of the electric-like pain is in direct relation to the suddenness and the amplitude of the flexion of the head.

This curious type of pain is not new in neurological symptomatology. It was described by Babinski and Dubois (Society of Neurology, 1918) in concussions of the spine, and one of us (Lhermitte) published two observations regarding it, inserted in the excellent thesis of J. Ribeton (*Clinical study of pains resembling electrical shock following injuries of the neck.* Thesis of [Univ. of] Paris, January 1919).

The electrical pains that one of us observed in several soldiers suffering from direct concussion of the cervical cord are identical to those found in our patient. Furthermore, it is probably not a coincidence that the spinal lesions of multiple sclerosis are especially marked in the lower cervical cord where the lesions were located in our concussion patients.

Previously, in the thesis of J. Ribeton, one of us

discussed the origin and the pathogenesis of the phenomenon we are considering. We do not wish to dwell on this here, but we would like to draw attention to two points. The first is that these shock-like pains in direct spinal concussion as well as in multiple sclerosis are related not to root changes but to *spinal lesions.* The second point concerns the mechanism of the phenomenon.

As we have explained in the work of M. Ribeton, the sensation of an electrical discharge, which occurs in many patients with spinal concussion, presents an analogy with the sensations produced by percussing (Tinel's sign), by compressing, or by elongating peripheral nerves affected by a slight injury. Thus, we were naturally led to seek a common explanation for them.

Tinel accurately observed that the tingling (and we add the electrical sensations) produced by percussion or elongation of a nerve requires that these nerves be composed largely of demyelinated fibers or fibers covered only by a thin insulating membrane. Now, our investigations with Claude and with Roussy on direct concussional lesions of the spinal cord have revealed much greater injury to the myelin than to the fibers themselves. Does this fact not support the relationship that one of us (Lhermitte) has established between the anatomical abnormalities and the appearance of electrical sensations in the two types of cases?

In multiple sclerosis also the basic anatomical change consists of disintegration of myelin with preservation of axons. To account for all the facts set forth here, it seems to us reasonable that the type of pain common to peripheral nerve lesions, concussional changes in the spinal cord, and the degeneration of multiple sclerosis represents the inherent excitability of sensory fibers stripped of their insulating myelin sheath. This excitability may be evoked by direct percussion, which one applies to a peripheral nerve, or by elongation brought about by flexion of the head on the trunk.

We should mention in closing that in spinal concussion, as well as in multiple sclerosis, the pains resembling electric shock are accompanied by paresthetic and dysesthetic disturbances probably related to the extent and depth of the alterations in sensory pathways.

XXIV Erb's Palsy

E RB'S description of paralysis of the upper portion of the brachial plexus is remembered mainly for its postscript. As an afterthought to his discussion, Erb noted that birth trauma is one of the causes of such paralysis, and the term Erb's (or more properly Duchenne-Erb's) palsy now usually refers to this phenomenon.

Wilhelm Heinrich Erb (1840 to 1921) was the foremost German neurologist of his time and the first neurologist to wield a reflex hammer.[1] His original account of the tendon reflexes[2] advanced the art of neurologic diagnosis and was a great stimulus to physiologic research. Erb also pioneered in applying electrodiagnosis and electrotherapy to neurology, and it was he who first described the "reaction of degeneration" of muscle.[3] Not the least of Erb's accomplishments was his successful campaign to introduce neurologic instruction into the curriculum at Heidelberg.[4] He thus gained a place for neurology in medical education.

Obstetrical paralyses such as the upper brachial-plexus injury of Erb and the lower brachial-plexus injury of Klumpke[5] have become less common with improved management of cephalopelvic disproportion.[6]

When Erb's palsy does occur, the employment of physical therapy can help prevent contractures, and mobility can be improved with orthopedic reconstructive procedures.[6,7] The "bellhop's tip" position of the hand may develop in untreated cases.

Erb's description of upper brachial-plexus palsy displays his extraordinary talent for physical diagnosis and his interest in the techniques of electrical stimulation. Nevertheless, it is ironic that his name is commemorated for one of his lesser contributions to neurology, a contribution which he himself attributed to Duchenne.

References

1. Schiller, F.: The Reflex Hammer: In Memoriam Robert Wartenberg (1887-1956), Med Hist 11:75-85 (Jan) 1967.
2. Erb, W.: Ueber Sehnenreflexe bei Gesunden und bei Rückenmarkskranken, Arch Psychiat Nervenkr 5:792-802, 1875.
3. Erb, W.: Zur Pathologie und pathologischen Anatomie peripherischer Paralysen, Deutsch Arch Klin Med 4:535-578 et seq., 1868.
4. Viets, H.R.: "Wilhelm Heinrich Erb (1840-1921)," in Haymaker, W. (ed.): The Founders of Neurology, Springfield, Ill: Charles C Thomas, Publisher, 1953, pp 364-367.
5. Klumpke, A.: Contribution a l'Etude des Paralysies Radiculaires du Plexus Brachial. Paralysies Radiculaires Totales. Paralysies Radiculaires Inférieures. De la Participation des Filets Sympathiques Oculo-Pupillaires dans ces Paralysies, Rev Med 5:591-616, 1885.
6. Adler, J.B., and Patterson, R.L.: Erb's Palsy: Long-Term Results of Treatment in Eighty-Eight Cases, J Bone Joint Surg 49:1052-1064 (Sept) 1967.
7. Wickstrom, J.: Birth Injuries of the Brachial Plexus: Treatment of Defects in the Shoulder, Clin Orthop 23:187-196, 1962.

ON A CHARACTERISTIC SITE OF INJURY IN THE
BRACHIAL PLEXUS.*

BY: Dr. W. Erb, Professor at the University of Heidelberg

Presented on November 10, 1874

On reviewing the charts of patients with paralysis of the upper extremity, I found a number of cases characterized by a striking uniformity in the pattern of muscles affected. The paralysis was not localized to a main branch of the brachial plexus but involved several smaller branches (exclusive of the ulnar nerve) and always affected the same muscles.

The paralyses of the individual branches of the brachial plexus (the axillary nerve, median, radial, etc.) are well known, and their symptomatology has been investigated sufficiently. The same is not true of paralyses affecting the individual roots of the brachial plexus (the anterior branches of the cervical nerves). Yet, it would be desirable to know their symptomatology in order to localize lesions more accurately. It must be assumed that each root of the brachial plexus always, or nearly always, contains the same motor and sensory fibers. Thus, one can localize a lesion to a particular root by the pattern of the motor and sensory disturbances.

I believe that the following brief cases make a small contribution to our knowledge of this subject and therefore are worthy of publication even if only as a stimulus for further studies.

Case #1. Konrad Sauer, 52 years old, ropemaker. Became ill five weeks ago after carrying a heavy load on his head. The illness began with pain and stiffness in the left half of the neck and the left shoulder down to the fingers. The thumb and index finger seemed asleep, and the arm was so weak that it could not be lifted. The examination revealed: complete paralysis of the left deltoid, biceps, brachialis, and brachioradialis. The supinator also seemed very weak. The remaining shoulder muscles, the triceps, and all forearm muscles and small muscles of the hand were normal.

In the thumb and index finger there was a "furry" feeling; their sense of touch was somewhat diminished. The electrical examination demonstrated an incomplete reaction of degeneration. The muscles were somewhat tender on pressure and underwent atrophy during the course of the illness. The patient was treated by galvanism and was discharged as cured after seven weeks.

Apparently, this was a case of traumatic neuritis of a portion of the brachial plexus.

[Three other case reports follow.]

A review of the above cases reveals that they all have involvement of the same muscles and that these muscles are supplied by various nerves and various branches of the brachial plexus.

In all four cases the deltoid, biceps, and brachialis were involved. Usually the brachioradialis was involved too, and less frequently the supinator and the muscles supplied by the median nerve. This pattern of muscle paralysis cannot be accidental. It must have an anatomic basis since we see the same combination of paralyzed muscles resulting from the most varied etiologies.

Anatomy tells us that the muscles mentioned are supplied by different nerves. Thus, the deltoid receives its motor fibers from the axillary nerve; the biceps and brachialis from the musculocutaneous nerve (which frequently is a branch of the median); the brachioradialis and supinator from the radial nerve; and finally, we saw that the median nerve was involved in one case. The ulnar nerve, on the contrary, was not involved in any case.

Consideration of the anatomic relationships makes it clear that the responsible lesion in these cases cannot be located where the four named nerves have separated completely from the brachial plexus. The special arrangement of the nerves would forbid such an assumption. Even more strongly against this assumption is the fact that in several of these nerves only some fibers were affected and these were always the same. Furthermore, their sensory fibers were nearly always spared. We must therefore look for the lesion proximalward in the brachial plexus itself or more likely in one or several of its roots, where the motor fibers for the appropriate muscles are still united and have not yet separated into the various nerve trunks. The etiology of several of my cases

---

*Translation of: Ueber eine eigenthümliche Localisation von Lähmungen im Plexus brachialis, *Verhandlungen des Naturhistorisch-medizinischer Vereins Heidelberg* 1:130-136, 1874-1877.

also indicates that one has to search for the site of the lesion in the neck, in the supraclavicular area.

The anatomy textbooks give little detailed information on the arrangement of the muscle branches in the roots of the brachial plexus. Particularly in the human being it has not been determined precisely which muscles of the upper extremity are supplied by each of the anterior branches of the four lower cervical and the first thoracic nerves. What can be concluded from the descriptions (and I have confirmed this by inspection of anatomic preparations) is that the fifth and sixth cervical nerves participate in forming those branches of the brachial plexus that are of interest to us here. The ulnar nerve, which was unaffected in all cases, contains only the lower roots of the brachial plexus. I have found neither time nor opportunity to decide this issue by personal anatomic investigation.

However, I have attempted to fill this gap with detailed faradic examination of the brachial plexus. I found in several suitable individuals that, with a fine electrode, careful stimulation of a single area—which corresponds approximately with the exit of the fifth and sixth cervical nerves between the scalene muscles—causes simultaneous contraction of the deltoid, biceps, brachialis, brachioradialis, and supinator, while the remaining muscles are unaffected. . . . This shows that at one area of the brachial plexus, near the scalene muscles, those motor fibers that were always affected in the above cases are united. Therefore, it seems possible that the lesion in these cases is located in the fifth or sixth cervical nerve (anterior branches) or possibly at their site of union. When processes, such as neuritis, spread within the plexus, other branches of the brachial plexus (the median nerve, for instance) may also be affected, and thus the paralysis will attain larger dimensions. However, there is always the characteristic concomitant paralysis of the deltoid, biceps, brachialis, and brachioradialis—thus all forearm flexors.

When one finds this characteristic combination of paralyzed muscles, one will be justified—presuming confirmation of the above observations and interpretations—to look for a lesion in the roots of the brachial plexus and more specifically in the two superior ones. It is obvious that such precise localization of the source of the paralysis is of great importance for therapy, and especially for electrotherapy.

A further category of similar cases comprises certain types of delivery paralyses noted not uncommonly in newborns. Duchenne originally described them in an excellent manner (Electrisat. Localisée, 3rd ed., p 357 ff.). In deliveries attended by a difficult presentation of the arm or prolonged traction by an index finger inserted into the child's axilla, Duchenne found paralysis of the deltoid, biceps, and brachialis, as well as the infraspinatus. Frequently, secondary contractures occur, and the posture of the arm is characteristic.

I have personally observed a similar case in a child who two months earlier had been brought into the world by a difficult delivery (version followed by extraction). I found the arm rather immobile, flaccid and extended, hanging down at the side, strongly rotated internally, wrist and fingers bent and only slightly moveable. More detailed observation, which is naturally difficult in such little children, showed complete paralysis of the deltoid, biceps, and brachialis (and probably the brachioradialis too). Furthermore, the infraspinatus was probably paralyzed, and significant weakness was present in all muscles supplied by the radial nerve. Finally, a secondary contracture of the pectoralis major had developed.

It is obvious that this case strongly resembles the above cases. How and when the lesion comes about is difficult to say. However, it seems unlikely to me that the insertion of the finger into the axilla could lead to this characteristic pattern of muscle paralyses since the suprascapular nerve, which supplies the infraspinatus, cannot be involved in such trauma. It seems to me more probable that the version and extraction usually necessary for carrying out the so-called "Prague manipulation" is the most frequent cause of this type of "delivery paralysis." The fork-like grip of the fingers on the neck, with moderately energetic manipulation by the obstetrician, can easily compress the roots of the brachial plexus and the plexus itself so that a more or less persistent paralysis ensues. The participation in the paralysis of the infraspinatus, the nerve of which originates from the fifth and sixth cervical nerves in the uppermost portion of the plexus, provides decisive evidence that the source of the paralysis lies above the arm and in the neck, close to the scalene muscles (at the space indicated previously in more detail). The paralysis of the infraspinatus may become another important criterion for the localization of the lesion in the plexus, and it is recommended that future cases be studied with this in mind. Unfortunately, this was not done in my previous cases, which were all from the years 1866-1868.

XXV   Sturge-Weber Syndrome

THE Sturge-Weber syndrome is usually easy to recognize. It consists of angiomatosis of the upper portion of the face and the cerebral leptomeninges, with progressive calcification in the underlying cerebral cortex.[1] These abnormalities are usually unilateral. Atrophy of the involved cerebral hemisphere may be present, along with contralateral hemiparesis, focal seizures, and mental retardation. Buphthalmos or glaucoma may also occur.

Information about this unusual condition has been compiled slowly during the past century through individual case reports by many physicians. William Allen Sturge (1850 to 1919)[2] and Frederick Parkes Weber (1863 to 1962)[3] were English clinicians whose separate reports, published 43 years apart, illustrated different facets of the syndrome.

In 1860, Schirmer[4] published a brief description of a patient with a facial vascular nevus and buphthalmos, but he made no mention of any neurological abnormalities. Then in 1879, at a meeting of the Clinical Society of London, Sturge called attention to the main clinical features of the syndrome by describing a 6½-year-old girl with an hemangioma on the right side of the face, buphthalmos, and focal seizures.[5] Sturge's analysis of the seizures, which shows the influence of Hughlings Jackson's ideas, led him to predict the presence of a "port-wine mark" on the surface of the right side of the brain. However, he did not have the opportunity to carry out a pathological examination. Postmortem studies of other patients by Kalischer and others later proved that Sturge was right.[1,6]

In 1922, Parkes Weber, who is also remembered for his description of familial telangiectasis or Rendu-Osler-Weber disease,[7] reported a young woman with an extensive cutaneous angioma, spastic hemiplegia with "hemi-hypotrophy," buphthalmos, and glaucoma.[8,9] He reproduced crude skiagrams of the patient's skull and was, thus, the first to publish a roentgenogram of the intracranial calcifications in this syndrome. With better radiographic technique, Dimitri[10] later demonstrated the typical gyriform pattern of the intracranial calcifications, and Krabbe[11] established that the majority of these radiopaque calcium deposits are located in the cerebral cortex rather than in the leptomeningeal angioma.

The Sturge-Weber syndrome, or encephalofacial angiomatosis, is now often classified with the "phakomatoses"—the group of conditions in which there is maldevelopment of neural and other ectodermal structures. However, unlike Lindau's syndrome, tuberous sclerosis, and von Recklinghausen's disease, the Sturge-Weber syndrome is not inherited and is not associated with intracranial neoplasms.

Despite the ease with which it can be identified clinically, the Sturge-Weber syndrome remains a puzzle. The medical and surgical techniques that have been developed to control seizures and glaucoma have helped considerably, but since the etiology of the syndrome is not yet understood, its prevention remains a challenge.

References

1. Alexander, G.L., and Norman, R.M.: *The Sturge-Weber Syndrome,* Bristol, England: John Wright & Sons Ltd., 1960.
2. Barlow, T.:. William Allen Sturge, M.V.O., M.D. Lond., F.R.C.P., *Brit Med J* 1:468-469 (April 12) 1919.
3. MacNalty, A.: F. Parkes Weber, M.D., F.R.C.P., *Brit Med J* 1:1630-1631 (June 9) 1962.
4. Schirmer, R.: Ein Fall von Teleangiektasie, *v. Graefe's Arch Ophthal* 7:119-121, 1860.
5. Sturge, W.A.: A Case of Partial Epilepsy, Apparently Due to a Lesion of One of the Vaso-Motor Centres of the Brain, *Trans Clin Soc London* 12:162-167, 1879.
6. Kalischer, S.: Demonstration des Gehirns eines Kindes mit Teleangiektasie der linksseitigen Gesichts-Kopfhaut und Hirnoberfläche, *Berl Klin Wschr* 34:1059 (Nov 29) 1897.
7. Weber, F.P.: Multiple Hereditary Developmental Angiomata (Telangiectases) of the Skin and Mucous Membranes Associated with Recurring Haemorrhages, *Lancet* 2:160-162 (July 20) 1907.
8. Weber, F.P.· Right-Sided Hemi-Hypotrophy

Resulting From Right-Sided Congenital Spastic Hemiplegia, With a Morbid Condition of the Left Side of the Brain, Revealed by Radiograms, *J Neurol Psychopathol* 3:134-139 (Aug) 1922.

9. Weber, F.P.: A Note on the Association of Extensive Haemangiomatous Naevus of the Skin With Cerebral (Meningeal) Haemangioma, Especially Cases of Facial Vascular Naevus With Con-tralateral Hemiplegia, *Proc Roy Soc Med* 22:431-442 (Feb) 1929.

10. Dimitri, V.: Tumor cerebral congénito. (Angioma cavernoso), *Rev Assoc Med Argent* 36:1029-1037 (Dec) 1923.

11. Krabbe, K.H.: Facial and Meningeal Angiomatosis Associated With Calcifications of the Brain Cortex, *Arch Neurol Psychiat* 32:737-755 (Oct) 1934.

A Case of *Partial Epilepsy,* apparently due to a Lesion of one of the *Vaso-motor Centres of the Brain.**

By W. ALLEN STURGE, M.D. Read April 18, 1879.

ADA BROOK, aet. 6½. Both father and mother are living and healthy; both are steady; there is no blood-relationship between them. Two other children are living and healthy; three are dead, one by an accident, and the other two, who were twins, in early infancy. The mother never miscarried. The father had an uncle who is said to have died 'out of his mind;' he was not, however, in an asylum, but died in his own house. There is no other history of insanity, and no history of fits in the family. Several members of the father's family are said to have died of consumption.

The patient was born with a very extensive mother's mark' on the right side of the head and face. The mark is bounded pretty accurately by the middle line in the upper lip, nose, forehead, scalp, and back of the neck, extending a little beyond the middle line on the chin and on the upper part of the sternum. It extends as low as the third or fourth dorsal vertebra behind, and the second costal cartilage in front. The lips, gums, tongue, roof of mouth, floor of mouth, uvula, and pharynx are all similarly affected, to a greater or less extent, on the right side. There is in addition a patch about the size of the palm of the hand over the left eye, frontal, and temporal regions. The mark is everywhere of a deep purple colour, the colour partially disappearing on firm pressure. All the parts affected are distinctly larger than the corresponding parts on the opposite side.

The right eye is affected in a similar way both in its superficial and deep structures. It is larger than the left; the sclerotic is more vascular than usual, and with the ophthalmoscope it can be seen that the retina and choroid are involved. Mr. Nettleship has kindly examined the patient for me, and he has furnished me with the following most interesting and valuable report: . . . .

'*Ophthalmoscope.*—Right disc much redder than left; some of the right retinal veins are very tortuous, chiefly some of the large upward subdivisions: the tortuosity affects certain large branches or parts, and not the whole of any primary division; nor does it go so far as the disc. In the inverted image all the parts look smaller in the right than in the left eye, because of the difference of refraction.

'*Choroid.*—The general colour is very markedly darker and at the same time redder in the right than the left eye. The difference is not what we should expect if it were due to the pigment being more abundant in one eye than the other; it is suggestive of venous or venous and capillary hypertrophy like that on the skin.'

After her birth the child enjoyed good health till she was six months old. She then began to have attacks of twitching in her left side, affecting the face, arm, and leg. The mother describes the fits as lasting for ten or twelve minutes, and consisting of little jerks which occurred every two or three seconds during the period. She had several of these attacks every day. As time went on the attacks became stronger, but the child did not seem to lose consciousness. When she got older her mother found that after the attacks she was weak in the left side, and could not walk so well as at other times. The fits continued to get stronger, the shaking of the left side was more severe, and after a time the right side began to be affected also. About eighteen months or two years ago she began to lose consciousness, and now the fits did not recur so often. The twitchings which occurred without loss of consciousness disappeared, and their place was taken by severe fits in which consciousness was lost, and there was very marked convulsion. These fits only occurred about once in every three, four or six months.

Her mother describes the fits as she now has them as follows:—She first complains of a feeling in the palm of the left hand; the feeling appears to be a sort of painful tingling. She tells her mother a fit is coming on. The sensation in the hand lasts for several minutes, and she then clenches the hand firmly and bends up the arm.

*Reprinted from *Transactions of the Clinical Society of London* 12:162-167, 1879.

Sometimes both hands are clenched. A few seconds afterwards she falls down unconscious, but is not much more convulsed. After the fit is over the child sleeps soundly for some hours.

Sometimes the child tells her mother that she has a fit, but without any outward signs being seen. When asked what she feels, she says that it is a 'funny feeling' in the left hand.

She is troublesome and very restless.

Under the influence of bromide of potassium the patient has considerably improved. She has had fewer fits, and has been less restless.

Remarks.—I have no intention of going into the difficult question of the pathology of the port-wine mark. The point to which I wish to call particular attention is the probable relationship between the mark and the fits. It will have been observed that the fits were for a long time very partial, being confined to the left side only, and apparently unattended by loss of consciousness. Now fits of this kind are rare in connection with very young children, and I shall be able to show their significance more easily by saying a few words on the nature of epilepsy. It is becoming more and more certain that the phenomena of an epileptic fit or of an infantile convulsion are due to a liberation of force in an irregular and ungoverned manner in the nerve-cells of some part of the grey matter of the cerebro-spinal system. This irregular liberation of force is very well described under the term, now so commonly used, of 'nerve-discharge.' A nerve-discharge which gives rise to convulsions is evidently due to some instability in those groups of cells where it takes place. This instability may be due to some inherent fault of construction (so to speak) of the grey matter, whether from a hereditary tendency to badly-formed nerve-tissues, or as the result of bad conditions in the parent at the times of conception and development, or from other causes. In such a case the tendency is for large tracts of grey matter to be affected in the same way, and for the two sides of the brain to resemble one another more or less in this respect. Hence in these cases of idiopathic epilepsy we usually meet with the severer forms of an epileptic fit, where there is instantaneous loss of consciousness, with little or no warning, accompanied by rigid contraction of nearly every muscle in the body. Sometimes, however, even in cases of widespread tendency to instability of grey matter, some small tract may be more unstable than the rest. In such a case it alone discharges at the beginning of the fit, producing the phenomenon of the warning, which may be

mental, sensory, or motor, according to the seat of the discharging tract. Nerve-cells, however, intercommunicate freely with one another by connecting fibres, and when one cell is in action it tends to excite a similar state of activity in those with which it is brought into connection. It can easily be understood, then, that a disturbance such as that which is produced by a sudden and irregular discharge in a group of cells, propagates itself rapidly to neighbouring tracts. These being themselves over-excitable, though to a less extent than those cells where the discharge has begun, an irregular discharge takes place in them, producing the phenomenon of the fit following the warning.

Epileptic fits may, however, be due not only to an idiopathic morbid excitability of grey matter, but grey matter which is in itself quite healthy may be induced to discharge irregularly under the influence of external irritation, such as results, for instance, from the presence of tumours, of masses of fibrous tissue growing down into the cortical substance from the meninges, after attacks of sub-acute or chronic meningitis; or again, from increased blood supply, as in acute meningitis. . . .

Now everyone knows that, *caeteris paribus,* the grey matter is less stable in children than in adults; where an adult has a rigor, a child has a convulsion From this it results that it is much rarer for fits to begin slowly in a young child than in an adult, especially where the fits are due to a hereditary instability of nerve-tissue. Whenever in a child partial fits occur, or fits preceded by a considerable warning, they may be taken as indicative of some external morbid influence acting on grey matter which is naturally healthy. In the patient I have shown, the fits for a long time were confined to the left side opposite to the port-wine mark; and the mother says that there appeared to be no loss of consciousness until she was three or four years old. They then involved the right side as well, and had become more severe. Even now, however, they begin in the left hand with a sensory warning of considerable duration, and sometimes appear to consist only of a sensation of some kind in that hand. From the nature of the fits, and from their mode of onset, I think there can be no doubt that they are due to some cause external to the nerve-tissue, rather than to an inherent instability of grey matter, and this external cause is in all probability to be found in the presence of a 'port-wine mark' on the surface of the right side of the brain, just as we have found it in the skin, mucous membranes, and retina of that side.

XXVI Bell's Palsy and Bell's Phenomenon

I SEEMS appropriate that Sir Charles Bell (1774 to 1842) should have described the syndrome and the phenomenon that now bear his name.[1-4] He was trained in anatomy, surgery, and art; he made a detailed study of facial expression; he discovered the separate actions of the trigeminal and facial nerves; and because of these interests, he saw an unusual number of patients with facial paralysis in his clinical practice.

Early in the course of his medical education in Edinburgh, Charles Bell received instruction from his older brother John, one of the foremost anatomists and surgeons of the time. His contribution to John's textbook of anatomy[5] was one of the first of Charles' numerous publications, which included textbooks and atlases of neuroanatomy and surgery. A gifted artist, he illustrated many of these works himself.

Bell's training in anatomy and his interest in art led him to a comprehensive study of facial expression, first published in 1806.[6] The following year, Bell began his classical studies of nerve function, and became the first to distinguish between sensory and motor nerves.[7] Though he misinterpreted his observations initially,[3,8] Bell's basic discovery was verified and expanded by several other investigators, including François Magendie.[9,10] The fact that sensory nerves enter the spinal cord by the posterior roots and motor nerves leave it by the anterior roots is now known as the Bell-Magendie law.[11]

Like most anatomists of his time, Bell recognized only nine sets of cranial nerves.[3,12,13] The fifth pair were the trigeminal nerves, as in the present nomenclature, but the seventh nerve was divided into a portio dura (facial nerve) and a portio mollis (acoustic nerve). As his research into the anatomy and physiology of the nerves progressed, Bell established that the trigeminal and facial nerves have separate functions.[14-17] Bell proceeded to introduce a new method of classifying the nerves according to their function as well as their form. Thus he grouped the trigeminal nerve with the spinal nerves, since it subserves both sensation and motion and since it has a ganglion on its sensory root. In contrast, he classified the facial nerve (respiratory nerve of the face) with other nerves that he thought were concerned with respiration. These included the long thoracic (external respiratory) nerve, now known as the nerve of Bell.

In his practice of surgery in London, Bell encountered many cases of unilateral paralysis of the facial muscles.[18] This syndrome had been noted previously by others,[19,20] but Bell deserves the credit for differentiating peripheral from central facial paralysis. He also noted that the eyeball on the paralyzed side invariably rotates upward when the patient tries to close his eyelids. Bell pursued the matter further and observed the same event in normal individuals.[21] The palpebral-oculogyric reflex, which is more noticeable when eyelid closure is incomplete, has become known as Bell's phenomenon.

Bell's patients had developed facial paralysis from a variety of causes. However, the term Bell's palsy is now restricted to cases of cryptogenic impairment of the facial nerve.[22,23] In one such case, Bell appeared to inculpate draughts on the face, but the etiology remains uncertain. Most patients with cryptogenic paralysis recover, as noted by Bell, but some degree of residual weakness may persist and contractures may develop. Also, sequelae such as intrafacial synkinesis

or unilateral lacrimation on eating ("croco-
dile tears") may occur, perhaps as a result
of misdirection of regenerating axons.[24] Although Bell thought that electrical stimulation was beneficial, no form of therapy yet
devised has unequivocally improved the already favorable prognosis of Bell's palsy.

By virtue of his talents and his training,
Charles Bell was uniquely qualified to advance our knowledge of nerve functions.[25]
His several eponyms are but minor indications of his success in his chosen fields.

References

1. [Kelly, E.C.]: Sir Charles Bell: Scotch Physiologist, Physician and Surgeon in London, 1774-1842,
Med Classics 1:81-103 (Oct) 1936.
2. Graham, H.: Surgeons All, ed 2, London: Rich
& Cowan, 1956, pp 279-283.
3. Gordon-Taylor, G., and Walls, E.W.: Sir
Charles Bell: His Life and Times, Edinburgh: E. &
S. Livingstone, Ltd., 1958.
4. Zimmerman, L.M., and Veith, I.: Great Ideas
in the History of Surgery, Baltimore: Williams &
Wilkins Co., 1961, pp 410-423.
5. Bell, J., and Bell, C.: The Anatomy of the
Human Body, Edinburgh: Mudie, 4 vol, 1797-1804.
6. Bell, C.: Essays on the Anatomy of Expression
in Painting, London: Longman, Rees, Hurst and
Orme, 1806.
7. Bell, C.: Idea of a New Anatomy of the Brain:
Submitted for the Observations of his Friends,
London: Strahan & Preston, 1811.
8. Olmsted, J.M.D.: The Aftermath of Charles
Bell's Famous "Idea," Bull Hist Med 14:341-351
(Oct) 1943.
9. Magendie, F.: Expériences sur les fonctions
des racines des nerfs rachidiens, J Physiol Exper
Path 2:276-279, 1822.
10. Fulton, J.F.: Selected Readings in the History
of Physiology, Springfield, Ill: Charles C Thomas,
Publisher, 1930, pp 251-265.
11. Brazier, M.: "The Historical Development of
Neurophysiology," in Field, J.; Magoun, H.W.; and
Hall, V.E. (eds.): Handbook of Physiology: A
Critical, Comprehensive Presentation of Physiological Knowledge and Concepts: Section I. Neurophysiology, Washington, DC: American Physiological
Society, 1959, pp 1-58.
12. Rucker, C.W.: History of the Numbering of
the Cranial Nerves, Mayo Clin Proc 41:453-461
(July) 1966.
13. Flamm, E.S.: Historical Observations on the
Cranial Nerves, J Neurosurg 27:285-297 (Oct) 1967.
14. Bell, C.: On the Nerves: Giving an Account of
Some Experiments on Their Structure and Functions, Which Lead to a New Arrangement of the
System, Phil Trans Roy Soc Lond 111:398-424,
1821.
15. Bell, C.: On the Nerves Which Associate the
Muscles of the Chest in the Actions of Breathing,
Speaking and Expression: Being a Continuation of
the Paper on the Structure and Functions of the
Nerves, Phil Trans Roy Soc Lond 112:284-312, 1822.
16. Bell, C.: On the Nerves of the Face; Second
Part, Phil Trans Roy Soc Lond 119:317-330, 1829.
17. Bell, C.: The Nervous System of the Human
Body, Embracing the Papers Delivered to the Royal
Society on the Subject of the Nerves (With)
Appendix, Containing Cases and Letters of Consultation on Nervous Diseases, Submitted to the Author Since the Publication of His Papers on the
Functions of the Nerves, in the Transactions of the
Royal Society, and Illustrative of the Facts Announced in the Preceding Pages, London: Longman,
1830.
18. Power, D'A.: Eponyms: XI. Bell's Palsy, Brit
J Surg 11:405-409 (Jan) 1924.
19. Thomas, K.B.: Facial Palsy Before Bell, Middlesex Hosp J 63:254-256 (Dec) 1963.
20. Goldman, L., and Schechter, C.G.: Art in
Medicine: Peripheral Facial Palsy Throughout the
Ages, New York J Med 67:1331-1334 (May 15)
1967.
21. Bell, C.: On the Motions of the Eye in
Illustration of the Uses of the Muscles and Nerves
of the Orbit, Phil Trans Roy Soc Lond 113:166-186,
1823.
22. Taverner, D.: Bell's Palsy: A Clinical and
Electromyographic Study, Brain 78:209-228 (June)
1955.
23. Kettel, K.: Peripheral Facial Palsy: Pathology and Surgery, Springfield, Ill: Charles C Thomas,
Publisher, 1959.
24. Schwarz, G.A.: A Note on an Unusual Fa-
cio-Ocular Synkinesis, Arch Neurol 6:358-365
(May) 1962.
25. Thomson, H.C.: The Work of Sir Charles Bell
in Relation to Modern Neurology, Brain 48:449-457
(Dec) 1925.

THE NERVOUS SYSTEM OF THE HUMAN BODY*

by Sir Charles Bell

EXPERIMENTS ON THE NERVES OF THE FACE, WITH A VIEW TO ASCERTAIN THE USES OF THE PORTIO DURA

If an ass be thrown, and the *portio dura* be cut
across where it emerges upon the face, before the
ear, all the muscles of the face, except those of the
jaws, will be paralysed. If its nostrils be confined
for a few seconds, so as to make it pant and
forcibly dilate the nostrils at each inspiration, and
if the *portio dura* be now divided on one side of

*Reprinted from Bell, C.: The Nervous System
of the Human Body: As Explained in a Series of Papers
Read Before the Royal Society of London, With an Appendix of Cases and Consultations on Nervous Diseases,
ed 3, London: Henry Renshaw, 1844, pp 52-57, 148-
152, 250, 252-255, 258, 259, 283, 318, 319.

the head, the motion of the nostril of the same side will instantly cease, while the other nostril will continue to expand and contract in unison with the motions of the chest. . . .

If an ass be tied and thrown, and the superior maxillary branch of the fifth nerve exposed, touching this nerve gives acute pain. When it is divided, no change takes place in the motion of the nostril; the cartilages continue to expand regularly in time with the other parts which combine in the act of respiration; but the sensibility is entirely lost. If the same branch of the fifth be divided on the opposite side, and the animal let loose, the parts will be deprived of sensibility, and he will not pick up his corn: the power of elevating and projecting the lip, as in gathering food, will appear to be lost. He will press the mouth against the ground, and at length lick the oats from the ground with his tongue. In my first experiments the loss of sensibility of the lips was so obvious, that it was thought a useless cruelty to cut the other branches of the fifth.*

The experiment of cutting the *portio dura*, gave so little pain, that it was several times repeated on the ass and dog, and uniformly with the same effect. The side of the face remained at rest and placid, during the highest excitement of the other parts of the respiratory organs.

When the ass, on which this muscular nerve of the face had been cut, was killed by bleeding, an unexpected opportunity was offered of ascertaining its influence, by the negation of its powers on the side of the face where it was cut across.

When an animal becomes insensible from loss of blood, the impression at the heart extends its influence in violent convulsions over all the muscles of respiration; not only is the air drawn into the chest with sudden and powerful effort, but at the same instant the muscles of the mouth, nostrils, and eyelids, and all the side of the face, are in a violent state of spasm. In the ass, where the *portio dura* had been cut, the most remarkable contrast was exhibited in the two sides of the face;

for whilst the one side was in universal and powerful contraction, the other, of which the nerve was divided, remained quite placid. . . .

From these facts we are entitled to conclude, that the *portio dura* of the seventh is the nerve of motion to the muscles of the forehead, eyebrow, eyelids, nostril, lips, and ear; that is, to all the muscles of the face except those of mastication—that it is the respiratory nerve of the face; that the motions of the lips, the nostrils, and the velum palati, are governed by its influence, when the muscles of these parts are in associated action with the other organs of respiration. . . .

On cutting the respiratory nerve on one side of the face of a monkey, the very peculiar activity of his features on that side ceased altogether. The timid motions of his eye-lids and eyebrows were lost, and he could not wink on that side; and his lips were drawn to the other side, like a paralytic drunkard, whenever he shewed his teeth in rage. Considering these facts, the conclusion is inevitable, that the motions of the lips, nostrils, and eye-lids, and forehead, in expression, have nothing to do with the fifth pair of nerves, nor with the nervi molles, branches of the sympathetic nerve, which accompany the blood-vessels of the face.

In the Appendix we have proofs equal to experiments, that in the human face the actions of the muscles which produce smiling and laughing are a consequence of the influence of this respiratory nerve. A man had the trunk of the respiratory nerve of the face injured by a suppuration which took place before to the ear, and through which the nerve passed in its course to the face. It was observed, that in smiling and laughing, his mouth was drawn in a very remarkable manner to the opposite side. The attempt to whistle was attended with a ludicrous distortion of the lips: when he took snuff and sneezed, the side on which the suppuration had affected the nerve remained placid, while the opposite side exhibited the usual distortion.

Thus it appears, that whenever the action of any of the muscles of the face is associated with the act of breathing, it is performed through the operation of this respiratory nerve, or *portio dura*. I cut a tumour from before the ear of a coachman: a branch of the nerve which goes to the angle of the mouth was divided. Some time after, he returned to thank me for ridding him of a formidable disease, but complained that he could not whistle to his horses. . . .

*. . . . My late excellent brother-in-law, Mr. John Shaw, repeated my experiments on the roots of the spinal nerves, and when I had stated my conviction that it would be found that those two nerves of the face differ in their functions: and when the proofs came out so satisfactorily under his own hands in these experiments, nothing could exceed his delight. It is well known with what interest he prosecuted the subject, at once honourable to himself, and to me.

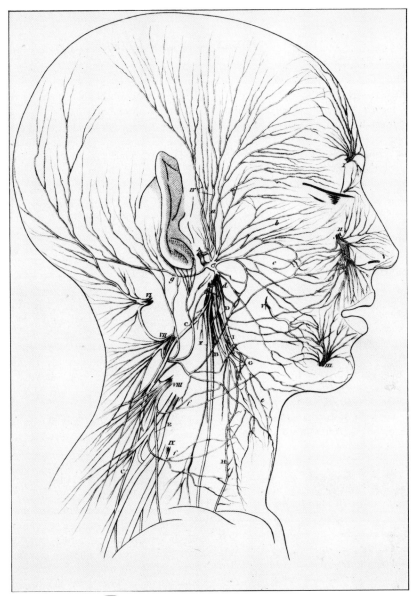

Drawn by C. Bell.

PLATE VI.

A VIEW OF THE NERVES OF THE FACE.

In this Plate the two distinct classes of nerves which go to the Face are represented; the one to bestow sensibility, and the other motion, that is, the motions connected with the respiratory organs.

The nerves on the side of the neck are also represented. These I have discovered to be double nerves, performing two functions; they control the muscular frame, and bestow sensibility on the skin. Besides these regular spinal nerves, which are for the common endowments, the nerves of the throat are represented. These latter nerves are the chords of sympathy which connect the motions of the neck and throat with the motions of the nostrils and lips, not merely in swallowing and during excited respiration, but in the expression of passion, &c.

A The Respiratory nerve of the face, or, according to authors, the portio dura of the seventh nerve.

    a Branches ascending to the temple and side of the head.

b Branches which supply the eye-lids.

c Branches going to the muscles which move the nostrils.

d Branches going down upon the side of the neck and throat.

e Superficial cervical plexus.

ff Connections formed with the cervical nerves.

 g A nerve to the muscles on the back of the ear.

B The eighth nerve, par vagum, or grand respiratory nerve.

C The superior respiratory nerve, or spinal accessory nerve.

D Ninth nerve, or lingualis.

E Diaphragmatic or phrenic nerve.

F Sympathetic nerve.

G Laryngeal nerve.

H Recurrent laryngeal nerve.

I Glosso-pharyngeal nerve.

MOTIONS OF THE EYE-BALL AND EYE-LIDS

. . . . There is a motion of the eye-ball, which, from its rapidity, has escaped observation. At the instant in which the eye-lids are closed, the eye-ball makes a movement which raises the cornea under the upper eye-lid.

If we fix one eye upon an object, and close the other with the finger in such a manner as to feel the convexity of the cornea through the eye-lid, and shut the eye that is open, we shall feel that the cornea of the other eye is instantly elevated; and that it thus rises and falls in sympathy with the eye that is closed and opened. This change of the position of the eye-ball takes place during the most rapid winking motions of the eye-lids. When a dog was deprived of the power of closing the eye-lids of one eye by the division of the nerve of the eye-lids, the eye did not cease to turn up when he was threatened, and when he winked with the eye-lids of the other side. . . .

Nearly the same thing I observed in a girl whose eye-lids were attached to the surrounding skin, owing to a burn; for the fore part of the eye-ball being completely uncovered, when she would have winked, instead of the eye-lids descending, the eye-balls were turned up, and the cornea was moistened by coming into contact with the mouths of the lacrymal ducts. . . .

The purpose of this rapid insensible motion of the eye-ball will be understood on observing the form of the eye-lids and the place of the lacrymal gland. The margins of the eye-lids are flat, and when they meet, they touch only at their outer edges, so that, when closed, there is a gutter left between them and the cornea. If the eye-balls were to remain without motion, the margins of the eye-lids would meet in such a manner on the surface of the cornea, that a certain portion would be left untouched, and the eye would have no power of clearing off what obscured the vision, at that principal part of the lucid cornea which is in the very axis of the eye; and if the tears flowed they would be left accumulated on the centre of the cornea, and winking, instead of clearing the eye, would suffuse it. To avoid these effects, and to sweep and clear the surface of the cornea, at the same time that the eye-lids are closed, the eye-ball revolves, and the cornea is rapidly elevated under the eye-lid.

Another effect of this motion of the eye-ball is, to procure the discharge from the lacrymal ducts; for by the simultaneous ascent of the cornea and descent of the upper eye-lid, the membrane on which the ducts open is stretched, and the effect is like the elongation of the nipple, to facilitate the discharge of secretion.

By the double motion, the descent of the eye-lid and the ascent of the cornea at the same time, the rapidity with which the eye escapes from injury is increased. Even creatures which have imperfect eye-lids, as fishes, by possessing this rapid revolving motion of the eye, are enabled to avoid injury and clear off impurities.

I may observe in passing, that, in the manner in which the eye-lids close, there is a provision for the preservation of the eye, which has not been noticed. While the upper eye-lid falls, the lower eye-lid is moved towards the nose. This is a part of that curious provision for collecting offensive particles towards the inner corner of the eye. If the edges of the eye-lids be marked with black spots, it will be seen that when the eye-lids are opened and closed, the spot on the upper eye-lid will descend and rise perpendicularly, while the spot on the lower eye-lid will play horizontally like a shuttle. . . .

We already see that two objects are attained through the motion of the eye-lids and eye-ball; the moistening the eye with the clear fluid of the lacrymal gland, and the extraction or rather the protrusion, of offensive particles.

There is another division of this subject no less curious: the different conditions of the eye during the waking and sleeping state remain to be considered. If we approach a person in disturbed sleep when the eye-lids are a little apart, we shall not see the pupil nor the dark part of the eye, as we should were he awake, for the cornea is turned upwards under the upper eye-lid. If a person be fainting, as insensibility comes over him the eyes cease to have speculation; that is they want direction, and are vacant, and presently the white part of the eye is disclosed by the revolving of the eye-ball upwards. Look to a blind beggar; these white balls are not turned up in the fervour of prayer or entreaty; it is the natural state of the eye-balls, which are totally blind, and from which the attention has been withdrawn. So it is on the approach of death; for, although the eye-lids be open, the pupils are in part hid, being turned up with a seeming agony, which however is only the mark of increasing insensibility. . . .

APPENDIX,

CONTAINING CONSULTATIONS AND CASES ILLUSTRATIVE OF THE FACTS ANNOUNCED IN THE PRECEDING PAPERS

.... No. XI.—*Clinical Lecture on partial Paralysis
of the Face, delivered by Sir Charles Bell,
at the Middlesex Hospital.*

Case.—Daniel Quick, aet. 70. . . .

Gentlemen, I have brought this man to you, that you might yourselves examine him, and be satisfied as to certain facts, which men, high in science, and respectable in our profession, have denied with a heat and pertinacity which I can never understand, and which surely ought not to belong to such an inquiry.

For years I had the conviction that the nerves, and especially the nerves of the face, had distinct functions. I was deterred from announcing my opinions, because I conceived it impossible but that experience and observation must have long ago ascertained the fact. Yes, gentlemen, from the dissection, I conceived that the branches of the fifth nerve, and of the *portio dura* of the seventh nerve, must have distinct offices. But then, I said, if it were so, the fact could not be so long concealed; these nerves are cut by surgeons every day; they are exposed in wounds; and yet I find no surmise to countenance this idea. Were I to refer to my note-books, I could prove to you how anxiously I looked around for some circumstance to support this opinion; and although of late years many such cases as the present have been submitted to me, there was a time in which I would have given all that I was worth to have had such proofs as you have now before you.

Some will contend about the propriety of making experiments on the living—none will hesitate to say that it is our duty to observe accurately when an accident may be converted into an experiment. This poor man was tossed by a bull: the horn went in here, at the angle of the jaw, and he hung suspended upon it, until the integuments before the ear giving way, he dropped. The blood flowed copiously, and he will tell you he heard it splashing upon the ground; notwithstanding, he expresses, with gratitude, that his doctor made a famous cure of it. The point of the horn had entered behind the upright portion of the jaw, and had hooked up and torn across the portio dura of the seventh, where it comes forwards from the stylo-mastoid foramen. I wish you to direct your whole attention to the effects of the division of

this nerve; since it is as much of the nature of an experiment as if you had tied an animal neck and heel, and had divided the nerve with your scalpel.

You have observed the remarkable distortion of the whole face; and that one side is become, as it were, a dead mass, incapable of motion or of expression of any kind; an effect which, heretofore, any medical man would have supposed could only be produced by the division of all the six nerves that go to the side of the face; whereas you see that the effect has been produced by the destruction of one only. You observe, by the answers to my questions, that whilst motion is gone, sensibility remains. And you cannot resist the conviction that the remaining sensibility is owing to the entireness of the branches of the fifth pair, which come out through the orbit, and through the upper and lower maxillary bones; whilst the loss of motion has resulted from the tearing of the portio dura. Nor is this a solitary case in this hospital. A patient was brought in who had put a pistol to his ear; which, strange to say, did not immediately destroy him, nor at once deprive him of his sense; although ultimately he died. The temporal bone was shattered, and the portio dura torn: and the paralysis of the muscles of the face was as complete as it is here.

[Sir Charles Bell.—Now, my friend, shut this left eye.

Patient.—No, Sir, I cannot do that: my wife says I never shut my eye.

Sir C.—But make an attempt: close both your eyes, as if you were going to sleep.

The patient makes the attempt, but still adds—it is needless; "my wife says I never shut this eye. In the attempt, we observed that, when the eyelids were closed, the left eye-ball was rolled up, so as to be concealed under the upper eye-lid.]

Sir C. continued—You witness the fact, then, gentlemen, that there is this very remarkable turning up of the cornea in the attempt to close the eye-lids; and you comprehend how this takes place. The imperfection is only in the eye-lids; and although the will cannot reach them, owing to the division of the portio dura, yet the rolling of the eye is performed, because the nerves to the oblique muscles within the orbit are entire. Before you, then, there can be no denying this revolving of the eye; in future you will allow no question about it.

If you will take the trouble to inquire, this man will tell you that he is not at all aware of the eye being turned up; although he can turn it up by a voluntary act, and be conscious of it at the same time. This is altogether an instinctive or involuntary action in the eye-ball; and you do not observe it in the ordinary case, merely because it is a part of the protecting action accompanying the rapid closing of the eye-lid which conceals it. You may, however, feel it at any time, by putting your finger gently upon the closed eye-lid; and then, acting with the eye-lids to close them more firmly, you will feel the convexity of the cornea slip upwards: or, spread out the eye-lid upon a friend's eye with your fingers, until you see the cornea under the tense skin: then ask him to make the effort to wink, and you will see the convex body slip up and disappear. . . .

The next thing that is curious is the condition of this man's eye in sleep. You find it stated that the cornea goes up during sleep; for his wife being asked, whether, since the eye-lid remained open, he continued looking at her when asleep, she answered, "that cannot be, for only the white of the eye is seen." You have here, then, all but ocular demonstration of what I have elsewhere affirmed, that there is a particular position of the eye-ball, or, in other words, another condition of the muscles of the eye-ball, peculiar to the state of sleep. Indeed, it must be obvious to you that if in this man the pupil were not covered, and the cornea moistened during sleep, there would be an incessant irritation upon the eye, from the entrance of the light, and the evaporation of the moisture from the cornea. But, however interesting in a philosophical light, this is not practical; and, therefore, I am not at liberty to detain you longer upon it in this place.

[Sir C.—Now, my friend, let us see you take a snuff—(the patient put the pinch to the right nostril). But why do you not snuff with the left side?

Patient.—Because it does not go high enough to let me feel it.

Sir C.—Can you breathe through that left nostril?

Patient.—My wife says I cannot.

A bottle of carbonate of ammonia being put to this nostril, he said, with some emphasis, "I can feel that."]

You see, gentlemen, that this honest fellow bids fair to have domestic peace: he confides more in his wife's authority than in his own sensations. But you will have no difficulty in understanding how the destruction of the portio dura affects the sense of smelling, and destroys, in a great measure, the gratification of snuffing. The cartilages of the nose form a very curious structure; and, you know, are moved by four appropriate muscles, these muscles being governed by the respiratory nerve of the face or portio dura. Every violent inspiration is attended with an excitement of these muscles, and an expansion of the tube: were this wanting, you see what the effect would be. At the moment of a sudden inspiration, instead of the tubes for the passage of the air being enlarged proportionally, they would hang, like this man's nostril upon the left side, which, you see, forms a loose membranous slit; and be more apt to close and cause a sniffling, in drawing the breath, than to become inflated to admit the air freely. In smelling, or in snuffing, there is such an action of these muscles as to produce both a narrowing and a new direction of the lower part of the tube of the nostril; by which the air, and whatever that air has suspended in it, is drawn forcibly upwards to the part of the Schneiderian membrane where the olfactory nerve is expanded. Our friend here finds it a mere waste of snuff to put it into this nostril: he tells you it does not go high enough: he can draw it in, but he cannot make it mount. You perceive, then, that although the function of the olfactory nerve remains entire, the loss of the portio dura is attended with a destruction of that apparatus which is made subservient to the organ of smelling.

[Sir C.—Do you put the morsel into the left side of your mouth?

Patient.—Yes; but I *wumble* it over to the other side.

He now got a pot of porter, and, as he swallowed, there was a flapping of the paralyzed cheek; he said that he required time, or it would fall out of his mouth again. Sir Charles thought he felt a stringy or active condition of the buccinator, but recommended us to give him a pot some other day, and ascertain this.

He was now asked if he could laugh: and, quaintly enough, he answered, "Yes, when he got something to laugh at;" and on this he exhibited a very singular distortion of countenance: at each cachinnation his left cheek was puffed out, flapping like a loose sail; and the forehead and eye-lids on this side remained perfectly still; whilst upon the right side the whole mouth was drawn upwards, the cheeks were strongly wrinkled, and the eye-lids puckered.] . . . .

No. XIV.—*Proposal to divide the branches of the Fifth Pair.*

A gentleman, in the vigour of life, came into my room to consult me, having the most remarkable distortion of countenance I had ever seen. He proceeded to state to me what he conceived to be the cause of this paralytic affection of one side of his face: he had been knocked down by a blow upon the ear, and had remained a whole night insensible, with bleeding from the ear, from which time his features had been thus drawn to the opposite side. I thought I should give him comfort by stating to him that this was a paralysis attributable to the injury of the bone, and that, as it had not preceded from an apoplectic tendency, there was no danger of a future attack, or of increase of the paralysis. But this was not what he expected from me; he had consulted my brother, then at Rome, who had proposed to cure him by an operation.

I was quite at a loss to conceive what operation my brother's ingenuity had contrived to relieve so remarkable a deformity. The gentleman mentioned that it had been intended to make three small incisions on different parts of his face, so as to restore the balance of his features: and he was obviously disappointed in finding me less intelligent, or less able than he had expected, and we parted.

On reflecting on the conversation of this gentleman, it occurred to me, that my brother, believing that the paralysis had arisen from an injury of the fifth nerve, had proposed to restore the features to an equilibrium by dividing the branches of the same nerve on the opposite side; trusting, no doubt, to the features being still animated by the seventh pair of nerves, according to the received doctrine. A singular consequence would have resulted from such an operation. The features would have remained drawn to the same side as before, and he would have been deprived of all sensibility of that side! If it was designed to cut the *portio dura* of the side contracted, a more unhappy consequence would have resulted; for he could never afterwards have spoken, or even have kept his lips to his teeth, or retained the saliva. The features of both sides would have fallen in relaxation; the eyes would have remained uncovered; and he would have lost his sight by the inflammation and opacity consequent on their continual exposure!

It must, indeed, appear a singular circumstance now, that so many surgeons were cutting the branches of the fifth pair of nerves for the tic douloureux, without being led to inquire more particularly into the functions of the several nerves of the face. We see how nearly my brother's ingenuity had led him wrong, from having often cut the fifth pair without producing horrible distortion. And I believe that the very same mistake led a gentleman to say that I had not cut the frontal branch of the fifth pair of nerves on the face of a nobleman, when in fact I had only cut that branch, and had not interfered with the branches of the *portio dura*, and, consequently, had produced no effect on the muscles of the eye-brow. All these circumstances, I hope, tend to enforce the importance of anatomy. . . . .

No. XXIV.

"When we see a person alarmed without cause, and there is no danger in the case, there is something approaching to the ludicrous in the scene. A physician paid me a visit who had come up from the country in the mail, and had fallen asleep in the night-time, with his cheek exposed at the open window to the east wind. On the morning of his arrival, when preparing to go abroad, he found, upon looking into his glass, that his face was all twisted. His alarm gave more expression to one side of his face, and produced more horrible distortion. Both laughing and crying, you know, depend on the function of the portio dura, but when he came to me he considered it no laughing matter: I never saw distortion more complete. It was difficult to comfort him; but I am happy to add, that the paralysis gradually left him, as I told him it would. I have at present a young lady under my care who has paralysis of the face, and who has received great benefit from galvanism. And I have lately seen an instance of the same kind; the more remarkable only as shewing how the want of expression will injure the finest countenance. I mention these things to remind you of the frequency of the occurrence, and of the necessity of your distinguishing the slighter cases, where the exterior branches of the nerve are affected, from those wherein the cause is deeper seated, and more formidable. . . .

No. XLVII

"J. Cooper.—This man's general appearance is completely that of an old paralytic, but the distortion of his face is more remarkable than usual, in consequence of the right, or paralysed side, being marked with a red blotch.

"The arm and leg of the same side are nearly powerless, his intellect is much impaired, and his memory gone. The history of his case was given very clearly by his wife. According to her account, her husband was for the first time, attacked with apoplexy about seven years ago; from this attack he gradually recovered, but at the end of twelve months he was a second time seized, and, since that period, he has had two distinct attacks every year; for the last two or three years he has been nearly in the same condition as at present.

"*State of the cheeks and mouth.*—When he is made to laugh, the right cheek rises in the same degree with the left; when he blows (he always bursts into a laugh when asked to whistle), the buccinator of the right cheek is in as much action as on the other side. When his nose is irritated by snuffing ammonia, the actions of the muscles, preparatory to sneezing, are equal on both sides of the face. The right cheek, and the right side of the mouth, fall lower than the left. When a piece of bread was put between the teeth and right cheek, the patient could not push it from its place, but was obliged to pick it out with his tongue. The saliva constantly flows from the right side of his mouth, and when drinking, part of the fluid escapes from the same side. The loss of the sensibility of the orbicularis oris was farther shewn by the inability to hold a pencil, or a tobacco-pipe, in the right side of his mouth.

"The comparative degree of sensibility in the two cheeks was next examined; when he was pricked on the right cheek with a needle he seemed perfectly insensible, even though I drew blood; but on giving the least prick to the left side he immediately started; the same difference in the degree of sensibility was observable in pulling a hair from each whisker. The sensibility of the right and left limb corresponded with that of the cheeks.

"On putting hartshorn to the right nostril he inhaled it as well as with the left, and immediately all the symptoms observable in a person about to sneeze were presented.* As the nose was turned up, and the alae nasi of both sides were equally in action, this was a sufficient proof of the state of the paralysed side being here very different from the condition described in the foregoing cases. The power of the fifth over the nose was tried, by tickling the inside of the right nostril no effect was produced; but tickling the left nostril the symptoms of sneezing were again evident.

"The motion of the eye was perfect.

"He could close the eye-lid of the paralysed side as well as the other; and when his nose was irritated by the hartshorn, or when he laughed, the orbicularis oculi and corrugator supercilii were in complete action, so that there was not here that heaviness in the expression of the upper part of the face, which is so remarkable in paralytic persons. Here, then, was proof that those actions of the eye-brows which we find to be deficient, when the portio dura is affected, are, in a case of common palsy, left entire; indeed, we may have daily opportunities, while walking in the streets, of observing that patients with palsy of one side of the body, have no difficulty in closing the eye-lids." . . . .

---

*The apparent sensibility of the nostril over which the fifth had lost its influence may be explained, by supposing that the fumes of the ammonia passed by the posterior nares to the other nostril, and thus caused sneezing.

XXVII Causalgia

CHANCE led Silas Weir Mitchell (1829 to 1914) into the field of neurology during the Civil War.[1] While treating battlefield casualties, the versatile and industrious Mitchell undertook the first major study of peripheral nerve injuries, in the course of which he recognized and described the syndrome of causalgia.

Weir Mitchell was an experimental physiologist with no experience in neurology when he enlisted in the United States Army in 1862. He was initially assigned to a general military hospital, where he soon developed an interest in patients with neurological disorders. As the numbers of these cases increased, Surgeon General William A. Hammond,[2] who with Mitchell was a founder of American neurology,[3,4] established a special neurological hospital in Philadelphia, first on Christian Street and then on Turner's Lane.[5] Weir Mitchell and George R. Morehouse were placed in charge of the hospital, and William W. Keen was added to the staff as resident surgeon.

The three men recognized the unique opportunity these cases provided, and they spent many hours making detailed notes. Mitchell wrote the following:

"Keen, Morehouse, and I worked on at notetaking often as late as 12 or 1 at night, and when we got through walked home, talking over our cases. . . . I have worked with many men since, but never with men who took more delight to repay opportunity with labor. . . . The cases were of amazing interest. Here at one time were eighty epileptics, and every kind of nerve wound, palsies, choreas, stump disorders. . . .

"Thousands of pages of notes were taken. . . . About midway we planned the ultimate essays which were to record our work. . . . There was a small book on neural injuries full of novelty, a short essay on reflex palsies, etc. One of the most notable was Keen's essay on malingering. Others on epilepsy, muscular disorders, and on acute exhaustion were never written because of accidental destruction of notes by fire. . . ."[6]   ,

The classic work of Mitchell, Morehouse, and Keen on peripheral nerve injuries[7] was summarized in two books, in 1864 and 1872, and in a follow-up report of 20 of the original cases by Weir Mitchell's son John in 1895.[8-10] These three volumes provided the foundation for similar detailed studies during the two World Wars, on which our present understanding of nerve injuries is based.[11,12]

A few individual cases with some of the features of causalgia had been reported before Weir Mitchell's Civil War experience,[13] but Mitchell gave the first full description of the syndrome, based on numerous cases, and he applied the name causalgia (from the Greek words for heat and pain) at the suggestion of his friend, Professor Robley Dunglison.[5,14] Causalgia, seen most commonly following a partial injury to a major nerve trunk caused by a high velocity missile, is defined as a severe persistent pain, usually with a burning quality, felt in the distribution of the involved nerve, and accentuated by various environmental and emotional stimuli.[12,15]

The pathogenesis is still uncertain, but it has been proposed that causalgia results from an interaction between efferent sympathetic and afferent sensory fibers.[16] However, the most notable advance since Weir Mitchell's original description of causalgia occurred during World War II when sympathectomy was found to be an effective treatment.[15]

References

1. McHenry, L.C., Jr.: "Introduction to the Dover Edition," in Mitchell, S.W.: *Injuries of Nerves and Their Consequences,* New York: Dover Publications, Inc., 1965, pp ix-xxii.

2. Walter, R.D.: Historical Note: William A. Hammond and His Enemies, *Bull Los Angeles Neurol Soc* 33:31-37 (Jan) 1968.

3. Jelliffe, S.E.: "Fifty Years of American Neurology: Fragments of an Historical Retrospect," in Tilney, F., and Jelliffe, S.E. (eds.): *Semi-Centennial Anniversary Volume of the American Neurological Association 1875-1924,* Albany, NY: American Neurological Association, 1924, pp 386-438.

4. DeJong, R.N.: The Founding of the American Neurological Association and Its Relationship to Neurology as a Specialty in 1875, *Trans Amer Neurol Assoc* 90:3-11, 1965.

5. Middleton, W.S.: Turner's Lane Hospital, *Bull Hist Med* 40:14-42 (Jan-Feb) 1966.

6. Mitchell, S.W.: Some Personal Recollections of the Civil War, *Trans Coll Physicians Phila* 27:87-94, 1905.

7. LaFia, D.J.: S. Weir Mitchell on Gunshot Wounds and Other Injuries of Nerves, *Neurology* 5:468-471 (July) 1955.

8. Mitchell, S.W.; Morehouse, G.R.; and Keen, W.W.: *Gunshot Wounds and Other Injuries of Nerves,* Philadelphia: J. B. Lippincott & Co., 1864.

9. Mitchell, S.W.: *Injuries of Nerves and Their Consequences,* Philadelphia: J. B. Lippincott & Co., 1872.

10. Mitchell, J.K.: *Remote Consequences of Injuries of Nerves and Their Treatment: An Examination of the Present Condition of Wounds Received 1863-65, With Additional Illustrative Cases.* Philadelphia: Lea Brothers & Co., 1895.

11. Woodhall, B., and Beebe, G.W.: *Peripheral Nerve Regeneration: A Follow-Up Study of 3,656 World War II Injuries,* Washington, DC: US Government Printing Office, 1956.

12. Sunderland, S.: *Nerves and Nerve Injuries,* Baltimore: Williams & Wilkins Co., 1968.

13. Ross, J.P.: Causalgia, *St. Barth Hosp Rep* 65:103-118, 1932.

14. Richards, R.L.: The Term 'Causalgia', *Med Hist* 11:97-99 (Jan) 1967.

15. Richards, R.L.: Causalgia: A Centennial Review, *Arch Neurol* 16:339-350 (April) 1967.

16. Doupe, J.; Cullen, C.H.; and Chance, G.Q.: Post-Traumatic Pain and the Causalgic Syndrome, *J Neurol Neurosurg Psychiat* 7:33-48 (Jan-April) 1944.

INJURIES OF NERVES AND THEIR CONSEQUENCES

by S. Weir Mitchell, M. D.*

Chapter VIII. Sensory Lesions

. . . . Usually the pains from nerve hurts are either aching, shooting, or burning, or perhaps all three at once. Looking carefully through my notes as to this point, I find that in a considerable proportion of gunshot wounds of nerves there is principally burning pain, or at least that this is the prominent symptom, while in slight injuries of nerves from compression or contusions, the other forms of pain are more apt to prevail.

---

*Reprinted from Mitchell, S.W.: *Injuries of Nerves and Their Consequences,* Philadelphia: J. B. Lippincott & Co., 1872, pp 195-201, 272, 292-295, 302-303, and 306.

Perhaps few persons who are not physicians can realize the influence which long-continued and unendurable pain may have upon both body and mind. The older books are full of cases in which, after lancet wounds, the most terrible pain and local spasms resulted. When these had lasted for days or weeks, the whole surface became hyperaesthetic, and the senses grew to be only avenues for fresh and increasing tortures, until every vibration, every change of light, and even, as in Miss Willson's case, the effort to read brought on new agony. Under such torments the temper changes, the most amiable grow irritable, the soldier becomes a coward, and the strongest man is scarcely less nervous than the most hysterical girl. Perhaps nothing can better illustrate the extent to which these statements may be true than the cases of burning pain, or, as I prefer to term it, causalgia, the most terrible of all the tortures which a nerve wound may inflict. In delineating this form of pain, perhaps I cannot do better than transfer to these pages the account originally written while I was seeing almost daily numbers of persons suffering as I have described them:

"In our early experience of nerve wounds, we met with a small number of men who were suffering from a pain which they described as a 'burning,' or as 'mustard red-hot,' or as a 'red-hot file rasping the skin.' In all of these patients, and in many later cases, this pain was an associate of the glossy skin previously described. In fact, this state of skin never existed without burning pain. Recently we have seen numbers of men who had burning pain without glossy skin, and in some we have seen this latter condition commencing. The burning comes first, the visible skin-change afterwards; but in no case of great depravity in the nutrient condition of the skin have we failed to meet with it, and that in its forms of almost unendurable anguish.

"We have some doubt as to whether this form of pain ever originates at the moment of the wounding; but we have been so informed as regards two or three cases. Certain it is that, as a rule, the burning arises later, but almost always during the healing of the wound. Of the special cause which provokes it, we know nothing, except that it has sometimes followed the transfer of pathological changes from a wounded nerve to unwounded nerves, and has then been felt in their distribution, so that we do not need a direct wound to bring it about. The seat of burning pain is very various; but it never attacks the trunk, rarely the arm or thigh, and not often the forearm or leg. Its favorite site is the foot or hand. In these parts it is to be found most often where the nutritive skin-changes are met with; that is to say, on the palm of the hand, or palmar face of the fingers, and on the dorsum of the foot: scarcely ever on the sole of the foot, or the back of the hand. When it first existed in the whole foot or hand, it always remained last in the parts above referred to, as its favorite seats. The great mass of sufferers described this pain as superficial, but others said it was also in the joints, and deep in the palm. If it lasted long it was finally referred to the skin alone.

"Its intensity varies from the most trivial burn-ing to a state of torture, which can hardly be credited, but which reacts on the whole economy, until the general health is seriously affected. The part itself is not alone subject to an intense burning sensation, but becomes exquisitely hyper-aesthetic, so that a touch or a tap of the finger increases the pain. Exposure to the air is avoided by the patient with a care which seems absurd, and most of the bad cases keep the hand constant-ly wet, finding relief in the moisture rather than in the coolness of the application. Two of these sufferers carried a bottle of water and a sponge, and never permitted the part to become dry for a moment. As the pain increases, the general sympa-thy becomes more marked. The temper changes and grows irritable, the face becomes anxious and has a look of weariness and suffering. The sleep is restless, and the constitutional condition, reacting on the wounded limb, exasperates the hyperaesthe-tic state, so that the rattling of a newspaper, a breath of air, the step of another across the ward, the vibrations caused by a military band, or the shock of the feet in walking, gives rise to increase of pain. At last the patient grows hysterical, if we may use the only term which describes the facts. He walks carefully, carries the limb with the sound hand, is tremulous, nervous, and has all kinds of expedients for lessening his pain. In two cases, at least, the skin of the entire body became hyperaesthetic when dry, and the men found some ease from pouring water into their boots. They said, when questioned, that it made walking hurt less; but how, or why, unless by diminishing vibration, we cannot explain. One of these men went so far as to wet the sound hand when he was obliged to touch the other, and insisted that the observer should also wet his hand before touching him, complaining that dry touch always exasperat-ed his pain. Cold weather usually eased these pains; heat, and the hanging down of the limb, made them worse. Motion of the part was unen-durable in some of the very worst cases; but, for the most part, it did no harm, unless so excessive as to flush the injured region.

"The rationale of the production of this form of pain was at first sought for among reflex phenom-ena. It then seemed to us probable that a traumatic irritation existing in some part of a nerve trunk was simply referred by the mind to the extreme distribution of this nerve, agreeably to the well-known law of the reference of sensations.

"Further study led us to suspect that the irrita-tion of a nerve, at the point of wound, might give rise to changes in the circulation and nutrition of parts in its distribution, and that these alterations might be themselves of a pain-producing nature. The following considerations tend to strengthen the view, that the immediate cause of burning pain lies in the part where the burning is felt:

"If the burning were a referred sensation, it would sometimes be met with in cases of complete division of nerves, and, therefore, in parts devoid of tactile sensation. But we have encountered no such cases; and, on the other hand, the burning pain is often accompanied with hyperaesthesia, while motion and touch may remain unaltered. Is it not probable that the depraved nutrition, often so marked in the congested, denuded, and altered skin, may give rise to a disease of the ultimate fibres of the sensitive nerves? Just such a pain comes when we attack the cutis with irritants; and let us add, that the agents which help these cases of burning are those addressed to the spot where the pain is felt, and not to the cicatrix."

Since this description was written, several years have gone by, but new experience has only strengthened my belief that the explanation just given is physiologically correct, because in a large number of amputated cases—many of them neuralgic—I have never yet seen a case of subjective burning pain. . . .

Case 33.—Wound of right arm; glossy skin; causalgia and neuralgia; joint disease; acid sweats; slight loss of tact; constitutional symptoms. H., aged thirty-nine, New York, was shot July 2, 1863, through the inner edge of the right biceps, half an inch above the internal condyle of the humerus; the ball passed backward and downward. The musket fell from his left hand, and the right, grasping the rod, was twisted towards the chest and bent at the elbow. He walked to the rear. He cannot tell how much motion was lost, but he knows that he had instant pain in the median distribution, with tenderness of the palm, even on the first day, and a sense of numbness. My notes describe him on entering our wards as presenting the following symptoms: the temperature of the two palms is alike. The back of the hand looks as usual, but the skin of the palm is delicate and thin, and without any eruption. The joints of the fingers are swollen, and the hand secretes freely a sour, ill-smelling sweat. The pain is, in the first place, neuralgic, and darting down the median nerve track into the fingers; while, in the second place, there is burning in the palm and up the anterior face of the fingers.

Pressure on the cicatrix gave no pain, but the median nerve below that point was tender, and pressure upon it caused pain in the hand. There was slight want of tactile sensibility in the median distribution in the hand, but the parts receiving the ulnar nerve presented no sign of injury. The hyperaesthesia of the palm was excessive, so that even to blow on it seemed to give pain. He kept it wrapped up and wet, but could not endure to pour water on to the palm, preferring to wet the dorsum of the hand and allow the fluid to run around, so as by degrees to soak the palm. After a few weeks of this torment he became so sensitive that the rustle of a paper or of a woman's dress, the sound of feet, the noise of a band, all appeared to increase his pain. His countenance at this time was worn, pinched, and anaemic, his temper irritable, and his manner so odd that some of the attendants believed him insane. When questioned as to his condition he assured me that every strong moral emotion made him worse,—anger or disappointment expressing themselves cruelly in the aching limb. . . .

Chapter XI. Treatment

. . . *Causalgia or burning pain; water-dressings.* —A vast number of means were tried to ease or cure causalgia, but the one essential for comfort was the use of water-dressings which were unceasingly renewed, the sufferers carrying a bottle of water and a sponge and keeping the part covered. I have never known a man afflicted with causalgia who did not learn very soon the use of this agent, and I never knew one who could be induced to exchange it for any other permanent dressing. . . .

Chapter XII. Treatment

Case 47.—Injury of median and ulnar nerves by a bullet; loss of motion; excessive causalgia; exsection of four inches of median nerve; no relief. Jos. H. Corliss, late private Company B, 14th New York State Militia, aged twenty-seven, shingle-dresser, enlisted April, 1861, in good health. At the second battle of Bull Run, August 29, 1862, he was shot in the left arm, three inches directly above the internal condyle. The ball emerged one and a quarter inches higher, through the belly of the biceps, without touching the artery, but with injury to the median and ulnar nerves. He was ramming a cartridge when hit, and "thought he was struck on the crazy-bone by some of the boys for a joke." The fingers of both hands flexed and grasped the ramrod and gun tightly. Bringing the right hand, still clutching the ramrod, to the left elbow, he felt the blood, and knew he was wounded. He then shook the ramrod from his grasp with a strong effort, and unloosened with the freed hand the tight grip of the left hand on the gun. After walking some twenty paces he fell from loss of blood, but still conscious; attempted to walk several times, and as often failed. He was finally helped to the rear, taken prisoner, lay three days on the field without food, but with enough of water to drink, and had his wounds dressed for the first time on the fourth day, at Fairfax Court House.

On the second day the pain began. It was burning and darting. He states that at this time sensation was lost or lessened in the limb, and that paralysis of motion came on in the hand and forearm. Admitted to the Douglas Hospital, Washington, D. C., September 7, 1862. The pain was so severe that a touch anywhere, or shaking the bed, or a heavy step, caused it to increase. The suffering was in the median and ulnar distribution, especially at the palmar face of the knuckles and the ball of the thumb. Motion has varied little since the wound, and as to sensation he is not clear.

Peter Pineo, surgeon, U. S. V., Medical Inspector U.S.A., opened the wound and exsected two or three inches of the median nerve. The man states, very positively, that the pain in the median distribution did not cease, nor preceptibly lessen, but that he became more sensitive, so that even the rattling of a paper caused extreme suffering. He "thinks he was not himself" for a day or two after the operation. It seems quite certain that the pain afterwards gradually moderated, both in the ulnar and the median tracts. Meanwhile the hand lay over his chest, and the fingers, flexing, became stiffened in this position.

About a week after he was shot, the *right* arm grew weak, and finally so feeble that he could not feed himself. He can now (April, 1864) use it pretty well, but it is manifestly less strong than the other. The left leg also was weakened, but when this loss of power first showed itself he cannot tell. He gives the usual account of the pain, and of the use of water on the hands and in his boots, as a means of easing it.

Present condition, April 21, 1864.—Wound healed. Cicatrix of the operation two and a half inches long over median nerve. The forearm muscles do not seem to be greatly wasted. The interosseal muscles and hypothenar group are much atrophied, and the hand is thin and bony. The thenar muscles are partially wasted.

The skin of the palm is eczematous, thin, red, and shining. The second and third phalanges of the fingers are flexed and stiff; the first is extended. Nails extraordinarily curved, laterally and longitudinally, except that of the thumb.

Pain is stated to exist still in the median distribution, but much less than in the ulnar tract, where it is excessively great.

He keeps his hand wrapped in a rag, wetted with cold water, and covered with oiled silk, and even tucks the rag carefully under the flexed finger-tips. Moisture is more essential than cold. Friction outside of the clothes, at any point of the entire surface, "shoots" into the hand, increasing the burning in the median, sometimes, and more commonly, in the ulnar distribution. Deep pressure on the muscles has a like effect, and he will allow no one to touch his skin, save with a wetted hand, and even then is careful to exact tender manipulation. He keeps a bottle of water about him, and carries a wet sponge in the right hand. This hand he wets always before he handles anything; used dry, it hurts the other limb. At one time, when the suffering was severe, he poured water into his boots, he says, to lessen the pain which dry touch or friction causes in the injured hand. So cautious was he about exposing the sore hand, that it was impossible thoroughly to examine it; but it was clear to us that there was sensibility to touch in the ultimate median distribution, although he describes sensation as somewhat lessened in this region, and states that he has numbness on the inner side of the palm, and in the third and fourth fingers (ulnar tract). When the balls of the first and second fingers were touched, he said he felt it; but on touching those of the third and fourth fingers, he refused to permit us to experiment further, and insisted on wrapping up and wetting the hand. He thus describes the pain at its height: "It is as if a rough bar of iron were thrust to and fro through the knuckles, a red-hot iron placed at the junction of the palm and thenar eminence, with a heavy weight on it, and the skin was being rasped off my finger-ends." . . .

Case 51.—Gunshot wound of axillary nerves; paralysis of motion; slight loss of sensation; burning on tenth day; great atrophy and contracted muscles; subluxation of fingers; nutritive changes; eczema in both palms; great improvement; discharged; re-examined four years later. David Schiveley, aged seventeen, no trade, Pennsylvania, enlisted August, 1862, in Company E, 114th Pennsylvania Volunteers. Healthy before and after enlisting, except a slight attack of typhoid fever.

At Gettysburg, July 2, 1863, while aiming, a

ball entered one inch to the left of the middle line, and one inch above the sternal end of the clavicle. Exit on the posterior part of the right arm, at the middle line, two inches below the axilla. The ball passed in front of the trachea, broke the inner half of the right clavicle, went in front of the vessels of the neck and the subclavian artery, in front of the axillary artery, and below the humerus,—speaking of that bone as raised and abducted at the time. When hit, he thought his arm was shot off. It dropped, the gun fell, and, screaming that he was murdered, he staggered, bleeding freely, and soon fell unconscious. When a little later he revived and raised his head, a second ball struck him in the right temporal fossa, and emerged through the right eye. He jumped up, ran a little way, and fell once more. When hit, he lost all motion in the limb, which became numbed, but felt no pain. Two weeks later, feeble power to move returned gradually in the elbow, shoulder, and arm, and after two months in the wrist and hand.

Treatment.—Cold-water dressings and means to relieve burning, but all ineffectual. The joints became swollen early, and the arm bent at a right angle. The hand, dependent, lay across his chest during a long period. He made some attempts at passive motion as he found the hand becoming stiff, but no great good was thus gained; and, as the contractions took place and the joints grew worse, the wrist became moulded to the curve of the chest, on which it lay.

About the tenth day, burning pain began in the palm and fingers, especially in the cushions of the fingers and the knuckles. It was at its worst a month later, and remained thus another month, after which it grew less. When at its height, he suffered from loud sounds, vibrations, and dry contact. The rubbing of his boots on the floor was the greatest annoyance, and this he relieved by wetting his stockings. Since October, four months after he was wounded, it has been unaltered. Sensation, little affected at the outset, has undergone no change of moment. Voluntary motion, which grew better for awhile, suffered anew and increasingly as the nutritive changes developed themselves. When they first arose we have been unable to determine. . . .

Pain.—In August, 1864, he began to lose the violent pain. It was not gradual, but one day he noticed suddenly that his glove was dry, and yet he could use his hand well and without pain. It was not entirely gone, and he continued to wet his hand for some months; but it grew much better. Even now he feels dry rubbing in the palm of the hand and down to the finger-tips, and a loud noise, such as a wagon making a great noise in passing, or a sudden emotion, as seeing a person fall, etc., makes the same impression. In the left hand there is no pain. . . .

XXVIII   Jacksonian Epilepsy

J OHN Hughlings Jackson (1835 to 1911), the father of British neurology, had a special interest in focal motor epilepsy. As a reporter for the *Medical Times and Gazette* and later as a physician at the London Hospital and the National Hospital in Queen Square, he studied patients with this disorder and continued to ponder its meaning. His interest was reinforced by the fact that his wife suffered from focal convulsions before her early death.[1-4]

Proceeding from his analysis of focal epilepsy, Jackson was then able to formulate a series of remarkably astute philosophical inferences about the organization and function of the entire central nervous system.[5-16] These interpretations were based entirely on clinical observation and reasoning; he left the experimental proof of his assertions to others.

Epilepsy had been studied by physicians for more than 2,000 years before Jackson's time, and focal seizures had been described occasionally as medical curiosities.[17-25] In 1827, L. F. Bravais published a description of focal motor seizures in his thesis for the doctoral degree from the Faculty of Medicine of Paris, but he offered no suitable explanation for this phenomenon.[21,22,25-27] Subsequently, Richard Bright and Robert Bentley Todd observed similar cases in England,[22] but at that time epilepsy was generally thought to be spino-medullary in origin.[13] The electrical excitability of the cerebral cortex was not established until the pioneering research of Gustav Fritsch and Eduard Hitzig in 1870.[28]

Bentley Todd, who was a distinguished physician in London,[29,30] also described the occurrence of post-epileptic hemiplegia and monoplegia in some of his patients.[31] This phenomenon, though previously mentioned by Bravais and later studied by Alexander Robertson,[32] is now known as Todd's paralysis.[21,22,33,34]

Because of analogies with apoplectic hemiplegia, Hughlings Jackson reasoned that the lesion responsible for focal motor epilepsy lay within the territory of the middle cerebral artery. He erred in assigning too much importance to the corpus striatum, but he correctly deduced that focal convulsions are the result of sudden discharges of partly damaged and unstable gray matter in the contralateral cerebral hemisphere. In addition, he inferred that the movements of muscle groups are represented on the brain's surface.

The accuracy of Jackson's reasoning has been proven during the past century by extensive evidence from the fields of pathology, neurophysiology, and electroencephalography.[35-39] Although his writings show little interest in individual patients or in treatment, his insights into pathophysiology provided a rational basis for later advances in the understanding and control of epilepsy.

References

1. Taylor, J.: *Selected Writings of John Hughlings Jackson*, London: Hodder and Stoughton, Ltd., 1931 (also New York: Basic Books, Inc., 1958).

2. [Kelly, E.C.]: John Hughlings Jackson, *Med Classics* **3**:889-971 (June) 1939.

3. Critchley, M.: Hughlings Jackson, the Man; and the Early Days of the National Hospital, *Proc Roy Soc Med Sect Neurol* **53**:613-618 (Aug) 1960.

4. Greenblatt, S.H.: The Major Influences on the Early Life and Work of John Hughlings Jackson, *Bull Hist Med* **39**:346-376 (July-Aug) 1965.

5. Head, H.: Hughlings Jackson on Aphasia and Kindred Affections of Speech, *Brain* 38:1-190 (July) 1915.

6. Langworthy, O.R.: Hughlings Jackson—His Opinions Concerning Epilepsy, *J Nerv Ment Dis* 76:574-585 (Dec) 1932.

7. Riese, W.: The Sources of Jacksonian Neurology, *J Nerv Ment Dis* 124:125-134 (Aug) 1956.

8. Critchley, M.: Jacksonian Ideas and the Future, With Special Reference to Aphasia, *Brit Med J* 2:6-12 (July 2) 1960.

9. Jasper, H.H.: Evolution of Conceptions of Cerebral Localization Since Hughlings Jackson, *World Neurol* 1:97-112 (Aug) 1960.

10. Walshe, F.M.R.: Contributions of John Hughlings Jackson to Neurology: A Brief Introduction to His Teachings, *Arch Neurol* 5:119-131 (Aug) 1961.

11. Levin, M.: Our Debt to Hughlings Jackson, *JAMA* 191:991-996 (March 22) 1965.

12. Riese, W.: The Sources of Hughlings Jackson's View on Aphasia, *Brain* 88:811-822 (Nov) 1965.

13. Maurice-Williams, R.S.: The Achievement of Hughlings Jackson, *St. Thomas Hosp Gazette* 65:43-51, 1967.

14. Riese, W.: Changing Concepts of Cerebral Localization, *Clio Medica* 2:189-230 (Aug) 1967.

15. Clarke, E., and O'Malley, C.D.: *The Human Brain and Spinal Cord: A Historical Study Illustrated by Writings From Antiquity to the Twentieth Century*, Berkeley, Calif: University of California Press, 1968, pp 499-505.

16. McHenry, L.C., Jr.: *Garrison's History of Neurology: Revised and Enlarged With a Bibliography of Classical, Original and Standard Works in Neurology*, Springfield, Ill: Charles C Thomas, Publisher, 1969, pp 307-312.

17. Streeter, E.C.: A Note on the History of the Convulsive State Prior to Boerhaave, *Res Publ Assoc Nerv Ment Dis* 7:5-29, 1922.

18. Pirkner, E.H.: Epilepsy in the Light of History, *Ann Med Hist* 1:453-480 (July) 1929.

19. Kanner, L.: The Folklore and Cultural History of Epilepsy, *Med Life* 37:167-214 (April) 1930.

20. von Storch, T.C.: An Essay on the History of Epilepsy, *Ann Med Hist* 2:614-650 (Nov) 1930.

21. Jefferson, G.: Jacksonian Epilepsy: A Background and a Postscript, *Postgrad Med J* 11:150-162 (April) 1935.

22. Temkin, O.: *The Falling Sickness. A History of Epilepsy From the Greeks to the Beginnings of Modern Neurology*, Baltimore: Johns Hopkins Press, 1945, pp 288-323.

23. Lennox, W.G.: "Epilepsy," in Bett, W.R. (ed.): *The History and Conquest of Common Diseases*, Norman, Okla: University of Oklahoma Press, 1954, pp 243-259.

24. Penfield, W., and Jasper, H.: *Epilepsy and the Functional Anatomy of the Human Brain*, Boston: Little, Brown & Co., 1954, pp 3-19.

25. Fulton, J.F.: History of Focal Epilepsy, *Int J Neurol* 1:21-33 (Dec) 1959.

26. Bravais, L.F.: *Recherches sur les symptômes et le traitement de l' épilepsie hémiplégique; Thèse*, Paris: Faculté de Médecine de Paris, 1827.

27. Gibson, W.C.: *Young Endeavor: Contributions to Science by Medical Students of the Past Four Centuries*. Springfield, Ill: Charles C Thomas, Publisher, 1958, p 187.

28. Wilkins, R.H.: Neurosurgical Classic—XII. *J Neurosurg* 20:904-916 (Oct) 1963.

29. Collier, J.: Inventions and the Outlook in Neurology, *Lancet* 2:855-859 (Oct 20) 1934.

30. McIntyre, N.: Robert Bentley Todd, 1809-1860, *King's Coll Hosp Gazette* 35:79-91, 184-198, 1956.

31. Todd, R.B.: *Clinical Lectures on Paralysis, Certain Diseases of the Brain, and Other Affections of the Nervous System*, ed 2, London: John Churchill, 1856, pp 284-307.

32. Robertson, A.: On Unilateral Convulsions, Localization, etc., *Edinburgh Med J* 15:513-523 (Dec) 1869.

33. Jefferson, G.: The Prodromes to Cortical Localization, *J Neurol Neurosurg Psychiat* 16:59-72 (May) 1953.

34. Barrows, H.S.: Neurological Eponyms, *Arch Neurol* 3:91-97 (July) 1960.

35. Brazier, M.A.B.: "The Historical Development of Neurophysiology," in Field, J.; Magoun, H.W.; and Hall, V.E. (eds.): *Handbook of Physiology: A Critical, Comprehensive Presentation of Physiological Knowledge and Concepts*, Washington, D.C.: American Physiological Society, section 1, volume 1, 1959, pp 1-58.

36. Brazier, M.A.B.: The EEG in Epilepsy: A Historical Note, *Epilepsia* 1:328-336 (June) 1960.

37. Wilkins, R.H.: Neurosurgical Classic—I, *J Neurosurg* 19:700-710 (Aug) 1962.

38. Wilkins, R.H.: Neurosurgical Classics—II, *J Neurosurg* 19:801-805 (Sept) 1962.

39. Wilkins, R.H.: Neurosurgical Classics—XXII, *J Neurosurg* 21:724-733 (Aug) 1964.

A STUDY OF CONVULSIONS.*

By J. Hughlings Jackson, M.D., F.R.C.P.

A convulsion is but a symptom, and implies only that there is an occasional, an excessive, and a disorderly discharge of nerve tissue on muscles. This discharge occurs in all degrees; it occurs with all sorts of conditions of ill health, at all ages, and under innumerable circumstances. But in this article I shall narrow my task to the description of one class of *chronic* convulsive seizures. The great majority of chronic convulsions may be arranged in two classes.

*Reprinted from *Transactions of the Saint Andrews Medical Graduates Association* 3:162-204, 1870.

1. Those in which the spasm affects both sides of the body almost contemporaneously. In these cases there is either no warning, or a very general one, such as a sensation at or about the epigastrium, or an indescribable feeling in the head. These cases are usually called epileptic, and sometimes cases of "genuine" or "idiopathic" epilepsy.

2. Those in which the fit begins by deliberate spasm on one side of the body, and in which parts of the body are affected one after another.

It is with the second class only that I intend to deal in this article.

But although I thus limit myself to one class of cases, I contend that the title of my article is correct.* I trust I am studying the general subject of convulsion methodically when I work at the simplest varieties of occasional spasm I can find. Cases of unilateral convulsions are unquestionably the simplest. We can, when we are luckily present at a paroxysm, watch the march of the spasm. I have known a fit of this kind last ten minutes. . . . For instance, we may first see movement of the index finger, then of the hand, then of the whole arm, then of the face, leg, &c. Besides, patients can describe the onset and much of the march of such seizures. We can therefore compare and contrast these convulsions with hemiplegia— which form of palsy the convulsion not unfrequently leaves. In some of these cases we find *gross* disease of the brain . . . *post-mortem*, and thus we can infer the seat of the minute changes on which the discharge producing the spasm was dependent. This done, we have, . . . on the one hand a record of the events occurring in a certain kind of convulsion, and on the other hand a knowledge of the internal part diseased. We are freed, therefore, from the great vagueness of the word "epilepsy." We do not care to say that a tumour of the brain (or minute changes near it) had "caused epilepsy," but that changes in a particular region of the nervous system—say in the region of the left middle cerebral artery—led to convulsions, in which the spasm began in the right hand, spread to the arm, attacked next the face, then the leg, &c.

I chiefly wish to show in this article that the most common variety of hemispasm is a symptom of disease of the same region of the brain as in the symptom hemiplegia; *viz.* the "region of the corpus striatum." The loose term "region of the corpus striatum" is advisedly used. Hemiplegia shows damage (equivalent to destruction) of the motor tract, hemispasm shows damage (equivalent to changes of instability) of the convolutions which discharge through it. Palsy depends on destruction* of *fibres,* and convulsion on instability of *grey matter.* As the convolutions are rich in grey matter I suppose them to be to blame, in *severe* convulsions at all events; but as the corpus striatum also contains much grey matter I cannot deny that it may be sometimes the part to blame

in slighter convulsions. Indeed if the discharge does begin in convolutions, no doubt the grey matter of lower motor centres, even if these centres be healthy, will be discharged secondarily by the violent impulse received from the primary discharge. Now both these parts—the corpus striatum and many convolutions—are supplied by one artery, the middle cerebral or Sylvian, and this artery circumscribes the region I speak of. . . .

The muscles which suffer most are those which can act independently of their fellows of the opposite side. Those which must act along with their fellows of the other side—for instance the intercostals—do not suffer at all; and those which are, so to speak, half way in their action—*e.g.* muscles which turn the two eyes and the head to one side—suffer only in very large lesions, and then but for a short time, a few hours or days. It is but putting these facts in another way to say that parts suffer directly as the actions they engage in are voluntary, and inversely as the action they engage in are automatic. This is seen in the order of recovery. The muscles serving in the more automatic actions recover first. Now just the same principle applies to cases of hemispasm, so far as this at least, that the fit begins most frequently in those parts which suffer most in hemiplegia. This point is now to be considered in some detail.

Fits beginning unilaterally may doubtless begin by movement in any part of the region which is paralysed in hemiplegia, *i.e.* in the face, in the arm, or in the leg. But I know few cases of fits of this class which begin other than in the side of the face, (usually the cheek), in the hand, or in the foot. They very rarely begin in the upper arm, or in the calf. The fit usually begins, it is to be observed, in that part of the face, of the arm, and of the leg, which has *the most varied uses.* . . . Fits beginning in the hand are common, fits beginning in the cheek and tongue are less frequent, fits beginning in the foot are rare . . . . the fits which begin in the hand begin usually in the index finger and thumb; fits which begin in the foot begin usually in the great toe. . . .

---

*Those who say that the two classes differ "only in degree," make a remark the truth of which is admitted. . . . My speculation is that the first class differs from the second in that convolutions at a greater distance from the motor tract are discharged.

*The word "destruction" is scarcely the correct word to use. By it is not meant that the nerve fibres are necessarily broken up, although they often are in palsy, but simply that there is a change in them which *destroys their function.* Thus, . . . palsy is supposed to follow a convulsion because the axis cylinder of the nerve fibre has temporarily lost its function, from the effects of the excessive quantity of nerve force it has had to "carry." Here the nerve fibres are not physically destroyed, since the palsy quickly passes off. With this qualification the word destruction may conveniently be used.

Parts which have the most varied uses will be represented in the central nervous system by most ganglion* cells. I say most *varied* movements, as it is not only a question of number of movements, but also of number of *different* movements.

We shall speak of three varieties of convulsions beginning unilaterally:—

1. Those beginning in the hand.
2. Those beginning in the face and tongue.
3. Those beginning in the foot.

The seizures occur in all degrees. . . .

There are not merely degrees of more or less *quantity* of spasm. The point of significance is that the spasmodic movements are not contemporaneous, but follow a distinct march, and a different march according as the spasm begins in the hand or in the foot. The sequence is, however, not simple. The spasm does not affect the arm, then cease, next affect the face, &c. It is a *compound sequence*. For instance, the face begins to be affected before the spasm of the arm ceases.

When observing the paroxysms we have therefore to note two things.

First, the region affected; for instance, we say the face, arm, and leg of one side are in spasm.

Secondly, the order in which parts are involved; for instance, we say the spasm began in the hand, passed up the arm, then attacked the face and lastly went down the leg—"out at the toes," one of my patients said. . . .

REMARKS ON EPILEPTIC HEMIPLEGIA.

The cases I am describing are those cases of chronic convulsions which are so often followed by hemiplegia. It is the epileptic hemiplegia of Dr. Todd. I do not know how it is that some patients have no palsy after these seizures, and some have. The same patient is hemiplegic after some of his seizures, and not after others. The presumption is that the degree of palsy depends on the severity of the convulsions, *i.e.* on the *quantity* of discharge. When the convulsion is limited in range, the palsy left by it is limited in range. . . . I have recorded a case ("Medical Mirror," September 1869), in which palsy of the arm only followed a convulsive seizure—the spasm, according to the patient, being limited to that limb. In this case, there was a new growth in the hemisphere in the hinder part of the superior frontal convolution. . . . When the fit is severe, there may be hemiplegia complete in range, except perhaps for deviation of the head and eyes. But the hemiplegia, however complete in range, and however decided in degree, is transitory, and we may very safely tell our patient that it will pass off in a few days or weeks, and we may usually say so when we feel certain that the fits are the result of organic disease in the head. The palsy does not depend directly on the organic disease . . . but is doubtless the result of "overwork" of the nerve fibres which pass from the part discharged to the muscles convulsed. The nerves and the muscles require time to recover from the effects of the sudden and excessive discharge.

But although we can assure our patient that his palsy will pass off, we shall be obliged to confess that both his fits and the palsy will *probably* return again and again.

It is not said that hemiplegia after a convulsion is transitory, but that hemiplegia after a convulsion deliberately beginning unilaterally is transitory. Hemiplegia after a convulsion may signify large cerebral haemorrhage destroying the motor tract, and then the palsy is permanent, or it may signify plugging of the middle cerebral artery. . . .

ARREST OF FITS BY THE LIGATURE.

. . . . There can be no question that the ligature is a most valuable means of arresting such fits. I have known very great success from this procedure in Brown Séquard's practice, and also from another plan he adopted, founded on the same principle, viz., circular blisters—a garter of blister round the limb.* Probably the ligature, &c., merely put off the explosions; and patients the subjects of this, as of other varieties of fits, very often say that they feel better *after* a seizure—after a full discharge of that part of the nervous system which is unstable. It indeed occasionally happens that an epileptic complains more to his doctor when his fits are diminished in number. It may be that when his serious troubles are lessened, he thinks of the smaller ones. But I suppose that before the abrupt explosion which constitutes the severe fit there are frequent minute discharges—too trivial to produce any visible effects, but enough to cause discomfort to the patient. Never-

---

*Although both the nerve fibre (axis cylinder) and the ganglion cell "store up force," it is the latter which stores it up in large quantity, and to instability of grey matter, therefore, will be chiefly owing the excessive discharges in convulsions. . . .

*Pulling against the spasm, *e.g.*, opening the clenching hand, will sometimes put off the fits. In other kinds of seizures, when the fit begins by a general warning of confusion in the head, the patients can shake them off by walking about, stamping, &c. . . .

theless it is a gain to put off the fit—to save the patient from the *effects* of the discharge, especially to save him from the sudden violent stoppage of respiration and its secondary effects on the circulation in the head. . . .

I presume that the first outward spasm is the result of the beginning of the internal discharge. It is an interesting question how the sensation which so often precedes the spasm is related to the seizure, and how the ligature averts the seizure. . . .

ABSENCE OF INSENSIBILITY IN CONVULSIONS.

. . . . I shall now speak only of the absence of insensibility in the seizures. These are the very cases of convulsions in which so often there is no loss of consciousness. As before said, these seizures occur in all degrees, and when they are partial the patient may be conscious, although sometimes speechless, throughout. So far as I can ascertain, the rule is, that (when the fit begins in the hand) consciousness is lost as soon as, or just before, the leg is seized, but sometimes the whole side may be affected, and even, I believe, the thoracic muscles slightly, without any loss of consciousness. It has been said by the late Dr. Addison, of Guy's, that absence of insensibility in convulsions is some evidence that the internal lesion is organic, such for instance as tumour. I have had no autopsy in any case of the class of fits which I describe in this paper in which I have not found organic disease. For all that, I cannot hold the opinion which this great physician has expressed. *Such convulsions point only to minute changes involving instability in the opposite hemisphere.* If the reader will not admit this, it suffices for the present argument to say that they point only to *local* changes of instability. They tell us nothing of the pathological processes by which that local instability results. . . . To tell whether the changes are diffused from a foreign body, such as a syphilitic lump, a tumour, &c., we have to consider a very different kind of evidence. . . . If the patient have severe pain in the head—not the mere sequel of a convulsion,—if he have vomiting, above all if he have double optic neuritis, I should then think it probable that the convulsion depended on changes diffused from a foreign body in the brain. If he have no such symptoms, I should suppose the local change was not diffused from a foreign body.

Patients with minute local lesions of the brain are not likely to die under our care. A patient with a foreign body in his brain very often dies under our care. Partial fits—fits without insensibil-

ity—very often occur without symptoms implying a foreign body, and I can therefore place no value on absence of insensibility in such seizures towards the diagnosis of organic disease. If we work in the wards of a hospital only, where we find patients who are admitted for *severe* intracranial disease, we shall be misled. We must work also in the out-patient room, where we see patients year after year with fits of the kind above mentioned, and without any symptoms to lead us to suppose that there is "coarse" disease of the brain. . . .

CONVULSIONS BEGINNING IN THE FOOT.

The next group is of cases in which the spasm begins in the leg, and it usually begins in the great toe. Sometimes, however, the patient will say it starts from the calf. I shall relate no cases of this kind.* They are rare, and I have never witnessed a paroxysm. The point of great interest is the march of the spasm. Fits which begin in the foot have a different march from those which begin in the hand, although in each the same muscles are ultimately convulsed. When a fit begins in the hand it goes *up* the arm and *down* the leg. . . . Now patients who have fits beginning in the foot tell me that the spasm goes *up* the leg and *down* the arm. . . . Here we have two seizures, in each of which the same muscles are engaged, but in each in different order. The two sorts of fits are "isomeric." Another matter to observe is the kind of hemiplegia which follows fits beginning in the leg. This is a rare sequel of such fits, and I have no notes of any such cases. The leg is often partially paralysed for a time after fits so beginning, but of the condition of the arm and face I can say nothing. On these points I ask information.

Again, I have had no *post-mortem* examination of a patient who had had fits beginning in the foot, and I am very anxious to learn where lies the disease which causes such seizures. . . .

THE CAUSE OF CONVULSIONS BEGINNING UNILATERALLY.

We now come to the question of cause. The word "cause" is used in various senses in medical language, and we shall therefore discuss the following points. . . .

1.—*The seat of the internal lesion.* The fact that the symptoms are local, implies, I hold, that there *is* of necessity a *local* lesion. I submit that

---

*I have recorded a very striking case, ("Lancet," May 16, 1868), in which fits beginning in the great toe were stopped by rubbing the calf, &c.

one-sided spasm, or spasm beginning in one side, implies *local* change in the central nervous system as surely as one-sided palsy does. . . .

Let us suppose that a square inch of convolution is diseased. If this part were destroyed, there need be no symptoms; but if it be not destroyed, but unstable, there must be symptoms—for it will *discharge* on muscles when its tension reaches to unstable equilibrium. . . .

And even in those cases where we *do* find a lump in the brain . . . we do not discover the *very* changes on which the discharge depends. The lump does not discharge, but some ("softened") part of the brain near it—which part cannot be destroyed or it would not discharge at all, but which part must be diseased or it would not discharge so much, nor in so disorderly a manner, nor on slight provocation. . . .

It is held by some that the coarse disease, although it lies in the cerebral hemisphere, is quite as much an *eccentric* cause of a fit, as is a worm in the duodenum; and that in both the medulla oblongata and pons are the centres which discharge. (I do not deny that grey matter in these parts is *secondarily* discharged.) When we consider that the hemiplegia left by the fits I describe is like that following *destroying* lesions in the Sylvian region, and is not like that following destroying lesions in the pons or medulla oblongata, it becomes, I submit, infinitely more probable that the primary discharge is of grey matter in the region (Sylvian) in which the coarse disease is discovered. . . .

2.—The functional nature of the change in nerve tissue.

. . . . if I am told that hemispasm is "only a symptom," and may depend on "many causes," I admit it in the sense that various pathological processes may lead to that instability of nerve tissue which permits an occasional excessive discharge on muscles; but *from the point of view of function* there is but one cause of convulsion, *viz.*, instability of nerve tissue. Of course there will be varieties of range of convulsion, degrees of instability, degrees of quantity of nerve tissue unstable, and, more important than all, degrees of evolution of the nervous processes (nearer to and further from the motor tract) which the pathological change renders unstable.

3.—The pathological processes. . . .

(a) *Embolism.*—It is not very uncommon to find when a patient has recovered or is recovering from hemiplegia, the result of embolism of the middle cerebral artery, or of some branch of this

vessel, that he is attacked by convulsion beginning in some part of the paralysed region, almost always, I believe, the face or the hand. I have not, however, yet made a *post-mortem* examination on a patient whom I knew to have had fits *of this kind* after supposed embolism. It will be safer, then, to say that such seizures occur in patients who have recovered partially, or seemingly entirely, from hemiplegia occurring with heart disease, or with the parturient state. . . .

(b) *Coarse Disease.*—. . . It is admitted that it may be of any kind, but it so happens that in nearly all the chronic cases on which I have had autopsies, the examination has revealed *syphilitic* disease of the hemisphere. The foreign body has been a syphilitic nodule. . . .

4.—Circumstances which determine the paroxysm.

Many things may discharge nerve tissue. . . . But I speak here only of chronic cases in which there is a persistent local lesion and an occasional discharge.

I think . . . that there are two factors in the production of a paroxysm—1st, Permanent local instability; 2ndly, Something which determines the discharge of the part unstable.

The part unstable "stores up" force, and when it reaches a certain degree of instability discharge of it is easily provoked. It may be that when by continuous nutrition it has risen to a certain degree of instability—it explodes, either "spontaneously," or in some normal periodical change in the body, or in some abnormal disturbance, the result for instance of fright. . . . It falls then to a state of stable equilibrium, and once more by continouous nutrition rises to its former undue instability, when another explosion can occur. It is in short an exaltation of ordinary nutrition and function. I suppose that the provoking agents may be various—that many things will upset the equilibrium of the highly unstable nerve tissue. . . .

All these general causes, I presume, act by altering the circulation in the head, during which alteration the equilibrium of the unstable patch is upset. . . .

The usually accepted theory of the production of the paroxysm is that it is determined by contraction of arteries. (Brown-Séquard.) I have advanced the speculation that . . . the *liability* to the convulsions which I have described in this paper—those at least beginning in the hand—is due to persistent changes in the region of the middle cerebral artery, and that the *paroxysm* itself is owing to a *local* vascular contraction. . . .

XXIX Wernicke's Sensory Aphasia

oretical possibilities. Of the ten cases he presented, only four had autopsy examinations, and the lesions involved relatively large areas. Furthermore, the illustrations in Wernicke's monograph depicted the right side of the brain; he did not stress the importance of the left cerebral hemisphere, though all four of his patients examined postmortem had left-sided lesions.

Despite these inadequacies, some of Wernicke's deductions have proven correct. Subsequent studies have demonstrated that lesions in the posterior half of the left superior temporal gyrus and the adjacent part of the middle temporal gyrus (Wernicke's area) may give rise to a receptive dysphasia characterized by defective comprehension of spoken words, voluble but incorrect speech (jargon dysphasia), dysgraphia, and dyslexia.[11] The syndrome is now known as Wernicke's sensory aphasia, in honor of the man who first brought it to the attention of the medical world. Though the subject of aphasia is more complex than Wernicke envisioned, he shares with Broca the distinction of providing the first anatomical framework for our present knowledge of aphasia.[3,12-18]

I N THE Edwin Smith Surgical Papyrus, dating from the 17th century BC, an association was noted between temporal skull trauma and loss of speech.[1] Nevertheless, before the work of Broca, the brain was generally thought to act as a whole, with no anatomical localization of the different cerebral functions.[2,3] In 1861, Paul Broca presented two cases of dysphasia associated with lesions in the posterior portions of the second and third left frontal convolutions.[4,5] Although Broca underestimated the extent of the lesions in his first patient, his provocative presentations provided an early anatomical localization for the expressive aspects of speech.[3]

In 1874, the German neuropsychiatrist, Carl Wernicke (1848 to 1905),[6-9] published a short monograph in which he used simple anatomical diagrams to present a more comprehensive view of speech mechanisms.[10] Wernicke described five clinical syndromes that would be expected from lesions of (1) the afferent auditory pathways, (2) the speech reception center, (3) the association tracts between the speech reception and speech expression centers, (4) the speech expression center, and (5) the efferent speech pathways. However, he provided little pathological documentation of these the

References

1. Wilkins RH: Neurosurgical classic—XVII. *J Neurosurg* 21:240-244, 1964.
2. Wilkins RH: Neurosurgical classic—XII. *J Neurosurg* 20:904-916, 1963.
3. Wilkins RH: Neurosurgical classic—XIX. *J Neurosurg* 21:424-431, 1964.
4. Broca P: Perte de la parole, ramollisement chronique et destruction partielle du lobe antérieur gauche du cerveau. *Bull Soc Anthrop Paris* 2:235-238, 1861.
5. Broca P: Nouvelle observation d'aphémie produite par une lésion de la moitié postérieure des deuxiéme et troisième circonvolutions frontales. *Bull Soc Anat Paris* 6:398-407, 1861.
6. Goldstein K: Carl Wernicke (1848-1905), in Haymaker W (ed): *The Founders of Neurology.* Springfield, Ill, Charles C Thomas Publisher, 1953, pp 406-409.
7. Kleist K: Carl Wernicke (1848-1905), in Kolle K (ed): *Grosse Nervenärzte.* Stuttgart, Georg Thieme, 1959, vol 2, pp 106-128.

8. Hill D: The bridge between neurology and psychiatry. *Lancet* 1:509-514, 1964.

9. Brody IA, Wilkins RH: Neurological classics IX: Wernicke's encephalopathy. *Arch Neurol* 19:228-232, 1968.

10. Wernicke C: *Der aphasische Symptomencomplex: Eine psychologische Studie auf anatomischer Basis*. Breslau, Max Cohn & Weigert, 1874.

11. Wernicke C: The symptom-complex of aphasia, in Church A (ed): *Diseases of the Nervous System*. New York, D. Appleton and Co, 1908, pp 265-324.

12. Head H: Aphasia: An historical review (The Hughlings Jackson lecture for 1920). *Brain* 43:390-411, 1920.

13. Weisenburg T, McBride KE: *Aphasia: A Clinical and Psychological Study*. New York, The Commonwealth Fund, 1935, pp 6-27.

14. Nielsen JM: *Agnosia, Apraxia, Aphasia: Their Value in Cerebral Localization*, ed 2. New York, Paul B Hoeber Inc, 1946, pp 1-14.

15. Penfield W, Roberts L: *Speech and Brain Mechanisms*. Princeton, NJ, Princeton University Press, 1959, pp 56-81.

16. Brain R: *Speech Disorders: Aphasia, Apraxia and Agnosia*. London, Butterworth & Co Ltd, 1961, pp 30-53.

17. Leonhard K: Hatte Wernicke mit seiner lokalisationslehre unrecht? *J Neurol Sci* 3:434-438, 1966.

18. Marx OM: Aphasia studies and language theory in the 19th century. *Bull Hist Med* 40:328-349, 1966.

THE APHASIC SYMPTOM-COMPLEX

A Psychological Study on an Anatomical Basis*

by

Dr. C. Wernicke

. . . . That destruction of Broca's area causes aphasia appears to be established beyond doubt through such cases as the striking one of Simon, which actually resembled an experiment. However, other conscientious and experienced observers are also correct in insisting that Broca's area is not the only speech center, and that circumscribed lesions in the region of the Sylvian fissure can produce aphasia.

We may now ask what lies near the Sylvian fissure, and we note a gyrus on the convex surface of the cerebrum, running in a curve directed posteriorly and superiorly, almost enclosing the Sylvian fissure. From the central sulcus it runs anteriorly in a distinct longitudinal tract, the . . . first frontal gyrus. Its posterior peduncle is in the first temporal gyrus, just clearly discernible as the longitudinal tract. That the whole is to be considered as one gyrus is clear from comparison with the brains of animals, such as dogs. Comparative anatomy indicates . . . that the gyri describe a curve around the Sylvian fissure with the convexity toward the occiput and with two peduncles running more or less parallel to the Sylvian fissure in the frontal and temporal portions of the brain.

. . . . The whole area of the convolution encircling the Sylvian fissure, in association with the

*Translation of *Der aphasische Symptomencomplex: Eine Psychologische Studie auf anatomischer Basis*. Breslau, Max Cohn & Weigert, 1874, pp 15, 16, 18, 19, 21, 22, 24, 25, 43-45.

cortex of the insula, serves as a speech center. The first frontal gyrus, being motor, is the center for representation of movement, and the first temporal gyrus, being sensory, is the center for word-images. The fibrae propriae, which are confluent in the insular cortex, form the connecting psychic reflex arc. The first temporal gyrus consequently should be considered as the central end of the auditory nerve, and the first frontal gyrus (including Broca's area) as the central end of the nerves to the speech muscles.

[Figure 3]

Let F be the frontal, O the occipital, and T the temporal end of a schematically drawn brain. C is the central fissure; around the Sylvian fissure (S) extends the first primitive convolution. Within this convolution, a_1 is the central end of the acoustic nerve, a its site of entry into the medulla oblongata; b designates the representation of movements governing sound production, and is connected with the preceding through the association fibers a_1 b running in the cortex of the insula. From b the efferent pathways of the sound-producing motor nerves run to the oblongata and exit there for the most part (the accessory and the phrenic nerves extend still further caudally).

Aphasia can result from any interruption of the path a a_1 b b_1. The clinical picture will depend upon the segment of the path involved . . . .

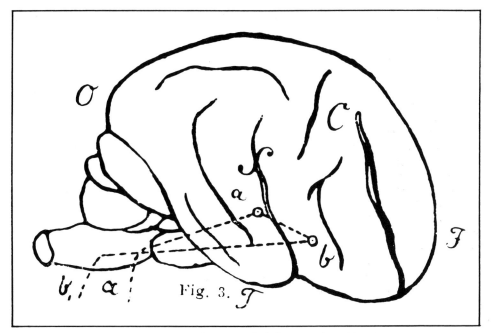

Fig. 3 [The speech areas and their connections. The "a"
near the Sylvian fissure should have been designated "a₁".]

II. A lesion may affect the center for word-images itself, a_1. This locus is not identical with the
central projection area of the acoustic nerve since
aphasia with complete loss of word-images has
been reported to occur in the presence of retained
hearing on both sides . . . .

Destruction of a_1, the cortex of the first temporal gyrus, leads to loss of memory for the sound-
images of the names of objects, while the concept
may persist in complete clarity. For the sound-im-
age of the name is usually incidental to the
concept of an object, while the feeling and tactile
images are essential to it. Impairments of the
visual and tactile images (Finkelnburg's asymbol-
ia) are thus not to be ascribed to a disturbance of
speech but to disturbance of the concept, consequently of the intelligence . . . .

Clearly, the preservation of the circuit a_1 b is
worthless once the word-images are lost. The
production of words is no longer initiated by
word-images. Moreover, the path is cut which
connects the sound that is heard with the remaining sensory image of an object (association fibers
running from the first temporal gyrus to the other
sensory areas of the occipital and temporal lobes).
The patient, therefore, cannot repeat the spoken
word—for that is indeed the particular function
of the path a a_1 b b_1—nor can he understand the
spoken word. Speech becomes a confused noise

devoid of sense—or at best a strange language, the
individual sounds of which he perceives and gradually learns to understand again.

There still remains a path by which speech
movements can be initiated. The patient with the
condition outlined has no disturbance of intelligence; he proves through his behaviour and
through his intelligent comprehension of signs
and gestures that the sensory images of the objects
surrounding him, as well as their concepts, remain
intact . . . .

The intensity of the symptoms varies with the
severity and extent of the disease process affecting
the first temporal gyrus. In the severe form, involving loss of word images of discrete objects
and actions as well as of the conjunctions necessary to form sentences, etc., the diagnosis will
depend on only two features; namely, the abundance of spoken words and the defect in understanding what is heard. That such obvious abnormalities have not been observed till now, or at
least have not been published, is attributable to
the rarity of the cases and to the fact that experienced and intelligent physicians have considered
this condition to be dementia . . . .

There are moderate degrees of the illness, in
which the important structural elements of sentences are retained and the general meaning of a
question can be properly conceived. The presence

of this defect must be established through suggestive questions. If the patient, for example, when asked: Is that a glass?, does not decide immediately but vacillates, considers, and finally utters a doubtful "yes" or "no", then he belongs in this category.

The following points deserve to be emphasized:

1. Partial lesions of the sensory speech center will limit the patient to a definite vocabulary, both in speaking and in hearing. This vocabulary can be ascertained through suggestive questions, but it requires a difficult and lengthy examination.

2. A large vocabulary is a prime feature of sensory aphasia. Conditions in which only a few simple words are retained always belong to the motor form of aphasia . . . .

3. There is no trace of hemiplegia.

4. There is agraphia. Writing is a conscious movement, learned with the most intimate dependence on sound and always executed under the guidance of it . . . . In cases of partial sensory aphasia, a partial agraphia may also be expected.

5. The situation is entirely different with respect to understanding written or printed characters . . . . The uneducated, slightly literate man understands what is written only when he hears it spoken. The educated man, accustomed to reading from early childhood, skims over a page and understands its meaning without being conscious of the wording. The former will show symptoms of alexia in addition to aphasia, but the latter, in marked contrast to his inability to understand what is spoken, will grasp everything written. On the other hand, he will be just as aphasic in reading aloud as in spontaneous speech.

Agraphia as well as alexia are caused by disease in an entirely different region; namely, in the visual cortex, for the visual memory of the characters is as indispensable for writing as for reading. . . .

Case 2

Susanne Rother, 75 years old, wife of a porter, was admitted to All-Saints' Hospital on 7 October 1873. She showed signs of marked senility and advanced atherosclerosis of all accessible vessels, and she had an expression of suffering . . . . She could walk only with assistance because of generalized weakness and a feeling of dizziness . . . . She usually lay moaning in bed, wrapped up deep in the covers; she was incontinent of feces and urine.

Her psychic state was considered at that time to be confusion, complicated by aphasia. She answered questions absurdly and failed to follow instructions, or else turned them around, thus giving the impression of apraxia.

In view of her failure to understand, the nurses believed she was deaf. She paid little attention to her surroundings and showed little need to communicate. Her spontaneous vocabulary seemed limited, but was still large enough that a motor aphasia could not be considered. The aphasia was recognizable in the confusions and distortions of the words she used. Thus, she very often said correctly: "I thank you right heartily" or "I thank you very much" etc. "I am very sick. Oh, I am so cold. You are a very good gentleman," were often used expressions. The physician, whom she had just called a good gentleman, she then would call "my little daughter" or "my little son," both in the same sense . . . .

Sensation appeared intact. The grasp was weak but equal on both sides. More exact examination of sensation and motor function was not made. . . .

There was no improvement in the psychic or somatic symptoms.

Death came on 1 December 1874 after a protracted intestinal catarrh, associated with vomiting and deep prostration during the last two days.

The history yielded that . . . the confused speech had appeared suddenly on 2 November 1873 . . . .

Autopsy revealed edema of the pia and slight internal hydrocephalus. The convolutions of both hemispheres and both insular regions were shrunken and atrophic throughout. Furthermore, all cerebral arteries showed atheromatous degeneration to an extreme degree. The branch of the artery of the left Sylvian fissure, running down into the inferior sulcus of Burdach, was occluded by a thrombus tightly adherent to the wall. The entire first temporal gyrus, including its junction with the second temporal gyrus and the origin of the latter from Bischof's inferior parietal lobule, were converted into a yellowish-white brei, to which opacified pia was tightly adherent. The connections of the temporal lobe into the insula were for the most part destroyed in the softened places. The insula itself and the brain stem ganglia showed no changes. The focus of softening was not bounded by inflammatory hardening but passed over directly into normal consistency . . . .

XXX Wallenberg's Syndrome

THE SYNDROME caused by infarction of the posterolateral portion of the medulla oblongata (the lateral medullary plate) is one of the most characteristic of the neurological syndromes following arterial occlusion. It was encountered occasionally by physicians over the years,[1] but its existence was firmly established in 1895 by Adolf Wallenberg (1862 to 1949), who published a detailed clinical report of a single case.[2]

Wallenberg was a physician and neuroanatomist of Danzig who fled Nazi persecution and spent his last years in the United States.[3] His expert knowledge of neuroanatomy, based in part on original research, permitted him to make sense of his patient's many symptoms and signs. He deduced the location of the infarct and postulated that it was caused by occlusion of the ipsilateral posterior inferior cerebellar artery. Furthermore, he reviewed several reports of similar cases and described the clinical picture common to all. His patient died in 1899, and Wallenberg verified the suspected arterial occlusion and medullary infarction at postmortem examination.[4]

Although Wallenberg thought the syndrome was due to embolization of the posterior inferior cerebellar artery, the most common cause is now known to be thrombosis of the vertebral artery.[5,6] Furthermore, a preexisting ocular lesion in his patient prevented Wallenberg from noting the ipsilateral miosis that usually accompanies the syndrome. Nevertheless, our present delight in expounding the anatomy of the brain stem at the bedside of a patient with the lateral medullary syndrome is a tribute to the pioneering efforts of Adolf Wallenberg.

References

1. Romano J, Merritt HH: The singular affection of Gaspard Vieusseux: An early description of the lateral medullary syndrome. *Bull Hist Med* 9:72-79, 1941.
2. Wallenberg A: Acute Bulbäraffection (Embolie der Art. cerebellar. post. inf. sinistr. ?). *Arch Psychiat Nervenkr* 27:504-540, 1895.
3. Wallenberg-Chermak M: Adolf Wallenberg (1862-1949), in Kolle K (ed): *Grosse Nervenärzte.* Stuttgart, Georg Thieme, 1963, vol 3, pp 191-196.
4. Wallenberg A: Anatomischer Befund in einem als "acute Bulbär-affection (Embolie der Art. cerebellar. post. inf. sinistr. ?)" beschriebenen Falle. *Arch Psychiat Nervenkr* 34:923-959, 1901.
5. Fisher CM, Karnes WE, Kubik CS: Lateral medullary infarction—the pattern of vascular occlusion. *J Neuropath Exp Neurol* 20:323-379, 1961.
6. Currier RD, DeJong RN: The lateral medullary (Wallenberg's) syndrome. *Univ Mich Med Bull* 28:106-113, 1962.

Acute Bulbar Disturbance (*Embolus of the Left Posterior Inferior Cerebellar Artery?*) [1]

by Adolf Wallenberg

of Danzig

This case report of an acute lesion in the medulla oblongata requires some justification since my observations thus far have been only clinical. However, the characteristic clinical picture, which can be easily recognized by a group of striking symptoms, will provide a certain interest in the following case history. . . .

[The detailed case history is presented, and then the following recapitulation:]

A 38-year-old man, with poor vision caused by a preexisting ocular condition (cataract on the left side, corneal scarring and anterior synechia on the right side. . .). . . .suffered an attack of vertigo without loss of consciousness. At the same time he developed pain and hyperesthesia on the left side of the face and body, hypesthesia of the right half of the face, and loss of pain and temperature sensitivity in the right extremities and the right half of the torso, with retention of the sense of touch. There was paralysis of swallowing; impaired sensation on the mucosa of the mouth, throat and palate; disturbed motility of the soft palate (on the first day bilateral, later left-sided); total paralysis of the left recurrent laryngeal nerve, and paresis of the left hypoglossal muscle. . . , with no disturbance in the innervation of the facial muscles. He also had ataxia of the left extremities without impairment of gross strength, and he fell to the left side. . . .The pulse became slower (from 96 to 76-82).

During the ensuing days the sensitivity of the right half of the face returned to normal. The hyperesthesia of the left half of the body disappeared, and that of the left trigeminal region changed to anesthesia predominantly for pain and temperature (less for proprioceptive and electrocutaneous sensations), with suppression of the corneal and conjunctival reflexes. . . .The pulse quickened again, but the other disturbances remained. On the eighth day an herpetic eruption appeared on some of the analgesic areas: the left face (including the nasal mucosa; the sensitivity of the mouth and throat had returned), right shoulder, and right inguinal region. . . .

Two to three months after the attack, the patient's status was as follows:

a) Subjective symptoms

1. Vertigo and a sense of falling to the left.

2. Numbness on the left half of the face and the right half of the body.

3. Difficulty in swallowing (very slight).

4. Pain in the nape of the neck and occasionally in the left eye.

b) Objective signs

1. Unsteadiness of gait, with veering toward the left.

2. Ataxia of the left extremities.

3. Paresis of the left half of the soft palate.

4. Paralysis of the left vocal cord; followed by paresis, suggesting atrophy.

5. Greater volume of the left half of the tongue while resting in the mouth.

6. Disturbance of sensation in the first and, to a lesser degree, in the second divisions of the left trigeminal nerve, especially affecting the eyes, eyelids, bridge of the nose and nasal mucosa. . . . The impairment mainly affects pain and temperature, but localization, electrocutaneous and pressure sensations are also involved to some extent.

7. Absence of the left corneal and conjunctival reflexes.

8. Disturbance of pain and temperature sensitivity on the right side of the body. . . .

9. Slight alteration of the other sensations (i.e., localization, faradocutaneous and pressure sensations). . . .

In the following weeks, the difficulty swallowing, the falling to the left, and the ataxia gradually disappeared. The other phenomena. . .remained unchanged. . . .

The localization of the lesion in this case is not difficult, in my opinion. . . .The diagnosis can be made on a secure foundation in view of certain pathological and experimental research. I may add that the patient's ocular disorders prevented an examination of the pupillary reflexes. . . .

The paralysis of the vocal cord and the paresis of the tongue and palate on the left side strongly suggest a lesion of the left half of the medulla oblongata. . . .

Only a few root fibers (or nuclear cells) of the hypoglossus may be involved since the mobility of the tongue was completely unimpaired and the hypoglossus suffered only a loss of tone. The bulbar portion of the left accessory nucleus[2] must

[1]Translation of: Acute Bulbäraffection (Embolie der Art. cerebellar. post. inf. sinistr. ?), *Archiv für Psychiatrie und Nervenkrankheiten* 27:504-540, 1895.

be greatly affected in view of the paralysis of the vocal cord and the paresis of the velum. The extent to which the vagus and the glossopharyngeus are responsible for the weakness of the palate and the vocal cord is difficult to state, since the anatomical and physiological investigation of the innervation of the pharyngeal and palatal musculature is still incomplete. . . .The region of the acoustic and facial nerves does not fall within the area of the lesion. . . .We can therefore assume that the left half of the medulla oblongata is involved by the lesion, perhaps from the termination of the decussation of the pyramids to the emergence of the upper vagal or lower glossopharyngeal roots, and that the extent of the anatomical changes diminishes from below to above.

I have intentionally not mentioned the left trigeminal, because we can use its disturbance to establish not only the level of the lesion but also its location in cross-section. . . .

Beginning from the ventral surface of the medulla: the fibers of the pyramid must be essentially intact, for all movements were normal in strength and extent (although the ataxia of the left extremities might be influenced by a lesion of the still uncrossed pyramidal fibers of the left side). . . .

Very near the exit of the accessorius lies the lateral (direct) cerebellar tract. A separation of this into anterior and posterior portions has no great value for our purposes. Therefore I will limit myself to a search for symptoms which indicate a permanent or transient interruption of this path of conduction between the spinal cord and the vermis cerebelli. It can hardly be disputed any more that these fibers are related to muscle sense, and specifically to the coordination of the movements of the same side. . . .Thus, in our case, we can attribute the marked ataxia of the left extremities to a temporary affection of the left lateral cerebellar tract. . . .

Besides ataxia. . .our patient had a remarkable tendency to fall to the left, a sign that still could be demonstrated at a meeting of the Danzig Medical Society two months after the attack. This phenomenon can be explained, in my opinion, only by involvement of the left restiform body. . . .Accordingly, we are forced to the assumption that the rostral extent of the lesion is higher on the dorsolateral aspect of the medulla than on the ventral aspect. . . .This disturbance of movement, like the ataxia, later disappeared. Therefore the

lesion did not destroy this tract but only interfered with its conduction temporarily.

If we return to our cross-section and focus our attention medial to the fibers of the lateral cerebellar tract that are coursing to the restiform body, we come to the "ascending" tract[3] of the fifth nerve and its nucleus. . . .In our patient the affection of the trigeminal was confined to a large part of the first and a smaller part of the second divisions. The branch to the mucous membrane of the mouth was only transiently involved. The nasociliary nerve suffered the most. Pathological observations[4] and experimental research[5] make it apparent that the branches from the oral mucosa and gustatory nerves end in the caudal part of the ascending fifth nucleus, and that the branches of the third division radiate farther up in the nucleus than the branches of the first two divisions. . . .If we accept these results[6], then we postulate a lesion of the lower and middle part of the ascending tract including the nucleus. . . .This assumption agrees fully with the extent of the lesion that we inferred earlier. I leave undecided whether the more marked involvement of pain and temperature point to a particular part of the nucleus, in order not to lose myself in empty hypotheses. . . .

The predominant involvement of these sensory modalities on the right half of the body may help to localize the lesion. The fibers for pain and temperature sensation enter the posterior horn on the same side. Their central continuations cross (mainly in the white commissure), ascend in the anterior column[7] of the opposite side, move medially at the level of the decussation of the pyramids, and more superiorly lie lateral to the medial lemniscus. The latter is derived from the internal arcuate fibers, which proceed out of the nuclei of the opposite posterior funiculus. . . .The fibers mediating touch, position, and pressure radiate from the nuclei of the posterior funiculus, so we must expect to find them in the medial lemniscus. . . .The lesion we assume in the left half of the medulla oblongata must therefore involve the

---

[2]This portion of the accessory nucleus is now designated as the "nucleus ambiguus" — Translator.

[3]The "ascending" tract is now known to be "descending" — Translator.

[4]Eisenlohr, This Archiv, Vol. XIX, p. 314.

[5]E. Bregmann, Ueber experimentelle aufsteigende Degeneration motorischer und sensibler Hirnnerven. Jahrb. f. Psychiatrie, 1892, p. 88.

[6]To establish the localization of the corneal reflex, I have partly destroyed the "ascending" tract of the fifth nerve in the cervical spinal cord in rabbits and cats. These studies are still incomplete, but have already revealed that damage to the tract or nucleus at the level of the opening of the central canal can destroy the corneal reflex on the same side in the rabbit.

projection of the anterior column[8] in toto, while the medial lemniscus forms its medial boundary and suffers only slight damage. . . .

It appears certain that the internal arcuate fibers of the left side were injured on their way to the crossing of the lemniscus. . . .The relatively small number of these fibers explains the small extent of the tactile deficit on the left side of the neck and shoulder and on the dorsum of the foot. . . .

This presentation would be entirely theoretical were there not several cases in the literature with strikingly similar clinical findings, in whom a bulbar lesion could be demonstrated in the region indicated above. . . .

[Cases from the literature are then reviewed, and a common clinical syndrome and its variations are outlined.]

. . . .The absence of any disturbance of consciousness speaks against hemorrhage, as does the improvement of most of the focal signs. Furthermore, an intrabulbar hemorrhage is almost always fatal. A thrombosis appears to me very improbable in view of the sudden onset. On the other hand, an embolism with circumscribed softening would satisfactorily explain the symptoms and the course. Whether the embolus came from the heart, the great vessels, or the cerebral arteries themselves, I leave undecided. It is hardly possible to establish its place of origin; the place where it lodges interests us more.

To determine which vessel is involved, it is necessary to consult analogous cases in the literature. The vertebral or basilar arteries were implicated most often, but the obstruction was not always complete. Wernicke suspected (*op. cit.,* Vol. 2, p. 227), "that an area of softening in the lateral region of the medulla oblongata is always related to changes in the posterior inferior cerebellar artery or its branches." However, Wernicke did not go on to explain the reasons for his hypothesis. . . .

I will now state the results of my own research on the course and the ramifications of the posterior inferior cerebellar artery from seven injected brains. . . .These results form the basis of my attempt to explain the symptom complex in our case. If we postulate an occlusion of the left posterior inferior cerebellar artery where it comes off the vertebral (perhaps through an embolus at the point of division), . . .what will be the result? For the. . .pathological consequences of

this interruption of blood flow, it will be necessary to examine three separate areas:

1. The dorsomedial area, adjacent to the floor of the rhomboid fossa, is supplied mainly by the medial artery and the posterior spinal arteries. There are adequate collaterals from the vertebral . . .so that a circulatory disturbance here can be compensated immediately and thus gives rise only to transient symptoms: hyperesthesia of the left side of the body, slowing of the pulse, and anesthesia of the pharynx and palate. Also the areas adjacent to the occluded vessel will suffer only transient changes in blood flow. Therefore, we can explain the involvement of the right half of the face, and the initial spreading of disturbances in sensibility to all branches of the trigeminal on the left side. . . .The paralysis of swallowing, which lasts for a longer time and in which both sensory and motor disturbances play a part, forms the transition to the second group of phenomena.

2. A renewal of normal blood-flow to the dorsolateral area of the medulla oblongata and the cerebellum (restiform body, direct cerebellar pathway, etc.) is less likely. Here the existing anastomoses between the terminal branches of the cerebellar arteries must enlarge, permitting blood to travel retrograde in the posterior inferior cerebellar artery with adequate force up to the site of the embolus. The focal symptoms here are thus more lasting, especially the tendency to fall to the left, and the ataxia of the left extremities. . . .

3. From the first portion of the cerebellar artery arise a few hypoglossal twigs, which supply the upper accessory, the lower vagus roots and motor nucleus, the ascending 5th root and nucleus (predominantly the ventral part), and the structures adjacent to the 5th nucleus medially. . . . With the postulated arterial occlusion, a small focus of softening will be established inside this zone. . . .To this focus correspond the permanent signs, especially those associated with trophic disturbances: Anesthesia in the first and second branches of the left trigeminal, with herpetic eruption; analgesia and thermal anesthesia on the right side of the body, also with herpes; slight left-sided hypoglossal and palatal paralysis, and nearly total paralysis of the left vocal cord (with subsequent atrophy?). . . .

How far such theoretical hypotheses are justified can only be decided in the future through a careful collection of clinical and anatomical reports. The purpose of this work is to provide a clinical contribution.

Danzig, 21 March 1894.

---

[7]More accurately, the lateral column—Translator.

[8] The lateral spinothalamic tract—Translator.

XXXI Tuberous Sclerosis

A QUIRK of fate led Désiré Magliore Bourneville (1840 to 1909)[1] to discover the disease that now bears his name. In 1879, while substituting for his teacher, L. J. F. Delasiauve, Bourneville attended a child with psychomotor retardation, seizures, and an eruption over the nose and cheeks. After the patient's death from pneumonia, Bourneville found peculiar firm enlargements in the cerebral convolutions, which led him to call the disease tuberous sclerosis.

If Bourneville had procrastinated in reporting this case, his disease would not have been "new." Simultaneously and independently, Hartdegen[2] described the same condition in a newborn in Germany.

In addition to the cerebral lesions, Bourneville found several small renal tumors in his patient. However, only after he and other physicians reported additional cases did it become apparent that tuberous sclerosis is a dysgenetic syndrome, frequently familial, involving many organ systems throughout the body.[3-7]

The development of radiology has facilitated the recognition of this disease, since scattered areas of calcification are often seen within the substance of the brain. Although Bourneville's patient had normal ventricles, pneumoencephalography may demonstrate small nodules lining the ventricular walls, giving a characteristic appearance called "candle gutterings."

Bourneville later studied cretinism and mongolism and became an authority on the subject of mental retardation in children.[1] But he is best remembered for his initial chance encounter with tuberous sclerosis.

References

1. Benda CE: Désiré Magliore Bourneville (1840-1909), in Haymaker W (ed): *The Founders of Neurology.* Springfield, Ill, Charles C Thomas Publisher, 1953, pp 250-252.

2. Hartdegen A: Ein Fall von multipler Verhärtung des Grosshirns nebst histologisch eigenartigen harten Geschwülsten der Seitenventrikel ("Glioma gangliocellulare") bei einem Neugeborenen. *Arch Psychiat* 11:117-131, 1880.

3. Critchley M, Earl CJC: Tuberose sclerosis and allied conditions. *Brain* 55:311-346, 1932.

4. Borberg A: Clinical and genetic investigations into tuberous sclerosis and Recklinghausen's neurofibromatosis: Contribution to elucidation of interrelationship and eugenics of the syndromes. *Acta Psychiat Neurol Scand* 71(suppl):3-239, 1951.

5. Paulson GW, Lyle CB: Tuberous sclerosis. *Develop Med Child Neurol* 8:571-586, 1966.

6. Pratt RTC: *The Genetics of Neurological Disorders.* London, Oxford University Press, 1967, pp 93-94.

7. Lagos JC, Gomez MR: Tuberous sclerosis: Reappraisal of a clinical entity. *Mayo Clin Proc* 42:26-49, 1967.

CONTRIBUTION TO THE STUDY OF IDIOCY*
by BOURNEVILLE, Physician at the Bicêtre
. . . Case III

Tuberous Sclerosis of Cerebral Convolutions:

Idiocy and Hemiplegic Epilepsy

. . . . L. Marie, three years old on arrival at the Salpêtrière on July 18, 1867 (Service of Mr. Delasiauve).[1]

*Translation of: Contribution à l'étude de l'idiotie. *Archives de Neurologie* 1:69-91, 670, 671, 1880.
1. I made this observation while replacing Mr. Delasiauve.

Information given by her mother (March 31, 1879).—*Father,* 45, in good health. . . . No neurologic illness in his family. *Mother,* 40, nervous. . . . Neither of her parents had neurologic diseases. No consanguinity.

Five children: 1. the patient; 2. and 3. two children who died while with a wet nurse (it is not known if they had convulsions); 4. a ten year old girl, and 5. a seven year old boy, in good health, having never had convulsions.

During *pregnancy,* the mother went through emotional crises due to the loss of her brother and frequent arguments with her mother-in-law. . . . The delivery was natural, at term. The child was breast fed by a wet nurse until 14 months of age. During this time she may have had several convulsions restricted to the eyes. At two years, *seizures* appeared, during which the arms shook and turned slightly. "It was especially in the head." . . . Marie never walked or talked. She gradually deteriorated. Brought to the children's hospital at 3, she was declared a hopeless case. . . .

Present status (March, 1879).—Large, regular *head;* low forehead, frontal bones not prominent. . . . The eyes are dull, there is no strabismus. Normal ears, flat nose. . . . Rosaceous and pustular acne of the face; also a confluent vesiculopapular eruption over the nose, cheeks and forehead; numerous small molluscums on the nape and surface of the neck, which is abnormally short. . . .

Upper Limbs.—The left limb is quite mobile. The right is paralyzed; the forearm is at a right angle to the arm, the hand is violaceous and turned outward, and the joints are more or less rigid. However, the paralysis is not complete, since she is able to bring her hand to her mouth to suck it, though less often than the left hand.

Lower limbs.—The left lower limb is longer and heavier than the right. . . . The foot is flat and violaceous. The right thigh is adducted and flexed on the pelvis; the leg is flexed on the thigh; the foot is flat, in varus, and violaceous. . . . The patient is incapable of standing on her legs. There are scars and ulcerations over the greater trochanters and the sacrum.

Attitude.—The lower limbs are bent and crossed, even in bed, as if the child is sitting on a chair. The upper limbs are close together, the hands almost always at the mouth. Constant slaver.

Seizures.—At the end of the examination she had a small *seizure:* the eyes moved up and to the left; the arms came together on the chest and were rigid, especially the right one. Then a few clonic convulsions appeared simultaneously in the right arm and leg with rapid convulsions of the eyelids; finally, stertorous breathing and bloody froth.

These *seizures* usually came in *series.* . . .

April 20.—30 seizures. . . . A quart enema of *bromide of camphor,* 2 gr.

April 21.—During the previous night, 40 seizures. . . .

Evening.—From half past eleven to one A. M., 47 seizures. Application of leeches behind the ears. From 1 to 6 A. M., 229 seizures. Permanent coma. . . .

April 22.—From 6 P. M. to 6 A. M., 340 seizures. Yesterday afternoon there was a brief cessation, after inhalation of *amyl nitrite.* . . .

The child died on May 7, at 3 A. M. . . .

Autopsy on *May* 8. . . . . The *brain* weighs 1000 grams. The *cerebellum* and the *isthmus,* 150 grams. The *right hemisphere* weighs 10 grams less than the left.

Left cerebral hemisphere.—The *pia mater* is very thin and is hard to take off, except at the site of the lesions that are present in many of the convolutions. These lesions consist of rounded islets, forming protuberances of variable size. They are whitish, opaque, and much denser than the neighboring areas, though still part of the convolutions. In other words, there is a sort of *hypertrophic sclerosis* of various portions of the convolutions.

Distribution. a) *Convex surface:* Islets are present in the mid portions of the *third and first frontal convolutions.* In the *ascending frontal and ascending parietal convolutions,* they are very irregular, very hard, and are united in their upper half. The mass is separated by a transverse sulcus from the lower portions of these two convolutions. . . . There are islets in the posterior part of the *third temporal convolution,* in the middle part of the *second temporal convolution,* in the *superior parietal lobule,* in the *angular gyrus,* and in the tip of the *occipital lobe.*

b) *Inferior surface:* Islets are present in both internal convolutions. . . .

c) *Internal surface:* The *convolution of the corpus callosum* is irregular and shows several islets: *The hippocampal convolution* is very irregular, and so is the *convolution of Ammon's horn.* The internal surface of the *first frontal convolution* is the site of several very distinct islets. The *paracentral lobule* is notably deformed; the end of the Rolandic fissure can be seen here. We also note deformation of the *precuneus and cuneiform lobules;* these parts contain numerous sites of induration.

The *cavity of the lateral ventricle* is normal. The *optic thalamus* is healthy, but the *corpus striatum* contains scattered sclerotic islets, their white color contrasting with the grey background of the corpus striatum. . . .

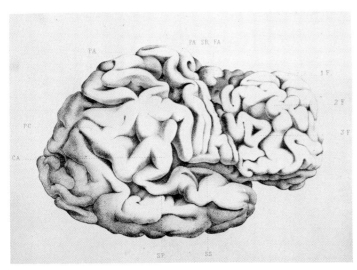

Fig. III

SS   Fissure of Sylvius, and S P, parallel fissure
SR   Fissure of Rolando
1 F   1st frontal gyrus
2 F   2nd frontal gyrus
3 F   3rd frontal gyrus
PA   Ascending parietal gyrus
FA   Ascending frontal gyrus
PC   Angular gyrus, situated posterior to the inferior frontal lobule, but
      far from the posterior termination of the fissure of Sylvius
CA   Supramarginal gyrus, vertically closing the fissure
      of Sylvius posteriorly

Fig. IV

Medial surface of the left hemisphere

Lp   Paracentral lobule
Lq   Precuneus lobule
L   Lateral ventricle
Cs   Corpus striatum
N, N, N   Foci of tuberous sclerosis

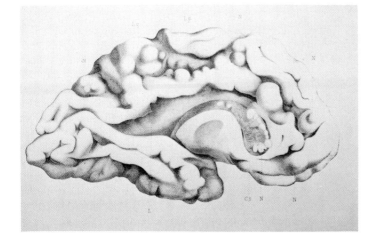

Right cerebral hemisphere. Pia mater appears the same. The same lesions in the convolutions, but less numerous. . . .

Thorax. Grey hepatization of the entire *right lung* and inferior part of the left lung. No tubercles. *Heart* (60 gr.), concentric hypertrophy of the left ventricle, the walls of which are 11 millimeters thick. No clots. . . .

Kidneys: The right weighs 70 gr. On its surface are three whitish, mammillary, hard masses, projecting 3 to 5 millimeters. One of these masses is the size of a walnut. In addition, 15 other small masses are found disseminated on both sides of the kidney, but they do not protrude. When cut, the principal masses have the appearance of cancerous tissue. The left kidney (60 gr.) shows similar but less numerous lesions.

The origin of this illness is obscure. . . . The abnormal areas are in the convolutions, which are hard and hypertrophied at these sites. . . . Multiple sclerosis tends to affect the more central parts of the brain, and the plaques, instead of being white, have a grey coloration. The comparison between Fig. IV and the figures in the *Leçons sur le système nerveux* of Mr. Charcot will demonstrate the difference in these lesions.

Does the site of the lesions explain the focal epilepsy? . . . . The *ascending frontal and parietal convolutions on the left side* contain, in their superior portions, a large islet of sclerosis, disposed in such a way that the two convolutions are united in that region. It is to this lesion that we attribute the convulsions which affected the limbs on the right side. . . .

XXXII Von Recklinghausen's Neurofibromatosis

F RIEDRICH Daniel von Recklinghausen (1833 to 1910) had a long career as professor of pathology at the University of Strassburg.[1] Among the many disease processes that occupied his interest was neurofibromatosis,[2-5] which he discussed at length in an 1882 Festschrift dedicated to his teacher, Rudolf Virchow.

Von Recklinghausen reviewed the previously reported cases and added the descriptions of two additional patients. He and his predecessors noted the multiple tumors of the skin and the peripheral and autonomic nerves, as well as the café au lait spots. Subsequently, it has been discovered that patients with this disease may also have a variety of neoplasms and malformations involving the brain, spinal cord, meninges, autonomic ganglia, and the roots of the cranial and spinal nerves, as well as anomalies in other tissues.[6,7] The disorder is typically familial, being transmitted as an autosomal dominant trait.[8,9]

Although he was not the first to describe neurofibromatosis, and his cases exhibited only a few of its numerous features, von Recklinghausen's prominence in the medical world and his influence as a teacher assured the firm attachment of his name to the disease.

References

1. Chiari H: Friedrich Daniel v. Recklinghausen. *Verh Deutsch Path Ges* 15:478-488, 1912.

2. Kelly EC: *Encyclopedia of Medical Sources*. Baltimore, Williams & Wilkins Co, 1948, p 339.

3. Long ES: *Selected Readings in Pathology*. Springfield, Ill, Charles C Thomas Publisher, 1961, pp 198-202.

4. Rang M: *Anthology of Orthopaedics*. Edinburgh, E & S Livingstone Ltd, 1966, pp 57-58.

5. Jablonski S: *Illustrated Dictionary of Eponymic Syndromes and Diseases and Their Synonyms*. Philadelphia, WB Saunders Co, 1969, p 256.

6. Lichtenstein BW: Neurofibromatosis (von Recklinghausen's disease of the nervous system): Analysis of the total pathologic picture. *Arch Neurol Psychiat* 62:822-839, 1949.

7. Aita JA: *Neurocutaneous Diseases*. Springfield, Ill, Charles C Thomas Publisher, 1966, pp 5-6, 57-59.

8. Pratt RTC: *The Genetics of Neurological Disorders*. London, Oxford University Press, 1967, pp 93-97.

9. Aita JA: Genetic aspects of tumors of the nervous system, in Lynch HT (ed): *Hereditary Factors in Carcinoma*. New York, Springer-Verlag, 1967, pp 86-110 (also in *Nebraska Med J* 53:121-124, 302-304, 1968).

Concerning Multiple Fibromas of the Skin and Their Relationship to Multiple Neuromas*

by F. v. Recklinghausen
Professor in Strassburg
Case I

Autopsy: 24 January 1879. Marie Kientz, 55 years old. . . . Innumerable nodules over almost the entire epidermis (Plate I), for the most part pedunculated, others sessile, most of them simply spherical, of all possible sizes. . . . The tumors were most numerous on the skin of the abdomen and the chest, though they were perhaps denser and even larger on the skin of the back. . . . They sent ramifications into the subcutaneous tissue, . . . but were easily palpable through the thinned-out cutis. In addition there were mobile tumors that were entirely subcutaneous. . . .

In general, the skin of the entire body had a dirty brown color, but when examined more closely, there were innumerable pea-sized brown pigmented spots, especially over the thorax and neck, and a larger one (4 × 3 cm.) in the left gluteal region. . . .

On the surface of the small intestine there were two small nodules, both firm. . . . A large tumor protruded into the abdominal cavity, growing out of the wall of the jejunum. . . . There were numerous nodules on the surface of the stomach. . . .

On the anterior surface of the left tibia, approximately at its middle, were two pale red, translucent tumors attached to the external surface of the periosteum. . . , and a third tumor was located above the middle. On the right tibia there was a large tumor . . . and three small nodules, also sitting flat on the periosteum. . . .

In the left femoral nerve . . . there was a

spindle-shaped tumor . . . with the nerve running on its posterior side. There was another small tumor on the saphenous nerve at the knee. . . . The lateral femoral cutaneous nerve had two tumors . . . , and in the muscular branches of the obturator nerve there were more nodules. . . . On the posterior branches of the right first and second intercostal nerves and along the course of the axillary branches were more nodules. . . . The olfactory, optic, oculomotor, trochlear and facial nerves were free of nodules. . . , but the frontal and supraorbital nerves had them. . . .

It was difficult to detect neuromas along the subcutaneous nerve fibers of the upper back . . . in spite of the numerous fibromas in that area. On the other hand, it was fairly easy to find them in the leg which had few fibromas. . . .

The sacral plexus was full of nodules. . . . These thickenings extended right up into the sacral canal, but not to the dura. The intraspinal roots of the sacral nerves were clear, as were the other nerve roots. The spinal cord and brain showed nothing unusual. . . . The origins of the cranial nerves were free, though the vagus showed two small asymmetrical swellings in the neck. . . . The cervical and thoracic sympathetics were clear . . . but there were neuromas in the superior mesenteric plexus . . . and in the gastric nerves. . . .

Death was from hemorrhage into the lung from an aneurysm of the pulmonary artery.

History: K. was brought into the hospital on 23 January, 1879, because of her pulmonary bleeding, but died there after only a few hours. She had stated to the female attendant that the tumors on her skin had existed since her third year and were completely painless. . . .

I learned from her 48 year old brother that she

*Translation of *Ueber die multiplen Fibrome der Haut und ihre Beziehung zu den multiplen Neuromen*. Berlin, August Hirschwald, 1882, pp 3-18.

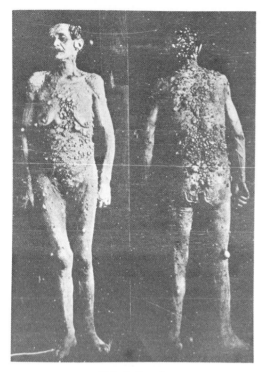

Plate I: Case I.

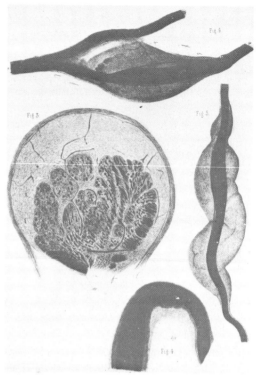

Plate III.

Fig. 3—Cross-section through a fibroneuroma blackened by treatment with osmium. . . .

Fig. 5—Spindle-shaped spiral fibroneuroma. The main body of the fibroma external, and only a small part of it within the nerve fiber bundle. . . .

Fig. 6—Spindle-shaped fibroneuroma. A nerve fiber bundle sectioned through the tumor mass. . . .

had been married twice and had borne 11 children. . . , but none of these children was still alive. . . . She had shown nothing unusual of a psychological nature except for a strong inclination for the male sex.

On the body of this brother. . . , I could find no pigmented spots. He had a flat tumor of the skin and subcutaneous tissue on the nape of his neck. . . , and a soft hemispheral tumor in the skin at the level of his lowest dorsal vertebra. . . . Along his nerves there was no palpable firmness.

Sections, strands and pieces of the tumors were studied using various techniques, such as staining with osmic acid, gold chloride, picrocarmine, or hematoxylin. . . .

In the neuromas . . . the nerve fibers were well preserved and easy to follow through the thick tumor. . . . There was an increased amount of connective tissue, especially in undulating longitudinal trabeculae. . . . The nerve fiber bundle was only slightly separated by this newly-formed connective tissue, which lay primarily between the nerve fiber bundles on one side and their lamellar sheaths on the other side (Plate III, Figs. 3, 5, and 6) . . . though the sheath layers in many neuro-

mas had merged into the newly-formed connective tissue. . . . In several soft translucent neuromas, resembling myxomas, the proliferated connective tissue was loosely woven and less trabecular. . . .

The cutaneous fibromas generally were composed of a tough translucent connective tissue. . . . This tissue, characterized by an abundance of cells and a paucity of fibrils, was separated . . . by irregular trabeculae . . . and a plexiform arrangement resulted. . . .

If one examined the projections that could be followed up into the interior surface of the skin tumors, one found for the most part that they contained altered sweat glands, but in some it was possible to perceive a nerve entering the tumor (Plate IV, Fig. 11). . . . If one peeled out the numerous small translucent clumps of tumor tissue in the pars reticularis, each was found to be the lower end of a cone which the projecting skin nodule sent down through the cutis. Frequently

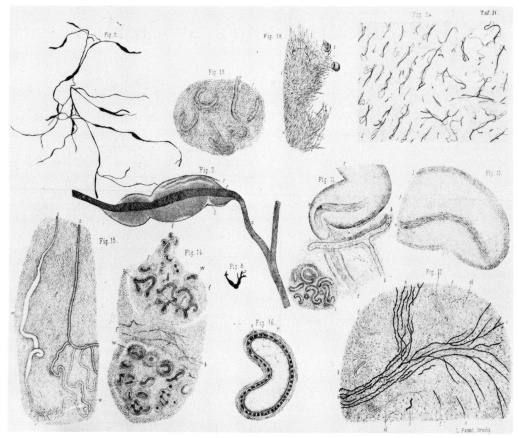

Plate IV.

Fig. 2—Ramifications of the nerves in the subcutaneous tissues of the thigh, occupied by neuromatous swellings, blackened by osmic acid. . . .

Fig. 8—Horseshoe-shaped fibroneuroma from the skin, with nerve fibers leaving it on the right. . . .

Fig. 11—The end of a soft fibroma of the skin . . .

with an axial nerve fiber bundle, crossed by a normal artery; beneath that, a sweat tubule with an incipient fibroma between its coils.

Fig. 12—Horizontal section of the soft basal portion of a cutaneous fibroma. . . . The nerve fiber bundles are disintegrated through the fibroma tissue. . . .

these cones projected 3-6 mm. into the subcutaneous fat. . . . It was often possible to place one of the cones on the stage of the microscope and to unfold it into a horseshoe shape. In this case one occasionally was able to see a curved neuroma (Plate IV, Fig. 8). . . . On the cross-sections through thicker portions of the tumors one saw 1 to 4 nerve fibers in the midst of the tissue, traceable for long distances. . . .

The nodules of the intestinal and gastric walls . . . were made up of fine connective tissue with small spindle-shaped cells like the skin tumors . . . , and were embedded in the interfascicular connective tissue of the muscularis. It was understandably difficult to demonstrate a connection with the pale, unmyelinated intestinal nerves. . . .

One of the large jejunal tumors . . . demonstrated internal degeneration, resulting in the diagnosis of sarcoma and the hypothesis that a fibroma became sarcomatous. . . .

In the periosteal tumors . . . it was very easy to find nerves in almost all bits of tumor. . . .

In the case presented . . . it appears that the multiple neuromas and cutaneous fibromas existed simultaneously. It also appears that this was not a fortuitous combination, but rather that the tumors were related structurally. . . . The evidence for the latter is: 1) the nature of the neoplastic tissue in both types of tumor was almost identical, 2) nerve tumors penetrated the under surface of the tumors of the skin and sometimes could be peeled out of them, and 3) the cutaneous fibromas presented an arrangement different from the usual multiple fibromatous neoplasms. . . .

XXXIII   Gerstmann's Syndrome

WHEN THE concept of cerebral localization was first established at the end of the 19th century, numerous cerebral "centers" for a wide variety of mental functions were described.[1-4] Subsequently, it has become apparent that the localization of the psyche is not so simple, but nevertheless, several disorders of mental function have persisted in neurological texts as indicators of pathological lesions in specific cerebral areas. One of these syndromes, the peculiar combination of finger agnosia, right-left confusion, dysgraphia, and dyscalculia, as described by Josef Gerstmann[5-10] and others,[11] has come to signify involvement of the posterior portion of the dominant parietal lobe.

Josef Gerstmann, born in 1887, spent the first half of his professional career in Vienna, where he rose to become Professor of Neurology and Psychiatry at the University and Director of the Institute of Nervous Diseases at the Maria-Theresien-Schlössel. In 1938, he fled to the United States, where he continued his work until his death in 1969.

Gerstmann's syndrome held his interest for many years. His first description of finger agnosia appeared in 1924, and as he accumulated further experience and discovered the other aspects of the syndrome, he published additional accounts over the ensuing 33 years.[5-10]

The Gerstmann syndrome was first recognized in adults, but in recent years it has been described in children as a developmental defect, causing a characteristic type of retardation of reading and writing.[12] However, various doubts have been raised concerning the autonomy of the Gerstmann syndrome and the specificity of its pathological localization.[11,13-15] In fact, it has been called

". . . an artifact of defective and biased observation" having ". . . little support for its alleged focal diagnostic significance."[13]

Despite these serious objections, Gerstmann's publications have served to focus attention on a constellation of phenomena, a varying number of which are encountered in patients with lesions in the dominant parietal lobe. Reference to Gerstmann's syndrome is often a point of departure when the gnostic functions are discussed in present-day neurology.

References

1. Wilkins RH: Neurosurgical classic—XII. *J Neurosurg* 20:904-916, 1963.
2. Wilkins RH: Neurosurgical classic—XIX. *J Neurosurg* 21:424-431, 1964.
3. Wilkins RH: Neurosurgical classic—XXII. *J Neurosurg* 21:724-733, 1964.
4. Wilkins RH, Brody IA: Wernicke's sensory aphasia. *Arch Neurol* 22:279-282, 1970.
5. Gerstmann J: Fingeragnosie: Eine umschriebene Störung der Orientierung am eigenen Körper. *Wien Klin Wschr* 37:1010-1012, 1924.
6. Gerstmann J: Fingeragnosie und isolierte Agraphie—ein neues Syndrom. *Z Ges Neurol Psychiat* 108:152-177, 1927.
7. Gerstmann J: Zur Symptomatologie der Hirnläsionen im Übergangsgebiet der unteren Parietal- und mittleren Occipital-Windung (Das Syndrom: Fingeragnosie, Rechts-Links-Störung, Agraphie, Akalkulie). *Nervenarzt* 3:691-695, 1930.
8. Gerstmann J: Zur lokaldiagnostischen Verwertbarkeit des Syndroms: Fingeragnosie, Rechts-Links-Störung, Agraphie, Akalkulie. *Jahrb Psychiat Neurol* 48:135-143, 1931-1932.
9. Gerstmann J: Syndrome of finger agnosia, disorientation for right and left, agraphia and acalculia: Local diagnostic value. *Arch Neurol Psychiat* 44:398-408, 1940.
10. Gerstmann J: Some notes on the Gerstmann syndrome. *Neurology* 7:866-869, 1957.
11. Critchley M: The enigma of Gerstmann's syndrome. *Brain* 89:183-198, 1966.
12. Kinsbourne M, Warrington EK: The developmental Gerstmann syndrome. *Arch Neurol* 8:490-501, 1963.
13. Benton AL: The fiction of the "Gerstmann syndrome" *J Neurol Neurosurg Psychiat* 24:176-181, 1961.
14. Heimburger RF, Demyer W, Reitan RM: Implications of Gerstmann's syndrome. *J Neurol Neurosurg Psychiat* 27:52-57, 1964.
15. Poeck K, Orgass B: An experimental investigation of finger agnosia. *Neurology* 19:801-807, 1969.

On the Symptomatology of Cerebral Lesions in the Transitional Area of the Lower Parietal and Middle Occipital Convolutions
(The Syndrome: Finger Agnosia, Right-Left Confusion, Agraphia and Acalculia) [*1]
by Professor Dr. Josef Gerstmann, Vienna

. . . The subject of this paper is the peculiar symptom that I first described several years ago (1924)[2] under the name of "finger agnosia." It manifests itself as an isolated disturbance in the recognition, naming, choosing, and differential exhibition of the various fingers of both hands—one's own fingers as well as those of another person. There is also a certain lack of freedom in the movements of individual fingers . . . . Furthermore, I will discuss the association that I noted between this symptom and a disturbance in right-left orientation (in one's own as well as in another's body), agraphia and acalculia.[3] And finally, I will relate the presence of this syndrome to focal lesions . . . in the transitional area between the angular and second occipital convolution.

Since my first observation, . . . I have established this syndrome with a considerable series of patients, in some of whom it existed as an independent condition from the beginning, while in others—though seldom—it was a residual syndrome after regression of a more complex deficit. The syndrome is obviously not rare . . . .

In its selective form, . . . my patients have not been affected conspicuously in their general psychic or intellectual function. Aphasia, apraxia, agnosia, or other disorders to which the symptom complex could be attributable have been lacking, or at least were not present during the period of observation. Furthermore, the other signs that have sometimes been associated with the syndrome (such as right hemianopsia, diminution of optokinetic nystagmus, amnestic disturbance of word-finding, impairment in reading ability, . . .) can be characterized as neighborhood or marginal symptoms because of their variable appearance and comparative mildness. The phenomenon of finger agnosia itself always appeared as an essential disturbance of recognition and orientation . . . , while the ability to recognize and orient has remained essentially undisturbed with regard to the other parts of the body and limbs . . . .

The most important corroboration of my statements concerning finger agnosia and its association with right-left confusion, agraphia and acalculia comes from Pötzl and Herrmann,[4] Schilder,[5] Kroll,[6] and most recently by Johannes Lange[7] . . . .

It has become evident that the syndrome of finger agnosia, agraphia, etc. can be related to focal disturbance in the area of transition between the angular gyrus and the second occipital convolution. In my first case of finger agnosia, I postulated a focal softening in the area of the left lower parietal lobe . . . but I could not undertake a more exact localization for lack of an anatomical study. Since the symptomatology of this case and my subsequent ones corresponds closely with the tumor case of Pötzl and Herrmann, I have assumed . . . a localization of the cerebral lesion analogous to that shown at autopsy of the tumor case . . . . Concrete confirmation has recently been found . . . in two further autopsy reports of patients with finger agnosia and agraphia from my personal material, and in the autopsy report of a case with the fully developed syndrome of finger agnosia, right-left confusion, agraphia and acalculia in Lange's material . . . .

It should be emphasized that with the exception of the tumor case of Pötzl and Herrmann, where the focal affection was localized in the right parieto-occipital region, . . . all other cases have had left cerebral lesions . . . . Therefore, it appears that the syndrome . . . is caused by a unilateral lesion in the left hemisphere in right-handed individuals.

In closing, gentlemen, may I direct your attention to the practical applicability of the knowledge of this syndrome . . . to the diagnosis of focal disorders in the parieto-occipital transition area. . . .

*Translation of: Zur Symptomatologie der Hirnläsionen im Übergangsgebiet der unteren Parietal—und mittleren Occipitalwindung. (Das Syndrom: Fingeragnosie, Rechts-Links-Störung, Agraphie, Akalkulie). *Nervenarzt* **3**:691-695, 1930.

1. A lecture presented at the 20th Annual Meeting of the "Gesellschaft deutscher Nervenärzte", September 18-20, 1930, in Dresden.
2. Fingeragnosie. Wien. klin. Wschr., 1924, Nr. 40.
3. Fingeragnosie und isolierte Agraphie—ein neues Syndrom. Z. Neur. 108 (1927).
4. Uber die Agraphie und ihre lokaldiagnostischen Beziehungen. Berlin: S. Karger 1926.—Mschr. Psychiatr. 70 (1928).
5. Z Neur. 113 (1928) (jointly with Isakower).
6. Die neuropathologischen Syndrome. Berlin: Julius Springer 1929.
7. Fingeragnosie und Agraphie. Mschr. Psychiatr. 76 (1930).

XXXIV Tinel's Sign

OUR KNOWLEDGE of peripheral nerve injuries has been accumulated primarily during the major wars.[1,2] In the First World War, an important clinical test[2,3] of nerve regeneration was first described independently in the same year by two physicians, each of whom was treating the casualties inflicted by the other's army. Since the war prevented free scientific communication between the opposing countries, each of the two physicians was unaware of the work of the other.

Paul Hoffmann,[4] who also first described the H reflex,[5,6] was born in Dorpat in 1884 and became Professor of Physiology in Würzburg. His publication, translated below, concerns a sign of nerve regeneration that he discovered in wounded German soldiers; it appeared in print on March 28, 1915. Jules Tinel, a French neurologist and the fifth in a line of distinguished physicians,[7] independently found the same sign in French soldiers and published his initial account on Oct 7, 1915. He mentioned it again in his book on nerve injuries, translated into English in 1917.[8]

Because of Tinel's greater experience in this field and his more comprehensive interpretation of the phenomenon, and perhaps because of the outcome of the war, this sign of nerve regeneration is usually referred to as Tinel's sign despite Hoffmann's priority.

In present-day neurologic practice the sign has particular usefulness in revealing a partial injury of the median nerve due to compression by the transverse carpal ligament. For eliciting the sign, the reflex hammer has tended to replace the tapping finger recommended by Hoffmann and Tinel.

References

1. Wilkins RH, Brody IA: Neurological classics XXVII: Causalgia. *Arch Neurol* 22:89-94, 1970.
2. Sunderland S: *Nerves and Nerve Injuries.* Baltimore, Williams & Wilkins Co, 1968.
3. Henderson WR: Clinical assessment of peripheral nerve injuries: Tinel's test. *Lancet* 2:801-805, 1948.
4. Jung R: Paul Hoffmann 1884-1962. *Ergebn Physiol* 61:1-17, 1969.
5. Hoffmann P: Über die Beziehungen der Sehnenreflexe zur willkürlichen Bewegung und zum Tonus. *Z Biol* 68:351-370, 1918.
6. Hoffmann P: *Untersuchungen über die Eigenreflexe (Sehnenreflexe) menschlicher Muskeln.* Berlin, J Springer, 1922.
7. Rang M: *Anthology of Orthopaedics.* Edinburgh, E & S Livingstone, 1966, pp 148-150.
8. Tinel J: *Nerve Wounds: Symptomatology of Peripheral Nerve Lesions Caused by War Wounds.* F Rothwell (trans), New York, Wood, 1917.

On a Method of Evaluating the Success of a Nerve Suture*
by
Priv. Doz. Dr. Paul Hoffmann
From the Medical Polyclinic of Wurzburg

This discussion concerns observations made on the wounded in military hospitals in Wurzburg, some of whom undergo electrical stimulation and regular observation at the Medical Polyclinic.

Nerve injuries impose a great demand on the patience of both doctor and patient. Even after a successful nerve suture, restitution of function can be expected only after several weeks. It would be a

great comfort to the patient if one could evaluate the success of the suture early in the course. The following will show that this is possible in many cases by a very simple technique.

Let us suppose that the radial nerve is severed by a bullet in the middle of the arm and that the nerve is then sutured. Naturally a long period of time must pass until movement can return to the paralyzed muscles, since the nerve fibers have to grow from the proximal stump to the muscles. During this time we simply watch and can say

*Translation of: Ueber eine Methode, den Erfolg einer Nervennaht zu beurteilen, *Medizinische Klinik* 11:359-360, 1915.

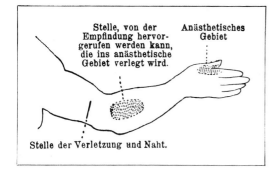

Stelle, von der Empfindung hervor-gerufen werden kann, die ins anästhetische Gebiet verlegt wird.

Anästhetisches Gebiet

Stelle der Verletzung und Naht.

nothing about the success of the suture. . . .

However, there are sensory fibers in the proximal nerve stump, and stimulation of these fibers should create a sensation referred to the insensitive cutaneous area. These fibers will grow after the nerve has been sutured. If stimulation of the growing fibers elicits a sensation in the anesthetic area, we can conclude that the suture site is conductive, i.e., growth of the fibers actually is taking place. The site of the suture is the critical location, and once the growing nerve has surmounted it, a restitution of function is very likely.

Experiments have convinced me that this method is quite practical in suitable cases. I would like to demonstrate its possibilities in two typical and comparable cases:

I. A noncommissioned officer, 22 years old, wounded on August 20, 1914. Shot through the right arm; transection of the radial nerve. Slight fragmentation of the humerus. The nerve injury is situated 8 cm. proximal to the elbow (see Fig. 1). In the hand, anesthesia in the distribution of the radial nerve. . . .

Nerve suture on October 8, 1914. Continuity established.

January 15, 1915. It is possible to create a prickling sensation radiating into the anesthetic area of the radial nerve in the hand by pressing with a finger on the area of the forearm depicted in Fig. 1. This sensation cannot be elicited further peripherally. The border of this area is relatively sharp. It is best to use finger pressure to elicit this sensation, faradic current also works, but not as well.

February 15. . . . The patient can extend the hand a little.

Thus, four weeks prior to the return of motor function it was determined with certainty that impulses could pass the sutured area. . . .

As can be seen from these facts, one is dealing with the stimulation of newly growing fibers. . . . It is not necessary to apply great pressure to elicit this sensation. One can do it best by tapping with the extended finger. . . .

It is also clear that one can use this technique in cases where restitution of nerve function takes place without nerve suture. The demonstration of such a pressure area peripheral to the site of injury proves that a nerve suture is not necessary.

The Sign of "Tingling" in Lesions of the Peripheral Nerves*
by
J. Tinel

Too often there is difficulty making a precise diagnosis in peripheral nerve lesions. Is the nerve divided, compressed, lacerated, or irritated? Is regeneration occurring? Is the palpable neuroma permeable to the axons? Has a sutured nerve reunited? . . . .

We think that the systematic study of *tingling provoked by pressure on a nerve* can help to answer these questions.

Pressure on a damaged nerve trunk often produces a *tingling* sensation, projected to the periphery of the nerve and localized to a very exact cutaneous area.

It is important to differentiate this tingling from the pain sometimes produced by pressure on an injured nerve. The *pain* is a sign of *irritation* of the nerve; tingling is a sign of *regeneration;* or more precisely, tingling indicates the presence of *young axons,* in the process of growing.

The *pain of nerve irritation* is almost always *local,* perceived at the point where the pressure is exerted on the nerve. When the pain radiates along the entire course of the nerve, it *is still most vivid at the place under pressure.* It almost always *coexists* with *pain on pressure of the muscle masses,* and usually the muscles are more tender than the nerve.

The *tingling of regeneration is not painful;* it is a vaguely disagreeable sensation that patients usually compare to electricity. It is barely perceived at the pressure point, and is appreciated *much more vividly in the corresponding cutaneous area.* The muscles adjoining the nerve that "tingles" are not painful.

These two kinds of phenomena aroused by

*Translation of: Le signe du "fourmillement" dans les lésions des nerfs périphériques. *La Presse Médicale* 23:388-389, 1915.

pressure on a nerve, pain and tingling, are easy to differentiate in almost all cases. They rarely coexist at the same site on the nerve, but we shall see that they may succeed one another on the same nerve trunk.

In addition to these two different signs aroused by pressure on the nerve, examination of the skin may reveal certain sensory abnormalities. Irritation of a nerve is often accompanied by a painful cutaneous hyperesthesia, while nerve regeneration is associated with hypesthesia and dysesthesias, most commonly a painful sensation of tingling aroused by touching, by pricking, and above all by lightly brushing the skin. . . .

---

1. *In complete transections,* we can find an exact spot along the course of the nerve trunk where pressure produces tingling in the cutaneous distribution of the nerve.

This area of tingling is *small;* no larger than 2 to 3 cm. It is *permanent, absolutely fixed;* it remains the same for weeks and months. It is *unique* along the course of the nerve, and we do not find any other point above or below the lesion where pressure can cause tingling.

This area indicates that here the interrupted axons have begun to regenerate and that, being unable to pass through an obstacle and to regain the peripheral segment, they are clumping up in a neuroma.

2. In *complete interruption of a nerve by* very tight *compression,* the same characteristics . . . are met with, but the area of tingling is larger. It may reach 6, 8, 10 cm. or more along the course of the nerve. . . .

3. We can, in certain cases, find *two different sites for eliciting tingling,* corresponding to *two lesions at different levels.*

For example, we have seen two men suffering from a radial paralysis due to injury in the upper arm. One area of tingling was on the radial nerve at the level of the exit wound of the bullet, on the posterior surface of the arm. A second larger area was on the external surface of the limb, at the level of a very large fracture callus. These two areas were stationary and delimited, with no trace of induced tingling encountered below the osseous callus. Operation showed that the nerve had been partly destroyed at the first area by the passage of the bullet and that the few fibers which escaped the damage had been compressed and interrupted in the fracture callus distally.

Furthermore, we can observe *partial tingling* of a nerve. Pressure on the sciatic, for example, may show a lesion limited to the internal or external part of the nerve when the tingling is localized to the cutaneous area of the lateral popliteal or of the medial popliteal. . . .

4. *Incomplete interruptions* of the nerve or, more exactly, *lesions permitting the passage of regenerating axons* are characterized by the gradual extension of the area arousing tingling sensations.

Thus, we see *tingling appearing below* the lesion and then progressively extending toward the periphery, along the course of the nerve. *A nerve that tingles below the lesion is a nerve that is regenerating* partly or completely. In this way we can, from week to week, follow the slow progression of the axons; we can appreciate the rapidity of nerve restoration; we can, above all, judge its degree by the intensity of the tingling evoked and the extent of the cutaneous area where it manifests itself.

The situation is the same in cases of *nerve suture,* where we can quickly judge the success of the operation by ascertaining the progressive extension of the area of tingling.

As the area of tingling extends and intensifies peripherally, it diminishes and finally disappears at the level of the injury. . . .

---

1. Tingling evoked by pressure on a nerve *rarely appears before the fourth or even the sixth week* following trauma. . . . The appearance of induced tingling corresponds to the period of axon sprouting.

2. The *tingling disappears as soon as the nerve has resumed its normal constitution* and the newly formed axons have reached a mature state. It is generally at the end of eight to ten months that tingling stops, though large variations exist. . . .

3. Finally, tingling may be absent in some cases. . . . In such cases the lesion may be very slight, not involving any major destruction of nerve fibers. Or, no regeneration may have taken place, as we sometimes see in elderly, sick or infected subjects with profoundly disturbed nutrition.

Induced tingling does not, then, constitute an absolutely constant sign, invariable and always easy to interpret. It cannot replace meticulous and repeated examination of the patient. . . . But, with all of these reservations, tingling appears to us to be capable of clarifying certain problems of neurological diagnosis and furnishing valuable information on the prognosis and treatment of peripheral nerve lesions.

XXXV   Down's Syndrome

DR. John Langdon Haydon Down (1828 to 1896) was a brilliant medical student from a distinguished family.[1] It therefore came as a surprise to his colleagues when he decided to devote his career to the study and care of the mentally retarded. Langdon Down became the first superintendent of the Earlswood Asylum for Idiots in Surrey, England, from 1858 until 1868, and then established his own private home at Normansfield in Teddington with the aid of his two sons, both physicians.

Among his many patients, Down discovered a group that exhibited a characteristic syndrome.[2,3] Certain of the features of the syndrome, such as prominent epicanthal folds, suggested a mongolian appearance to Down, and led him to advance an explanation. Apparently influenced by Charles Darwin's ideas of evolution, Down proposed an ethnic classification of mental retardation that viewed the so-called mongolian idiocy as a reversion to an earlier phylogenetic type, perhaps as a result of parental tuberculosis.[4,5]

It has subsequently been established that this syndrome does have a genetic basis.[6,7] The majority of the patients have 47 chromosomes with trisomy of a chromosome in the G-group, 21-22.[2,3] But the syndrome occurs in a variety of races,[2,3,8] and Down's use of the term mongolian can be interpreted as a racial slur.[9] Down's syndrome has been offered as a better designation, in honor of the man who first brought it to medical attention.

References

1. Brain [WR]: Chairman's opening remarks: Historical introduction, in Wolstenholme GEW, Porter R (eds): *Mongolism*. Boston, Little Brown & Co, 1967, pp 1-5.

2. Penrose LS, Smith GF: *Down's Anomaly*. Boston, Little Brown & Co, 1966.

3. Benda CE: *Down's Syndrome: Mongolism and Its Management*. New York, Grune & Stratton, 1969.

4. Down JLH: Observations on an ethnic classification of idiots. *London Hosp Clin Lects Reps* 3:259-262, 1866.

5. Down JL: *On Some of the Mental Affections of Childhood and Youth*. London, J & A Churchill, 1887.

6. Jacobs PA, Baikie AG, Court Brown WM, et al: The somatic chromosomes in mongolism. *Lancet* 1:710, 1959.

7. Lejeune J, Gautier M, Turpin R: Etude des chromosomes somatiques de neuf enfants mongoliens. *CR Acad Sci* 248:1721-1722, 1959.

8. Lilienfeld AM: *Epidemiology of Mongolism*. Baltimore, Johns Hopkins Press, 1969.

9. Matsunaga [E], in discussion, Wolstenholme GEW, Porter R (eds): *Mongolism*. Boston, Little Brown & Co, 1967, p 88.

OBSERVATIONS ON AN ETHNIC CLASSIFICATION OF IDIOTS.*

By J. LANGDON H. DOWN, M. D., Lond.

Those who have given any attention to congenital mental lesions, must have been frequently puzzled how to arrange, in any satisfactory way, the different classes of this defect which may have come under their observation. Nor will the difficulty be lessened by an appeal to what has been written on the subject. The systems of classification are generally so vague and artificial, that, not only do they assist but feebly, in any mental arrangement of the phenomena which are presented, but they completely fail in exerting any practical influence on the subject.

The medical practitioner who may be consulted in any given case, has, perhaps in a very early condition of the child's life, to give an opinion on points of vital importance as to the present condition and probable future of the little one. Moreover, he may be pressed as to the question, whether the supposed defect dates from any cause subsequent to the birth or not. Has the nurse dosed the child with opium? Has the little one met with any accident? Has the instrumental interference which maternal safety demanded, been the cause of what seems to the anxious parents, a vacant future? Can it be that when away from the family attendant the calomel powders were judiciously prescribed? Can, in fact, the strange anomalies which the child presents, be attributed to the numerous causes which maternal solicitude conjures to the imagination, in order to account for a condition, for which any cause is sought, rather than hereditary taint or parental influence. Will the systems of classification, either all together, or any one of them, assist the medical adviser in the opinion he is to present, or the suggestions which he is to tender to the anxious parent? I think that they will entirely fail him in the matter, and that he will have in many cases to make a *guarded* diagnosis and prognosis, so guarded, in fact, as to be almost valueless, or to venture an authoritative assertion which the future may *perhaps* confirm.

I have for some time had my attention directed to the possibility of making a classification of the feeble-minded, by arranging them around various ethnic standards,—in other words, framing a natural system to supplement the information to be

*Reprinted from *London Hospital Clinical Lectures and Reports* 3:259-262, 1866.

derived by an inquiry into the history of the case.

I have been able to find among the large number of idiots and imbeciles which come under my observation, both at Earlswood and the out-patient department of the Hospital, that a considerable portion can be fairly referred to one of the great divisions of the human family other than the class from which they have sprung. Of course, there are numerous representatives of the great Caucasian family. Several well-marked examples of the Ethiopian variety have come under my notice, presenting the characteristic malar bones, the prominent eyes, the puffy lips, and retreating chin. The woolly hair has also been present, although not always black, nor has the skin acquired pigmentary deposit. They have been specimens of white negroes, although of European descent.

Some arrange themselves around the Malay variety, and present in their soft, black, curly hair, their prominent upper jaws and capacious mouths, types of the family which people the South Sea Islands.

Nor have there been wanting the analogues of the people who with shortened foreheads, prominent cheeks, deep-set eyes, and slightly apish nose, originally inhabited the American Continent.

The great Mongolian family has numerous representatives, and it is to this division, I wish, in this paper, to call special attention. A very large number of congenital idiots are typical Mongols. So marked is this, that when placed side by side, it is difficult to believe that the specimens compared are not children of the same parents. The number of idiots who arrange themselves around the Mongolian type is so great, and they present such a close resemblance to one another in mental power, that I shall describe an idiot member of this racial division, selected from the large number that have fallen under my observation.

The hair is not black, as in the real Mongol, but of a brownish colour, straight and scanty. The face is flat and broad, and destitute of prominence. The cheeks are roundish, and extended laterally. The eyes are obliquely placed, and the internal canthi more than normally distant from one another. The palpebral fissure is very narrow. The forehead is wrinkled transversely from the constant assistance which the levatores palpebrarum derive from the occipito-frontalis muscle in the opening of the eyes. The lips are large and thick with transverse fissures. The tongue is long, thick, and is much roughened. The nose is small. The skin has a slight dirty yellowish tinge, and is deficient in elasticity, giving the appearance of being too large for the body.

The boy's aspect is such that it is difficult to realize that he is the child of Europeans, but so frequently are these characters presented, that there can be no doubt that these ethnic features are the result of degeneration.

The Mongolian type of idiocy occurs in more than ten per cent of the cases which are presented to me. They are always congenital idiots, and never result from accidents after uterine life. They are, for the most part, instances of degeneracy arising from tuberculosis in the parents. They are cases which very much repay judicious treatment. They require highly azotised food with a considerable amount of oleaginous material. They have considerable power of imitation, even bordering on being mimics. They are humorous, and a lively sense of the ridiculous often colours their mimicry. This faculty of imitation may be cultivated to a very great extent, and a practical direction given to the results obtained. They are usually able to speak; the speech is thick and indistinct, but may be improved very greatly by a well-directed scheme of tongue gymnastics. The co-ordinating faculty is abnormal, but not so defective that it cannot be greatly strengthened. By systematic training, considerable manipulative power may be obtained.

The circulation is feeble, and whatever advance is made intellectually in the summer, some amount of retrogression may be expected in the winter. Their mental and physical capabilities are, in fact, *directly* as the temperature.

The improvement which training effects in them is greatly in excess of what would be predicated if one did not know the characteristics of the type. The life expectancy, however, is far below the average, and the tendency is to the tuberculosis, which I believe to be the hereditary origin of the degeneracy.

Apart from the practical bearing of this attempt at an ethnic classification, considerable philosophical interest attaches to it. The tendency in the present day is to reject the opinion that the various races are merely varieties of the human family having a common origin, and to insist that climatic, or other influences, are insufficient to account for the different types of man. Here, however, we have examples of retrogression, or at all events, of departure from one type and the assumption of the characteristics of another. If these great racial divisions are fixed and definite, how comes it that disease is able to break down the barrier, and to simulate so closely the features of the members of another division. I cannot but think that the observations which I have recorded, are indications that the differences in the races are not specific but variable.

These examples of the result of degeneracy among mankind, appear to me to furnish some arguments in favour of the unity of the human species.

XXXVI   Wilson's Disease

T HE TALENTS of S. A. Kinnier Wilson (1878 to 1937) were most apparent at the bedside and in the lecture hall.[1,2] He had little interest in experimentation and confined his attention to clinical matters. Thus, during his long professional career at the National Hospital, Queen Square, London,[3-5] Wilson wrote on a variety of clinical topics, ending with a two-volume textbook of neurology that was edited and published after his death.[6]

Perhaps the best of these many contributions was a lengthy masterpiece that Wilson prepared for the MD degree at the University of Edinburgh.[7] In it, he reviewed a few previous reports and added four personal cases, crystallizing all of this information into a classic description of a distinct disease. But Wilson did not recognize the existence of the Kayser-Fleischer corneal ring[8-11] in his patients, and this sign was not appreciated as a manifestation of progressive lenticular degeneration until 1917.[12] Furthermore, Wilson erred in stating that this autosomal recessive disease[13] was not hereditary.

Though much has been learned about the nature of Wilson's disease and other types of hepatocerebral degeneration since 1912,[14-18] Wilson's original paper served to direct medical attention toward this disease. Moreover, this paper stimulated an awareness of the role of the basal ganglia in producing neurologic symptoms, and introduced the term "extrapyramidal" into neurologic parlance.

References

1. Critchley M: Wilson, Samuel Alexander Kinnier, in Legg LGW (ed): *The Dictionary of National Biography. 1931-1940.* Oxford, Oxford University Press, 1949, pp 914-915.
2. Haymaker W: Kinnier Wilson (1878-1937), in Haymaker W, Schiller F (eds): *The Founders of Neurology,* ed 2. Springfield, Ill, Charles C Thomas Publisher, 1970, pp 535-539.
3. Holmes G: *The National Hospital, Queen Square, 1860-1948.* Edinburgh, E & S Livingstone Ltd, 1954.
4. Blackwood W: The National Hospital, Queen Square, and the development of neuropathology. *World Neurol* 2:331-335, 1961.
5. Green JR: The origins of neurological institutes, in *Horizons in Neurological Education and Research.* Springfield, Ill, Charles C Thomas Publisher, 1965, pp 125-199.
6. Wilson SAK: *Neurology.* AN Bruce (ed), London, E Arnold & Co, 1940.
7. Wilson SAK: Progressive lenticular degeneration: A familial nervous disease associated with cirrhosis of the liver. *Brain* 34:295-509, 1912.
8. Kayser B: Ueber einen Fall von angeborener grünlicher Verfärbung der Cornea. *Klin Mbl Augenheilk* 40:22-25, 1902.
9. Fleischer B: Die periphere braun-grünliche Hornhautverfärbung, als Symptom einer eigenartigen Allgemeinerkrankung. *Munchen Med Wschr* 56:1120-1123, 1909.
10. Fleischer B: Über einen der "Pseudosklerose" nahestehende bisher unbekannte Krankheit (gekennzeichnet durch Tremor, psychische Störungen, bräunliche Pigmentierung bestimmter Gewebe, insbesondere auch der Hornhautperipherie, Lebercirrhose). *Deutsch Z Nervenheilk* 44:179-201, 1912.
11. Thornton SP: *Ophthalmic Eponyms.* Birmingham, Ala, Aesculapius Publishing Co, 1967, p 139.
12. Pollock LJ: The pathology of the nervous system in a case of progressive lenticular degeneration. *J Nerv Ment Dis* 46:401-420, 1917.
13. Bearn AG: A genetical analysis of 30 families with Wilson's disease (hepatolenticular degeneration). *Ann Hum Genet* 24:33-43, 1960.
14. Walshe JM, Cumings JN: *Wilson's Disease: Some Current Concepts.* Oxford, England, Blackwell Scientific Publications, 1961.
15. Victor M, Adams RD, Cole M: The acquired (non-Wilsonian) type of chronic hepatocerebral degeneration. *Medicine* 44:345-396, 1965.
16. Bearn AG: Wilson's disease, in Stanbury JB, Wyngaarden JB, Frederickson DS (eds): *The Metabolic Basis of Inherited Disease,* ed 2. New

York, McGraw-Hill, 1966, pp 761-779.

17. Adams RD: Hereditary hepatocerebral degeneration of Wilson-Westphal-Strümpell with reference to acquired hepatocerebral degeneration, in Bammer HG, Vogel P (eds): *Zukunft der Neurologie.* Stuttgart, Germany, Georg Thieme Verlag, 1967, pp 45-69.

18. Bergsma D: *Wilson's Disease: Birth Defects.* Original article series, vol 4, No. 2, New York, The National Foundation, 1968.

PROGRESSIVE LENTICULAR DEGENERATION:
A FAMILIAL NERVOUS DISEASE ASSOCIATED WITH
CIRRHOSIS OF THE LIVER[1]*

By S. A. Kinnier Wilson, M.D., B.Sc.EDIN., M.R.C.P.LOND.

Registrar to the National Hospital, Queen Square, London

(From the Laboratory of the National Hospital, Queen Square.)

Introduction

The object of this paper is to give a full description of a rare nervous disease, of which, as far as I am aware, no instance has been recorded during the last twenty years—a disease to which, for reasons which will hereinafter become evident, the name of "Progressive Lenticular Degeneration" may be conveniently applied . . . . This affection, where it occurs in an uncomplicated form, is *an extrapyramidal motor disease,* the importance of which is apparent not only because of its rarity, but also by reason of the light it sheds on such diseases as paralysis agitans. . . .

Progressive lenticular degeneration, as the disease may be called, is not one with which the medical profession is familiar. As far as I can discover, no case has been recorded since 1890, with the very doubtful exception of one reported by Anton, of Halle, under the title of "Dementia Choreo-asthenica, with Juvenile Nodular Cirrhosis of the Liver," some three years ago. In all probability this case was one of congenital syphilis. The total number of cases of the disease that have been published amounts to six only. Of these, two (brother and sister) were reported by Gowers in 1888 under the name of "Tetanoid Chorea, associated with Cirrhosis of the Liver"; one by Ormerod in 1890; three (two brothers and a sister) by Homén, of Helsingfors, also in 1890. . . .

In this paper will be described four cases of the affection which have been personally observed and diagnosed (in all but one the diagnosis was made during life), in three of which it has been possible to make a *post-mortem* examination.

The first patient (S.T.) came under observation in 1905, and died on July 28, 1908. At the autopsy bilateral degeneration of the lenticular nucleus was found, coupled with cirrhosis of the liver.

The second patient (D.P.) came under observation in 1906, and died on March 3, 1907. Here, also, cirrhosis of the liver and a slighter degree of lenticular change were discovered.

The third patient (E.P.), a brother of the above, came under notice in 1907. This patient was exhaustively examined in the summer of 1910. He died on September 20, 1910, and in his case identical findings were obtained at the autopsy.

The fourth patient (M. To.) came under observation in the autumn of 1911, and at the time of writing she is still living.

In addition to these four personal cases the record of two other cases of the disease has been obtained, one of which occurred in the family described by Gowers, but has not hitherto been published, as the notes were lost years ago. By a piece of good fortune I was able to trace the mother of the family, an old lady aged 70, and to obtain from her the clinical details of this new case. The other is one referred to by Ormerod in his paper of 1890; the notes, not hitherto published, are preserved in the National Hospital, Queen Square. . . .

Résumé of the
Clinical History of Case 1

A young woman, aged 21, whose family history is negative, and who has never suffered from any particular illness, who has always been intelligent and physically active, suffers from an attack of jaundice of about five weeks' duration, the exact

[1]This paper formed part of a thesis for the degree of MD of the University of Edinburgh, July 1911, for which a gold medal was awarded.

*Reprinted from *Brain* 34:295-509, 1912.

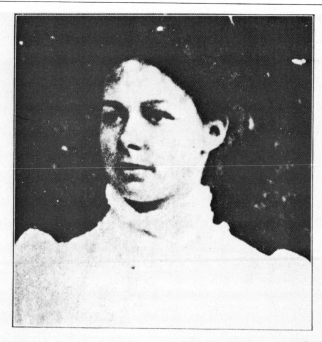

Fig. 12.—Photograph of S. T. before the onset of the symptoms of progressive lenticular degeneration.

details of which are not forthcoming, and at intervals thereafter, for about two or three years, has occasional swelling of the ankles, without being in any way incapacitated thereby. Four years after the icterus, at the age of 25, she notices that her right hand shakes a little as she is writing, and her articulation becomes a little slurring. In the course of a few months her friends notice a considerable alteration in her general condition; she is restless, unable to settle to anything, easily provoked to laughter, constantly smiling and unnaturally cheerful. At the same time the tremor spreads to both arms and hands, her writing deteriorates, her articulation is definitely impaired, and she has some trouble in swallowing.

At the age of 26 she is examined by a neurologist, who can find no signs of organic disease of the nervous system, notes that there is no nystagmus, and obtains a double flexor response. Nevertheless the condition is steadily progressive; the tremors are accentuated, the dysarthria and dysphagia increase, a generalized stiffness of the musculature reveals itself, and the fingers begin to assume certain attitudes of contracture. Her mental condition is one of facility; she is easily amused, and constantly laughing; her mouth is open and

saliva occasionally escapes involuntarily. In spite of the vacant expression on her face her memory and perception are quite good; she has neither delusions nor hallucinations; she is very observant and often makes apposite remarks about those with whom she is associated. The symptoms are characterized by a curious variability; articulation and the power of swallowing seem sometimes to improve, and there is no true paralysis, in the sense that all voluntary movements can be carried out, though slowly.

During the next two years the disease slowly progresses. While for a long time bodily nutrition is well maintained, the other symptoms increase in severity. The features are fixed in a perpetual smile; the mouth is wide open and the sialorrhoea is more marked; the patient is anarthric and dysphagic; yet with voluntary effort the mouth can be slowly closed, the tongue slowly protruded, while the palate rises on the attempt to articulate; the pupils react briskly to light, ocular movements are free, and the optic discs are normal. The muscles become more and more rigid, the arms, and to a less extent the legs, fixed in attitudes of contracture, which can be to some extent, but not entirely, overcome by passive movement; as a

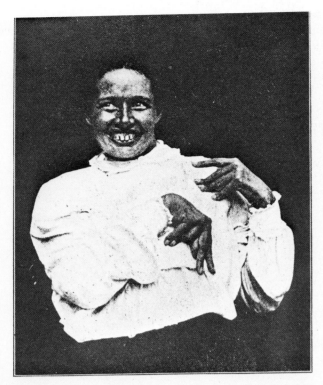

FIG. 13.—Photograph of S. T., taken at Virginia Water. Characteristic appearance of face and upper limbs. Compare with fig. 12. [For this photograph I am indebted to Dr. G. W. Smith.]

result the patient has become peculiarly helpless; but again on volitional effort a considerable range of movement is still possible. The tremor is absolutely constant, often wide in range and severe in degree; it affects all muscular groups in the limbs, especially the distal groups, but includes also the lower jaw, head, neck and trunk. No sensory change can be detected; the deep reflexes are present without being exaggerated, there is no ankle-clonus; the abdominal reflexes are diminished, and the flexor response on the left side has changed to extensor, the other remaining as before. Defect of control over the sphincters, probably of central origin, appears.

Eventually emaciation sets in; the patient is reduced to a profound degree of helplessness, is in a state of contracture, speechless, incontinent; nevertheless her mental condition remains clear, she understands everything and endeavours to express her wants. An acute attack of haematemesis ushers in the end, and she dies at the age of 29, after an illness of rather more than four years. With the exception of the initial symptoms nine years previously, there have never been either symptoms or signs referable to disease of the liver, but this is suspected during life and confirmed at the autopsy. . . .

[Figures 12 and 13]

Résumé of the Pathological Findings in Case 1

The brain is of good size, shape, and weight. The cerebral gyri are not atrophic, are of normal convolutional pattern, and present no obvious morbid appearance. The membranes are to all intents and purposes normal. The cerebral blood-vessels are not thickened or occluded, and show no patches of disease in their walls.

On Marie's *coupe d'élection*, the eye is at once

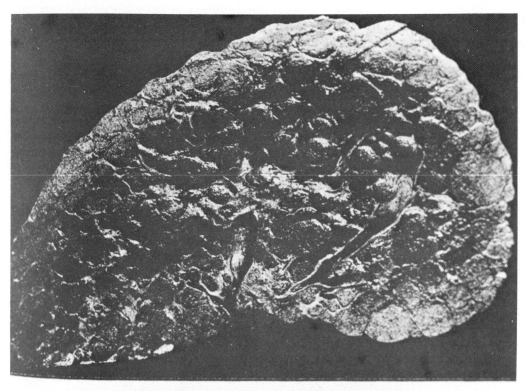

FIG. 26.—Liver (S. T., Case 1). Transverse section.

caught by a complete bilateral and symmetrical destruction of the lenticular nucleus. In place of the latter, on either side, and more especially in place of its outer and middle zones, is an elongated cavity, measuring $2\frac{1}{2}$ cm. long by $1\frac{1}{4}$ cm. wide, with dark-coloured crumbling walls, extending from the anterior to the posterior limit of the putamen, and from its extreme lower extremity almost to its upper limit. Only a small piece of the inner zone of the globus pallidus remains. Compared with this utter degeneration of the lenticular nucleus, the optic thalamus and the caudate nucleus are well preserved, except that in the former, on the left side, there is a small punched-out hole towards its posterior part, and the latter is on both sides a little shrunken, and less full and rounded than in a normal brain. The degenerated area extends close up to the internal capsule on both sides; on the right this seems quite intact throughout, although it is found to be somewhat undermined; on the left there is a small prolongation of the cavity across the genu of the capsule, the fibres of which are separated rather than destroyed. Microscopically, however, there is some descending degeneration in the genu fibres.

The external capsule is thinned on both sides, and degenerated in its middle third; the claustrum is very slightly invaded on the left side; the cortex of the island of Reil is well preserved on both sides, although microscopically there is some degeneration of the subcortical fibres of its convolutions towards its posterior part.

The white matter of the cerebral hemispheres is normal. The cortex is practically normal; in particular the origin of the pyramidal tracts in the Betz-cells of the motor area is carefully examined, and the great majority of the latter are found to present no morbid appearance, although some show chronic degenerative changes.

With the exception of the slight descending degeneration in some capsular genu fibres on the left side, the pyramidal tracts stain normally throughout, and, followed from the motor cortex through the capsule, crus, pons, medulla and cord, are perfectly normal.

On the other hand, the extrapyramidal system from the lenticular nucleus, viâ the ansa lenticularis, to the red nucleus, is degenerated on both sides; the lenticular bundle of Forel is partly degenerated, as are a large number of the strio-

Luysian fibres on both sides; the corpus Luysii is smaller than normal. The cells of the red nucleus do not appear changed, nor does the nucleus seem altered in its fibre-content. The striothalamic fibres are degenerated.

The external medullary lamina of the optic thalamus, the "zone grillagée," and the outer part of the thalamus generally, are to a certain extent altered.

The pons and medulla, and the cerebellum, are not the seat of any change that can be recognized microscopically.

The nuclei of the cranial nerves are unchanged, except for slight alterations of secondary significance.

The spinal cord (cells and fibres) is normal, except for certain slight alterations, also of secondary significance.

The same is true of the muscles.

The liver is in an advanced state of cirrhosis; the type is mainly multilobular, but some monolobular cirrhosis is found. In the cirrhotic tissue abundant bile-ducts ramify. The liver-cells are in many instances normal, others are necrosed, many show fatty infiltration and degeneration, others are actively regenerating. . . .

[Figures 26 and 29]

Chapter VII.—Syndrome of the Corpus Striatum

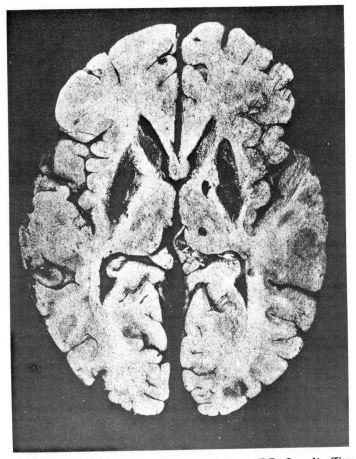

Fig 29.—Horizontal section through hemispheres (S.T., Case 1). (They are reversed in the figure, the left being at the right-hand side.)

The lenticular nucleus, and corpus striatum generally, occupy a considerable area in the middle third of the cerebral hemispheres; the arrangement of cells and fibres in them is somewhat complicated, and it is contrary to physiological conceptions to suppose that ganglia of such a size should be unimportant from a physiological standpoint. It is, however, undeniable that our knowledge of the functions and pathology of the corpus striatum has hitherto been curiously indefinite. On the one hand, small lesions of that body have often proved to have been entirely without effect, from a symptomatological point of view, and even larger lesions have sometimes, apparently, failed to reveal themselves by any recognizable symptoms during life. On the other hand, uncomplicated involvement of the corpus striatum is a comparative rarity, and the proximity and close relationship of the corticospinal paths have led observers to attribute to impairment of the function of the latter any symptoms which otherwise might have been associated with the lesion in the former region. For these, among other reasons, the prevailing opinion on the physiology of the corpus striatum has been one of uncertainty. Thus Monakow, in the latest edition of his well-known "Gehirnpathologie," is forced to adopt a negative attitude. "In spite of the investigations of numerous experimenters, we know as little of the clinical effects of lesions of the lenticular and caudate nuclei, or as much, as Nothnagel did twenty-five years ago."

In the disease which I propose to designate progressive lenticular degeneration three desiderata are fulfilled on which the establishment of a corpus striatum symptom-complex would seem to depend. The lesions are sufficiently large, in the first place; of sufficiently long duration, in the second place; and in the third they are confined to the ganglion itself. My Case 3 offers a perfect opportunity of differentiating lenticular from corticospinal symptoms. With integrity of the internal capsule and pyramidal paths generally there is bilateral degeneration of the lenticular nucleus, which reveals itself by a train of clinical symptoms amply corroborated by the results of the investigation of a number of other cases, all collected in this paper, so that a general review provides a striking confirmation of the general statement.

The syndrome of the corpus striatum, therefore, which is here put forward, may be expressed as follows:—

In pure, uncomplicated, bilateral lesions of the lenticular nucleus, and more generally of the corpus striatum, provided they are of sufficient size and of adequate duration, the clinical symptoms are bilateral involuntary movements, practically always of the tremor variety; weakness, spasticity or hypertonicity (sometimes spasmodic contractions) and eventually contracture of the skeletal musculature; dysarthria or anarthria and dysphagia, and a degree of emotionalism; but without any sensory disturbance, without any true paralysis, and without any alteration in the cutaneous reflexes. If the abdominal reflexes are absent (apart from muscular rigidity) or the plantars of extensor type, then the syndrome is no longer pure.

In view of this syndrome, thus differentiated for the first time from a study of progressive lenticular degeneration, the loose way, sometimes adopted, of considering "signs of organic nervous disease" and "signs of pyramidal nervous disease" as one and the same thing must be definitively abandoned. Pure cases of progressive lenticular degeneration show no signs of pyramidal defect of function (as estimated by the reflexes), but the disease is none the less one of the most serious organic diseases of the nervous system that the neurologist is likely to encounter. It is unfortunate that there is no expression in common use to indicate extrapyramidal motor disease.

It has been already remarked that the resemblance between progressive lenticular degeneration and paralysis agitans is considerable. In the latter there is a symptom-complex of tremor, rigidity, and weakness; sometimes there is a degree of emotional overaction, and, as in early cases of the former disease, the patient's utterance is monotonous and sometimes dysarthric; "il a perdu le chanson du langage," to use a picturesque French expression. The articulatory and phonatory defects of the Parkinsonian are in my opinion the result of rigidity of the corresponding musculatures, and not due to a true pseudobulbar condition. Hence the relation between the two conditions is very close, that is to say, as far as the clinical symptoms are concerned, for there are differences of age and etiology and duration which are obvious enough. It might be expected, then, that the pathology of the two conditions, or at least the localization of the lesions, should be more or less identical. Hitherto, in paralysis agitans, no certain pathology has been demonstrated. But within recent years various data have accumulated to show that its lesions will probably be found in the basal ganglia and regio subthalamica. What is paralysis agitans but an extrapyramidal motor disease? Its pathology must therefore be looked for along the lines that have been indicated in the last chapter. . . .

Chapter VIII.—Clinical Conclusions

(1) Progressive lenticular degeneration is a disease of the motor nervous system, occurring in young people and very often familial. It is not congenital or hereditary.

(2) It is progressive and fatal within a varying period; acute cases may last only a few months; one chronic case has as a maximum continued for seven years; the average duration of chronic cases is four years.

(3) It is characterized by a definite symptom-complex, whose chief features are: generalized tremor, dysarthria and dysphagia, muscular rigidity and hypertonicity, emaciation, spasmodic contractions, contractures, emotionalism. There are also certain mental symptoms, either transient and such as one sees in a toxic psychosis, but not severe, or more chronic, consisting in a general restriction of the mental horizon, and a certain facility or docility without delusions or hallucinations, and not necessarily as progressive as the somatic symptoms. The mental symptoms may be very slight and are sometimes absent.

(4) In pure cases the affection constitutes an extrapyramidal motor disease, for the reflexes are normal from the point of view of the function of the pyramidal tracts.

(5) The neurological symptoms constitute a syndrome of the corpus striatum, which has not hitherto been differentiated in this disease.

(6) In some ways the disease bears a resemblance to paralysis agitans, and throws light on the problem of that affection.

(7) Although cirrhosis of the liver is constantly found in this affection, and is an essential feature of it, there are no signs of liver disease during life.

Pathological Conclusions

(1) The chief pathological feature of the disease is bilateral symmetrical degeneration of the putamen and globus pallidus, in particular the former.

(2) This degeneration is the sequel to the selective operation of some morbid agent on the cells and fibres of the putamen and lenticular nucleus generally. The caudate nucleus is often somewhat atrophic, but never to the same extent, while other large collections of grey matter in the immediate neighbourhood of the lenticular nucleus —e.g., the optic thalamus, which has partially the same blood supply—is not affected at all in a pure case unless it be indirectly, and to a very slight extent.

(3) The morbid agent is probably of the nature of a toxin.

(4) A constant, essential, and in all probability primary feature of the pathology of the disease is cirrhosis of the liver, not syphilitic or alcoholic; it is multilobular or mixed in type, always pronounced, but presenting a varying pathological picture of necrosis, fatty degeneration, and regeneration.

(5) It is probable that the toxin is associated with the hepatic cirrhosis, and may be generated in connexion therewith. An important analogy may be drawn from the occurrence of "Kernikterus" in certain cases of familial icterus gravis neonatorum, where in spite of the universal bile-staining of the tissues of the body certain collections only of grey matter in the brain show a marked affinity for the circulating poison, while others do not. The parts that are stained deeply are in particular the nucleus lenticularis and the corpus Luysii (among others), while the optic thalamus, for instance, is scarcely stained at all.

(6) The pyramidal tracts are intact from Betz cells to muscles in a pure case; occasionally certain secondary changes occur of limited significance.

(7) Certain secondary degenerations in the subthalamic region, of physiological importance, follow on the lenticular disease.

Physiological Conclusions

(1) The corpus striatum exercises a steadying effect on the action of the corticospinal system.

(2) This is effected either by the lenticulo-rubrospinal system, or more indirectly viâ the optic thalamus and its cortical connections.

(3) When this influence is impaired pyramidal function is affected in its turn, and is seen in hypertonicity or rigidity, as well as in tremor on voluntary movement.

(4) There is not, however, any paralysis in the strict sense.

(5) The direct connexion of the corpus striatum with the cortex is minimal.

(6) There is no necessity to postulate articulatory "centres" in the putamen or globus pallidus.

(7) Dysarthria may result without any pyramidal involvement of genu fibres, and with intact cranial nuclei, from hypertonicity of the musculature concerned.

(8) Tremor is due more particularly to failure of function of the lenticulo-rubrospinal system.

(9) Hypertonicity or rigidity of the musculature, due to defect of the "inhibitory" action of the corpus striatum, is possibly associated with impairment of impulses from the body viâ the optic thalamus to the cerebral cortex. . . .

XXXVII   Infantile Spinal Muscular Atrophy

References

1. Bendheim OL: On the history of Hoffmann's sign. *Bull Inst Hist Med* 5:684-686, 1937.
2. Wartenberg R: Studies in reflexes: History, physiology, synthesis and nomenclature: Study I. *Arch Neurol Psychiat* 51:113-133, 1944.
3. Hoffmann J: Ueber chronische spinale Muskelatrophie im Kindesalter, auf familiärer Basis. *Deutsch Z Nervenheilk* 3:427-470, 1893.
4. Hoffmann J: Weiterer Beitrag zur Lehre von der hereditären progressiven spinalen Muskelatrophie im Kindesalter nebst Bemerkungen über den fortschreitenden Muskelschwund im Allgemeinen. *Deutsch Z Nervenheilk* 10:292-320, 1897.
5. Hoffmann J: Dritter Beitrag zur Lehre von der hereditären progressiven spinalen Muskelatrophie im Kindesalter. *Deutsch Z Nervenheilk* 18:217-224, 1900.
6. Hoffmann J: Ueber die hereditäre progressive spinale Muskelatrophie im Kindesalter. *Munchen Med Wschr* 47:1649-1651, 1900.
7. Pakesch E: Dr. Guido Werdnig, 1844-1919. Ein Nervenarzt in Graz. *Wien Klin Wschr* 77:445-447, 1965.
8. Werdnig G: Zwei frühinfantile hereditäre Fälle von progressiver Muskelatrophie unter dem Bilde der Dystrophie, aber auf neurotischer Grundlage. *Arch Psychiat Nervenkr* 22:437-480, 1891.
9. Werdnig G: Die frühinfantile progressive spinale Amyotrophie. *Arch Psychiat Nervenkr* 26:706-744, 1894.
10. Brandt S: *Werdnig-Hoffmann's Infantile Progressive Muscular Atrophy: Clinical Aspects, Pathology, Heredity and Relation to Oppenheim's Amyotonia Congenita and Other Morbid Conditions with Laxity of Joints or Muscles in Infants.* Copenhagen, Ejnar Munksgaard, 1950.
11. Byers RK, Banker BQ: Infantile muscular atrophy. *Arch Neurol* 5:140-164, 1961.
12. Oppenheim H: Ueber allgemeine und localisierte Atonie der Muskulatur (Myatonie) im frühen Kindesalter. *Mschr Psychiat Neurol* 8:232-233, 1900.
13. Walton JN: Amyotonia congenita: A follow-up study. *Lancet* 1:1023-1027, 1956.

WHEN Johann Hoffmann (1857 to 1919), professor of neurology at Heidelberg and discoverer of the digital reflex that bears his name,[1,2] published the first of his papers on infantile progressive muscular atrophy in 1893,[3-6] Guido Werdnig (1844 to 1919),[7] a neurologist in Graz, Austria, had already reported two such cases.[8,9] Both men described the same basic features of this familial degenerative disease, which usually leads to death by the age of 4 years.[10,11]

Hermann Oppenheim[12] then complicated the subject with his brief report in 1900 of a benign form of congenital muscular hypotonia (amyotonia congenita), and for many years, it was believed that amyotonia congenita began in the neonatal period, whereas progressive muscular atrophy began later in infancy. We now know that this distinction in terms of age of onset is not valid.[13] The term amyotonia congenita has generally been discarded in favor of the term benign congenital hypotonia, and the disease with the malignant course so well described by Werdnig is now referred to as infantile spinal muscular atrophy or Werdnig-Hoffmann disease.

Werdnig's discovery did not win him fame during his lifetime. He became paraplegic and was bedridden for 12 years before he died in a public sanitorium, a forgotten man.[7]

From the Pathological-Anatomical Institute of Graz
TWO EARLY INFANTILE HEREDITARY CASES OF PROGRESSIVE MUSCULAR ATROPHY SIMULATING DYSTROPHY, BUT ON A NEURAL BASIS*

by
Dr. G. Werdnig
Neurologist in Graz

...Case I
History of the Illness

*Translation of: Zwei frühinfantile hereditäre Fälle von progressiver Muskelatrophie unter dem Bilde der Dystrophie, aber auf neurotischer Grundlage. *Arch Psychiat Nervenkrank* 22:437-480, 1891.

Wilhelm Bauer, 3 years old, was born of healthy parents . . . . His 1¾-year-old brother, Georg, is paralyzed in his legs. (His case history follows this one.) A 10-month-old brother, Franz, is healthy.

The patient was born in May 1885 as a strong child, who carried out lively movements with his extremities. Soon after birth he was brought to the country, where he was fed cows' milk, went

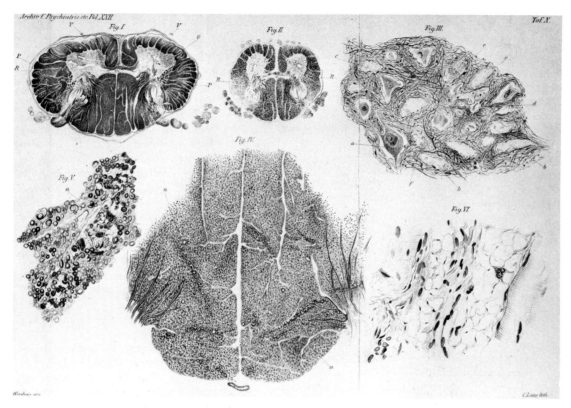

Explanation of the Illustrations (Table X)

Fig 1.—Cross-section at the level of the seventh cervical nerves. . . V = Anterior roots. G = Honey-combed anterior horn.

Fig II.—Cross-section at the level of the second-third lumbar nerves. . . .

Fig III.—Portion of the right anterior horn at L2-3. . . a. Normal ganglion cells. b. Empty cell beds. c. Empty cell beds with protoplasmic residues. d. Deiter's cells.

e. Vessels. f. Myelin droplets. Also various shrivelled ganglion cells.

Fig IV.—View of the posterior columns from the vicinity of the sixth cervical nerves. . . a. Arrangement of the empty network in the form of a pearl necklace.

Fig V.—A similar section at higher magnification. . . a. A small arterial vessel.

Fig VI.—Longitudinal section of the gastrocnemius muscle from Case I. . . .

through a mild gastro-intestinal catarrh after the first four weeks, and got his first teeth at 7 months. His mother stated that at each visit she had found the child wide-awake and kicking actively. Later, he tended to sit and hold his feeding-bottle with his hands. At the age of 10 months, the child returned to his mother. . . . At the end of his first year, he began to talk a little. It was at this time that weakness of the lower extremities appeared. In the summer of 1886 he was given back to acquaintances in the country, where he ate well and became very fat all over. But all the soft parts were like dough, and the mother commented that he seemed healthier and stronger when he was thin. The weakness of the lower extremities increased and extended to the back, so that it became difficult for the child to sit. In the autumn of 1886 the child had whooping cough. Soon after this, his mother took him back with her, and the cough subsided after a time. Nevertheless the weakness increased, and the hands began to tremble. . . . The child became unable to hold up his head. . . . His behavior became infantile. Voluntary movements ceased in

the lower extremities except for slight movements in the ankle joints and flexion and extension of the toes. He could no longer bring his hands to his mouth. . . . His eyes did not close fully during sleep, and swallowing became difficult. On April 4, 1888, the child was admitted to the Anna Children's Hospital here, and I draw on the observations made there by Prof. von Jaksh, which he kindly let me use in this case history.

Present status, recorded on April 4, 1888. The child is large for his age, has abundant adipose tissue, especially on the extremities, which have a doughy softness. . . . The musculature here is markedly atrophic. . . .

The boy holds the hip and knee joints flexed. Slight contractures in the flexors of the thigh and leg. . . . Both feet in equinovarus position. . . . Active movement of the lower and upper extremities is possible to a very slight degree, but takes place very slowly, with vermiform contractions of the muscles. . . .

Sensation is preserved in the trunk and extremities. Cutaneous reflexes are weak; patellar, biceps and triceps reflexes are absent. Faradic excitability is present in the muscles of the extremities, but is very weak. Galvanic current elicits more or less distinct twitching, but with very sluggish relaxation. . . .

April 26. Profuse rales. The intercostal spaces are strongly retracted in inspiration. Fever for two days.

April 28. Extreme dyspnea. Fever. . . .

May 1. . . . Death. . . .

Microscopic Examination

The spinal cord and portion of the gastrocnemius muscle were removed. The former remained for several weeks in Müller's solution, followed by soaking and storage for several days in weak alcohol.

A. The Spinal Cord

. . . . Level of the second and third cervical nerves. Cross-section of normal size and shape. Posterior bundles and lateral cerebellar tract intact. The other part of the lateral tracts, especially in the region of the pyramidal system, somewhat lacking in myelinated fibers, interspersed to a moderate extent with connective tissue. . . . The anterior funiculi are degenerated in the vicinity of the exit of the anterior roots. Posterior horns and posterior roots of normal appearance.

In both of the anterior horns most of the ganglion cells have indistinct processes, an indistinct nucleus or one with a fragmented border. Many cells are rounded, shrivelled, and reveal no further details. Finally, there are many entirely empty cell-beds, which contain only one or more granules. These empty cell-beds stand out from the surrounding tissue since they are still enclosed by the usual fiber network. All diseased cells are poor in pigment. Anterior roots on both sides present only thin bundles, which contain mostly supporting tissue, fibrous connective tissue, and only very few medullary fibers. Anterior commissure intact. . . . [Similar findings at the levels of the 4-5, 6-7, and 8 cervical, 1, 2-3, 5, 10 and 12 thoracic, and 2 and 5 lumbar nerves.]

B. The Gastrocnemius Muscle

The piece of muscle was placed in Müller's solution for some time, then in alcohol. It was examined both as a teased-out preparation and, after embedding it in paraffin, in longitudinal and cross-sections.

There was only simple atrophy in this muscle. The better preserved muscle fibers were 36μ in diameter, polygonal in cross-section and showed little disruption of fibrils. These fibers formed groups that were separated by moderately large masses of fatty tissue from other groups of round fibers, which had a diameter of only about 10μ, but which still exhibited cross-striations. Among the latter fibers were single fibers, the cross-striations of which were disrupted, with the contractile substance broken down into a formless mass. As these fibers degenerated, they could be traced as collapsed long tubes containing nuclei. . . . In addition to the hyperplasia of fat, there was a significant increase in the interfibrillary connective tissue. . . .

There are a few details of the anatomical findings still to be dealt with more closely. The atrophy of the anterior horn cells was especially marked in the cervical and lumbar enlargements. I found the lateral horn cells of the thoracic cord intact. . . .

I found the lateral funiculi to be normal in the upper and middle thoracic region, whereas they were pathologically altered in the cervical, and especially in the lowest thoracic and in the lumbar segments. In the last two regions, the degeneration involved the posterior parts of the lateral funiculi, but it differed from a secondary degeneration of the pyramidal system because it was not entirely restricted to this system (indeed, in the lumber cord it extended into the lateral parts of the posterior funiculi). Furthermore, there were a great many more intact nerve fibers in this region than is encountered in a secondary degeneration. . . .

The anterior roots corresponded to the condition of the anterior horn cells and were nearly completely degenerated in the cervical and lumbar cord and to a great extent in the thoracic cord. . . . Special cross-sections made it possible to establish the characteristics of this degeneration. From the thickened neurilemma a dense network branched off into the interior of the nerve, coalescing with the fibrous connective tissue that replaced the former nerve bundles. Sparse normal nerve fibers and fibers with thickened axis cylinders were enclosed by this network. . . .

We conclude that we are dealing, in both of our cases, with an early infantile, familial muscular atrophy, which resembles dystrophy only in its presentation and in the progressive nature of its development. In the rapidity of its course, however, it bears the distinct signs of a neural illness, and undoubtedly is due to a primary degeneration of the motor pathways of the spinal cord. . . .

XXXVIII   The Arnold-Chiari Malformation

THE ARNOLD-CHIARI malformation is more accurately designated the Chiari-Arnold malformation since Hans Chiari's first publication on this subject preceded Julius Arnold's by three years.[1-3] In his initial report, translated below, Chiari divided the hindbrain anomalies occurring in some hydrocephalic children into three types. Subsequently, two of Arnold's students gave the name Arnold-Chiari malformation to Chiari's second type, which they, like Chiari, found in association with meningomyelocele.[4] The eponymic error has been perpetuated ever since, though the term is now loosely applied to encompass a whole spectrum of related developmental defects.

There is considerable individual variation in the pathological composition of the Arnold-Chiari malformation, but in general, Chiari's type II changes are common in infants with hydrocephalus and meningomyelocele, and the type I changes are encountered occasionally in older children and adults. The detection of the latter cases has been aided greatly by the recent development of satisfactory techniques for air myelography and fractional pneumoencephalography.[5]

Chiari thought that the cerebellum and brain stem were pushed downward by the hydrocephalic cerebrum in the type II malformation, and there is some experimental evidence for this view.[6] However, the association of this malformation with meningomyelocele has led to the proposal that the cerebellum and brain stem are pulled down into the cervical spinal canal by the fixed spinal cord as the cerebrospinal axis of the developing embryo elongates.[7] This impaction then obstructs the outflow of cerebrospinal fluid from the fourth ventricle, causing the coexisting hydrocephalus.[8]

Valid objections have been raised to these hypotheses, and the actual pathogenesis of the Arnold-Chiari malformation may be more complex, involving a series of simultaneous developmental errors.[9,10] Similar processes also result in other developmental defects, such as syringomyelia and diastematomyelia, which may explain the occasional appearance of these entities in association with the Arnold-Chiari malformation.[10] Although the initial etiological factors in humans still elude detection, an identical malformation has been induced in the hamster with a viral agent.[6]

For many years the Arnold-Chiari malformation carried a grave prognosis. Now, most patients with the type I Chiari anomaly can be benefited by a direct surgical decompression at the level of the foramen magnum.[11] In contrast, it has been discovered that infants with a type II anomaly and an associated meningomyelocele often become more hydrocephalic after excision of the meningomyelocele, perhaps because a large absorptive surface has been removed.[12] However, with the development of successful operations for shunting cerebrospinal fluid,[11,13,14] the infants with the type II anomaly can also be salvaged and have a reasonably good chance for normal intelligence.[15,16]

References

1. Chiari H: Ueber Veränderungen des Kleinhirns infolge von Hydrocephalie des Grosshirns. *Deutsch Med Wschr* 17:1172-1175, 1891.

2. Arnold J: Myelocyste, Transposition von Gewebskeimen und Sympodie. *Beitr Path Anat* 16:1-28, 1894.

3. Chiari H: Über Veränderungen des Kleinhirns, des Pons und der Medulla oblongata in folge von congenitaler Hydrocephalie des Grosshirns. *Denkschr Akad Wiss Wien* 63:71-116, 1896.

4. Schwalbe E, Gredig M: Über Entwicklungsstörungen des Kleinhirns, Hirnstamms und Halsmarks bei Spina bifida. (Arnoldsche und Chiarische Missbildung.) *Beitr Path Anat* 40:132-194, 1970.

5. Jirout J: *Pneumomyelography.* JA Goree (trans-ed), Springfield, Ill, Charles C Thomas Publisher, 1969, pp 138-143.

6. Margolis G, Kilham L: Experimental virus-induced hydrocephalus: Relation to pathogenesis of the Arnold-Chiari malformation. *J Neurosurg* 31:1-9, 1969.

7. Lichtenstein BW: Distant neuroanatomic complications of spina bifida (spinal dysraphism): Hydrocephalus, Arnold-Chiari deformity, stenosis of the aqueduct of Sylvius, etc; pathogenesis and pathology. *Arch Neurol Psychiat* 47:195-214, 1942.

8. Russell DS, Donald C: The mechanism of internal hydrocephalus in spina bifida. *Brain* 58:203-215, 1935.

9. Peach B: The Arnold-Chiari malformation: Morphogenesis. *Arch Neurol* 12:527-535, 1965.

10. Gardner WJ: Myelocele: Rupture of the neural tube? *Clin Neurosurg* 15:57-79, 1968.

11. Matson DD: *Neurosurgery of Infancy and Childhood,* ed 2. Springfield, Ill, Charles C Thomas Publisher, 1969, pp 5-60, 76-83, 222-258.

12. Penfield W, Cone W: Spina bifida and cranium bifidum: Results of plastic repair of meningocele and myelomeningocele by a new method. *JAMA* 98:454-460, 1932.

13. Wilkins RH: Neurosurgical classic—XX. *J Neurosurg* 21:586-635, 1964.

14. Schulze A: Historische Entwicklung und gegenwärtiger Stand der Hydrozephalus-Operationen. *Deutsch Med J* 19:314-318, 1968.

15. Foltz EL: The first seven years of a hydrocephalus project, in Shulman K (ed): *Workshop in Hydrocephalus.* Philadelphia, University of Pennsylvania, 1966, pp 79-114.

16. Nulsen FE, Becker DP: The control of progressive hydrocephalus in infancy by valve-regulated venous shunt, in Shulman K (ed): *Workshop in Hydrocephalus.* Philadelphia, University of Pennsylvania, 1966, pp 115-137.

Concerning Changes in the Cerebellum

Due to Hydrocephalus of the Cerebrum[*][1]

By Dr. H. Chiari, Professor of Pathological Anatomy at

the German University in Prague

Despite the extensive literature on the pathology of hydrocephalus, little attention has been given to the sequential changes in the region of the cerebellum produced by cerebral hydrocephalus. . . . I will indicate several types of these changes in the following selected cases, and will reserve a full description for a later report.

The first type consists of elongation of the tonsils and the medial portions of the lobi inferiores . . . of the cerebellum into conical extensions that accompany the medulla oblongata and extend into the vertebral canal. . . .

It is my impression that this elongation results from hydrocephalus of the cerebrum, specifically the chronic hydrocephalus established early in life (congenital hydrocephalus). I never have found it in the absence of hydrocephalus, and never with

acute hydrocephalus or hydrocephalus of late onset. But I have found it in a large percentage of cases of chronic congenital hydrocephalus. Apparently we are dealing with a developmental anomaly of the cerebellum.

The substance of the elongated parts of the cerebellum may exhibit either normal texture, sclerosis, or softening. The fourth ventricle is either expanded very slightly or not at all, and the medulla oblongata is either unchanged or flattened symmetrically or asymmetrically by the lateral cerebellar elongations. . . . These elongations of the cerebellum usually extend only to the level of the atlas, but in several cases . . . their tips lay at the level of the origin of the 3rd cervical nerves.

I believe it is possible for bulbar symptoms to be caused by the described cerebellar elongation, but in none of the cases so far have I been able to settle this point clinically. . . .

[a brief case presentation follows]

A second type consists of the displacement of portions of the cerebellum into the enlarged verte-

[*]Translation of: Ueber Veränderungen des Kleinhirns infolge von Hydrocephalie des Grosshirns. *Deutsche Medicinische Wochenschrift* 17:1172-1175, 1891.
[1]Delivered in the Division for General Pathology and Pathological Anatomy of the 64th Meeting of the Association of German Naturalists and Physicians in Halle-on-the Saale on 22 September 1891.

*bral canal, the cerebellum lying within the fourth
ventricle, which is elongated and also extends
down into the vertebral canal.*

Since the anatomical relations are quite complicated in this type, I will deal at once with a
specific case.

A 6-month-old girl . . . was examined by autopsy on 17 November 1890 in the Kaiser Franz
Joseph Children's Hospital here. . . . She had been
extremely ill with pneumonia, and had complete
paralysis of both lower extremities, the bladder
and the rectum.

In addition to bilateral lobar pneumonia, the
autopsy showed a series of striking pathological
changes in the central nervous system. The cerebrum was very hydrocephalic, . . . with the most
noticeable dilatation involving the lateral ventricles, although the third ventricle was also considerably enlarged. . . . The tentorium cerebelli was
much less arched than usual, and the cerebellum
was flattened superiorly. . . .

The pons, 24 mm long, lay only partly within
the cranial cavity . . . and extended 6 mm into
the vertebral canal. Its ventral surface was notched,
corresponding to the anterior border of the foramen magnum and the superior end of the odontoid process. . . . The pons appeared flattened
asymmetrically from front to back. The medulla,
which was not sharply demarcated externally from
the pons, was entirely contained within the vertebral canal. It was 19 mm long, and its lower end
extended past the middle of the body of the third
vertebra. It appeared flat, and was asymmetrical to
the extent that on a cross-section through its
upper half, the raphe curved to the left, and the
left half was larger than the right half in the
dorso-ventral diameter. Corresponding to the elongation of the pons and medulla oblongata, the
cranial nerves arising from them were noticeably
stretched in their "intracranial" portions. At the
junction of the medulla and spinal cord, there was
a stepwise elevation . . . that dorsally produced a
protuberance . . . , and affected the upper 9 mm
of the spinal cord. . . .

Along the dorsal surface of the inferior end of
the pons . . . and the entire medulla oblongata,
there was a pocket-shaped elongation of the fourth
ventricle . . . , containing compressed portions of
the inferior vermis and part of the choroid plexus.
. . . The inferior vermis was no better developed
than the tonsils and the medial portion of the
inferior lobe of the cerebellum. In contrast, the
posterior and superior vermis, and the posterior

and superior lobes could be discerned very well
though they were smaller than usual. At the lower
end of the medulla, the central canal of the
cervical cord originated from the rhomboid fossa
in the usual manner.

The cervical cord measured only 24 mm in
length, and extended from the lower border of the
body of the third cervical vertebra to the middle
of the body of the seventh cervical vertebra. The
nerve roots arising from it were surprisingly close
together. . . .

The thoracic cord . . . contained a cylindrical
cavity in its dorsal half, extending from the . . .
first through the seventh segment, 6 mm at its
widest point, and filled with a clear fluid. A
second such cylindrical cavity, up to 4 mm wide,
was located in the area of the eleventh and twelfth
segments. In the upper lumbar area, the spinal
cord split along the midline into two halves . . .
and there was a myelomeningocele about the size
of a hen's egg. . . . Below the fifth lumbar segment, the two halves of the spinal cord . . . fused
again into a cylindrical cord. . . .

[a microscopic evaluation of the anomalous areas
follows]

. . . . In spite of the expansion of the skull, the
cranial cavity became too small for the hydrocephalic brain. The basal parts of the brain were
pressed downward into the widened vertebral canal, and the described changes in their architecture
and texture were gradually produced during their
further development. . . .

Of the *third type of consecutive changes in the
cerebellum caused by chronic congenital hydrocephalus* . . . I have seen only one case. It
demonstrated *the greatest degree of displacement
of the cerebellum, out of the cranial cavity
through the foramen magnum into the vertebral
canal* . . . , *involving the deposition of nearly the
entire cerebellum, which was itself hydrocephalic,
into a cervical spina bifida.*

This case likewise originated from the surgical
service of Dr. Bayer in the Kaiser Franz Joseph
Children's Hospital. The patient was a 5 month
old girl who was admitted in November 1890 for
operation on a spina bifida. The child had a large
head and a convergent strabismus. On her neck
was a fluctuant, tender, and easily compressible
tumor about the size of a hen's egg, extending
from the occiput to the seventh cervical vertebra.
It was covered with thin skin and was considered
to be a cervical hydromyelocele, at the base of

which a wide cleft in the upper vertebrae could be palpated. No paralysis was present.

On November 15, Dr. Bayer operated on the lesion by cutting around its base and pulling it away, during which a finger-sized central stalk was ligated and detached. On the first day after the operation, the wound remained free of reaction. But on 18 November, cerebrospinal fluid ran out, and the wound was again sutured. Meningitis developed on 21 November, and it killed the child on 23 November.

The tumor, given to me immediately after the operation, was hardened in Müller's solution. . . . It was a hemispheral sac with a wall of several layers. The most external layer was the cutis, with numerous sweat glands and sparse hair follicles and sebaceous glands. Next was a rather thick stratum subcutaneum, almost free of fatty tissue, to which dura was attached near the base of the tumor. The next layer was formed by a rather easily detached thin membrane with a smooth inner surface, which I must call arachnoid. The innermost portion of the sac . . . consisted of a vesicle with a thumb-sized opening, externally covered with a loose and heavily vascularized tissue. Its wall, on the average only 1 mm thick, consisted of a whitish gray firm tissue covered with numerous nodules . . . which microscopically was reminiscent of sclerotic central nervous tissue. . . .

At autopsy on 24 November . . . I found that the vesicle removed at operation had belonged to the cerebellum. . . . The lateral ventricles and the third ventricle appeared greatly expanded. . . . The tentorium cerebelli was absent . . . , and in place of the cerebellum there was only a walnut-sized knobby body, resting on the dorsal surface of the pons and medulla. . . . This residue of the cerebellum lay inside the widened foramen magnum. . . . The arches of the upper three vertebrae were split and widely separated. . . . The inferior margin of the ventral surface of the pons was located at the level of the tip of the odontoid process, and the medulla oblongata lay completely within the vertebral canal. . . .

Cross-sections through the pons and medulla showed them to be flattened. The Sylvian aqueduct and fourth ventricle had undergone marked dilatation. The remains of the cerebellum consisted of a vesicle opened at the amputation site, with walls about 1 mm thick, and knobby widenings up to 5 mm thick. The spinal cord was very hydromyelic. . . .

We are doubtlessly dealing here with a cervical cerebellar hydroencephalocele. Occipital encephaloceles often include the cerebellum . . . but what is noteworthy in the present case is the exit of the cerebellum from the cranial cavity . . . through the foramen magnum into a cervical spina bifida. . . . This extrusion of the cerebellum . . . was probably the result of the hydrocephalic enlargement of the cerebrum . . . , and from this I believe I have the right to offer this case as representative of a third type of the sequential changes of the cerebellum that are due to cerebral hydrocephalus.

XXXIX   Lindau's Disease

ARVID LINDAU (born in 1892), Swedish pathologist, made an important contribution to neurology with a detailed analysis of a unique disorder now known as Lindau's disease.[1] The fully developed disease includes cerebellar and retinal hemangioblastomas with cysts and neoplasms of the kidney, pancreas, and adrenal gland. Various manifestations of the disorder had been described as isolated findings for at least 50 years before Lindau's work, but he recognized them as variable features of a single underlying process.

Lindau's exhaustive study, published in 1926,[2] begins with a 24-page historical review of cerebellar cysts. The author's cases are then presented, with emphasis on the tumor subsequently named the hemangioblastoma, and the relevant medical literature is thoroughly reviewed. There follows a discussion of angiomatosis retinae (von Hippel's disease[3-5]) and its relationship to the intracranial hemangioblastomas, a topic that Lindau presented again the following year.[6]

Additional experience since 1926 has enlarged upon Lindau's perceptive analysis.[7-9] The intracranial or retinal hemangioblastomas typically occur as isolated abnormalities, but approximately 10% to 20% of the patients with one of these lesions will have both, or some other manifestation of Lindau's disease.[2,8,10] In at least 20% of the patients, there is evidence of familial transmission, which is apparently of the autosomal dominant type with a moderate degree of penetrance.[9-12] Thus, as Lindau pointed out, there is an underlying congenital disorder that is manifested by inconstant developmental abnormalities and neoplasms in various organs throughout the body in a fashion analogous to tuberous sclerosis or von Recklinghausen's disease.[9,10,13]

References

1. Cushing H, Bailey P: Hemangiomas of cerebellum and retina (Lindau's disease). *Arch Ophthal* 57:447-463, 1928.

2. Lindau A: Studien über Kleinhirncysten: Bau, Pathogenese und Beziehungen zur Angiomatosis retinae. *Acta Path Microbiol Scand* 1(suppl):3-128, 1926.

3. von Hippel E: Über eine sehr seltene Erkrankung der Netzhaut: Klinische Beobachtungen. *Graefe Arch Ophthal* 59:83-106, 1904.

4. von Hippel E: Die anatomische Grundlage der von mir beschriebenen "sehr seltenen Erkrankung der Netzhaut." *Graefe Arch Ophthal* 79:350-377, 1911.

5. von Hippel E: Über diffuse Gliose der Netzhaut und ihre Beziehungen zu der Angiomatosis retinae. *Graefe Arch Ophthal* 95:173-183, 1918.

6. Lindau A: Zur Frage der Angiomatosis retinae und ihrer Hirnkomplikationen. *Acta Ophthal* 4:193-226, 1927.

7. Lindau A: Discussion on vascular tumours of the brain and spinal cord. *Proc Roy Soc Med* 24:363-370, 1931.

8. Lindau A: Capillary angiomatosis of the central nervous system. *Acta Genet* 7:338-340, 1957.

9. Melmon KL, Rosen SW: Lindau's disease: Review of the literature and study of a large kindred. *Amer J Med* 36:595-617, 1964.

10. Aita JA: Genetic aspects of tumors of the nervous system, in Lynch HT (ed): *Hereditary Factors in Carcinoma*. New York, Springer-Verlag, 1967, pp 86-110.

11. van der Wiel HJ: *Inheritance of Glioma: The Genetic Aspects of Cerebral Glioma and its Relation to Status Dysraphicus*. Amsterdam, Elsevier Publishing Co, 1960, pp 20, 21.

12. Pratt RTC: *The Genetics of Neurological Disorders*. London, Oxford University Press, 1967, p 97.

13. Smith DW: *Recognizable Patterns of Human Malformation: Genetic, Embryologic, and Clinical Aspects*. Philadelphia, WB Saunders Co, 1970, p 158.

Studies of Cerebellar Cysts
Structure, Pathogenesis, and Relation to Angiomatosis Retinae*
by
Arvid Lindau
From the Pathological-Anatomical Institute of the University of Lund

.... A. Cyst with an Angioma in its Wall

.... Case 2. .... E. K., 26 year old woman. Father, mother and sister healthy. The patient was in good health until the age of 5, when she began to feel pressure and pain in her head. These symptoms were periodic, and there were months when she had few complaints. At Christmas, 1920, the headache increased in intensity and led to an attack, lasting approximately 15 minutes, in which the pain rose to a peak, and vomiting occurred, followed by relief for some hours. The

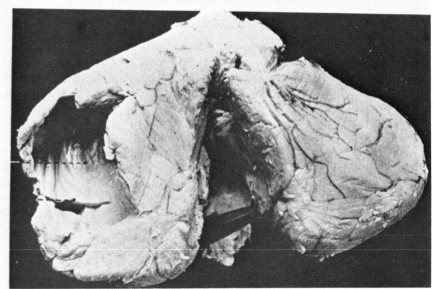

Cyste

Lage des
Angiomes

Fig. 32. Case 2 (2/3)

Fig. 71. Case 2. Cystic Pancreas (Reduced 2/3)

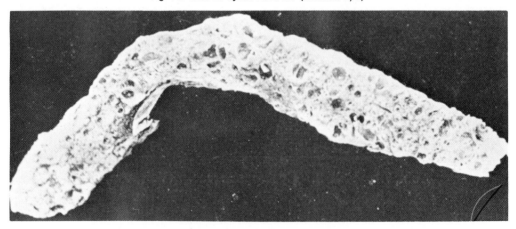

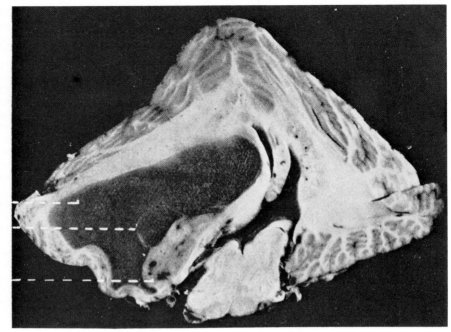

Cyste mit
fixiertem
Inhalt

Sekundäre
Cyste

Angiom

Fig. 34. Case 4. . . .

pain was localized to the forehead, but occasionally to the
occiput. In December 1920, the
patient's gait was unsteady and
she fell easily. By January 1921
she had become confined to bed.
She was seen in the medical
clinic on February 26, 1921.

Status: Her general condition
was markedly affected. . . .
Papilledema and diminished
corneal reflexes bilaterally. Pupils dilated, markedly unequal,
and reacting sluggishly to light.
Spontaneous nystagmus. The
finger to nose test was performed unsteadily, especially
with the left arm. Pointing was
altered at the shoulder joint,
with a distinct deviation of the
left arm toward the right.
Adiadokokinesis, especially of
the left hand. The patient wob-
bled and tended to fall. She had

*Translation of: Studien über Klein-
hirncysten. Bau, Pathogenese und
Beziehungen zur Angiomatosis retinae. *Acta Pathologica et Micro-
biologica Scandinavica* Supplement
1:3-128, 1926.

Fig. 58. Case 5 (Enlarged 175/1.) Hyperplastic angioma. Wide vascular
spaces.

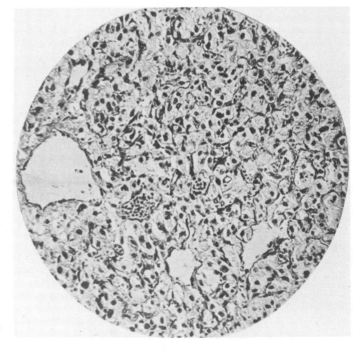

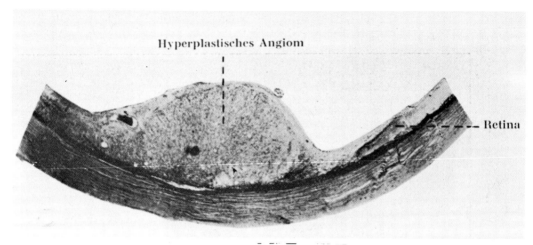

Fig. 68. Brandt's Case No. 2 (Enlarged 10/1.)

Fig. 69. Brandt's Case No. 2. (Enlarged 175/1.) Hyperplastic angioma, with a few prominent capillaries.

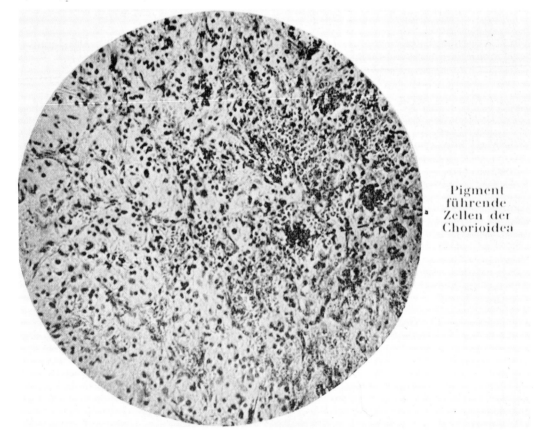

pain on forward flexion of the head. She was referred to the surgical clinic for operation. There she had a continual headache with episodic violent vomiting, and was given morphine daily. On March 8 a left facial paralysis was noticed, and shortly thereafter she died suddenly.

Autopsy (the author): Internal hydrocephalus with marked flattening of the cerebral convolutions. In the superior lateral portion of the left cerebellar hemisphere, a cyst (5 × 4 × 2 cm.) with a thin smooth wall was found. It occupied the lateral portions of the superior semilunar lobule and the quadrangular lobule, but left the vermis and ventral part of the cerebellum untouched. Nowhere was there a communication with the fourth ventricle. At the bottom of the cyst laterally was *a small mottled tumor the size of the kernel of a nut, and with a rounded shape.* This was well delimited from the adjacent cerebellar substance. The location of the tumor and the cyst, as well as the macroscopic appearance, is shown in figures 3 and 32.

At postmortem examination of the abdominal organs, the following abnormalities were discovered: *Pancreas* large and nodular throughout with *numerous small pea-sized cysts;* on the cut surface only a small amount of parenchyma was left untouched between the fibrotic cyst walls (Figs. 71-73). *The kidneys* contained *several cysts,* which had not attained the size of peas. In the left kidney was also found *a well-encapsulated hypernephroma, at least the size of a pea* (verified microscopically).

Pathological-Anatomical Diagnosis: Hemangioma and cyst of the cerebellum + internal hydrocephalus + cystic pancreas + renal cysts + hypernephroma of the left kidney....

Case 4. A. M., 37 year old man.

Presented to the medical clinic of the Serafimerkrankenhaus in Stockholm on September 5, 1922. Died September 29, 1922.

His father died at the age of 70 of a gastric disorder; his mother for many years had an undiagnosed illness. She was said to have had epilepsy. The patient had 4 sisters, all living and well. In 1914 the vision in his left eye began to deteriorate; he was seen in the ophthalmology clinic of the Serafimerkrankenhaus and given the diagnosis of *"arteriovenous aneurysm of the retina of the left eye"....*

According to his wife, the patient had frequently complained of headache, often beginning suddenly with a glittering before the eyes. He carried on his duties as superintendent of an insane asylum until July 1922, when he complained of continuous headache and fatigue, along with nausea and vomiting. During the second half of July, he nearly fell on repeated occasions, always to the right.... For 3 weeks before admission the patient lay in bed, and during this time his condition gradually deteriorated.

Status on September 6, 1922: The patient lay lethargic and somnolent, yet answered questions clearly, though slowly and somewhat haltingly. Complained of headache. Amaurotic left eye with

Fig. 70. Angiomatosis retinae (Seidel's Case)

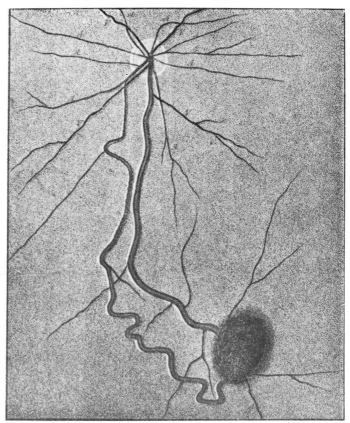

marked downward displacement. Papilledema in the right eye. Nystagmus in the primary position as well as to the right and left. Corneal reflexes were equal on both sides.

Strength was diminished somewhat in the legs as well as in the arms. Nothing remarkable about the finger-nose and knee-heel test. Adiadokokinesis not present. Neck stiff. Lasègue positive. At lumbar puncture the pressure was 190 mm. The fluid was clear. Pandy positive. Nonne negative. No cells.

During his stay in the hospital, the patient was lethargic and forgetful, and complained of severe headaches. . . . On September 28 a lumbar puncture was undertaken, with the simultaneous insufflation of air. The patient withstood the procedure well, but complained of pain in his head and neck. He died the next morning.

Autopsy (Dr. Wahlgren): Internal hydrocephalus with flattening of the cerebral convolutions. A somewhat bulging and fluctuant area was present in the left cerebellar hemisphere. Section of the cerebellum after fixation, revealed a cyst the size of a hen's egg (6 × 4.5 × 2.5 cm) in the left hemisphere, occupying the inferior portion of the lobe and extending somewhat beyond the midline. It was filled with a coagulated, jelly-like, brownish gray substance (formalin-fixed cyst fluid). In the inferomedial wall of the cyst, in the location of the cerebellar tonsils, *a bean-sized tumor* (1.5 × 1.4 × 0.7 cm) was found. The tumor was well delimited from the adjacent cerebellar tissue, and showed on its cut surface numerous blood-filled capillary spaces. The locations of the cyst and the tumor and their macroscopic appearance are shown in Figs. 5 and 34.

The autopsy protocol also gave the following information:

The *right adrenal* was the size of a goose egg. Its cut surface was red and fleshy, with dark red spots alternating with gray areas. Its boundaries were sharp. The *left adrenal* was about the size of a hen's egg. It showed similar changes when cut.

For the rest, no tumors were found.

The *pancreas* and the *kidneys* exhibited no abnormalities.

Pathological-Anatomical Diagnosis: Hemangioma and cyst of the cerebellum + internal hydrocephalus + bilateral adenomas of the suprarenal gland. . . .

Principal Conclusions

1. Cerebellar cysts are by no means rare. More than 275 cases have been reported. They make up almost 10% of all cerebellar tumors.

2. In the majority of cases, the cysts are either simple or are associated with a tumor, usually the latter.

3. The neoplasms associated with the cysts are of two types: angioplastic tumors (capillary angioma) or gliomas.

4. The angioplastic tumors have a characteristic appearance. They are small, well demarcated, situated cortically or subcortically, and are usually lateral and posterior in the cerebellum. The microscopic picture is that of a hyperplastic capillary angioma with pseudoxanthoma cells, small giant cells, and a plasma-like transudate.

5. In this group belong 24 cases from the literature and 16 of my own, as well as 4 cases of similar tumors in the medulla oblongata. . . .

8. Angiomatosis retinae (von Hippel's disease) is associated with intracranial lesions in 20%. In the cases studied anatomically, the lesions have turned out to be cerebellar cysts or angioplastic tumors in the cerebellum or medulla oblongata. . . .

10. An angioma occurring in the medulla oblongata or spinal cord can also develop a cystic cavity and bear a superficial resemblance to true syringomyelia.

11. The concept of angiomatosis can be enlarged to include angiomatosis of the central nervous system with tumors in the retina, rhombencephalon, or spinal cord. Fifteen cases of this pathological-anatomical complex have been collected, and I have observed 9 myself.

12. The mesenchymal vessels in the roof of the fourth ventricle may be considered to be the matrix for the development of an angioma in the rhombencephalon.

13. In 8 cases a cystic pancreas was present, which is a characteristic malformation in this condition. In 10 cases renal cysts developed, and hypernephromas in 6 cases.

14. All of these neoplasms may be due to a defect in mesodermal development during the third embryonic month.

15. Angiomatosis of the central nervous system can be classified as a nosological group analogous to tuberous sclerosis. . . .

18. In the case of the cyst having an angioma in its wall, the angioma is primary and the development of the cyst is secondary, caused by the tumor. . . .

XL   Creutzfeldt-Jakob Disease

I N 1920, Hans Gerhard Creutzfeldt of Berlin (1885 to 1964) published a detailed case report of a patient with an unusual combination of neurological signs and pathological findings.[1,2] Then within three years, the neuropathologist Alfons Jakob of Hamburg (1884 to 1931), a student of Nissl and Alzheimer,[3] described five similar cases and established this condition as a distinct disease entity.[4-7] Despite Creutzfeldt's priority, the disorder is often called Jakob-Creutzfeldt disease because of Jakob's greater contribution to its delineation.[8]

It is now recognized that this disease or group of diseases is manifested by a rapidly progressive dementia combined with pyramidal and extrapyramidal signs, myoclonus, and often with amyotrophy.[9-10] The disease affects middle aged individuals of both sexes and is usually fatal in a few months to a few years. Neuronal degeneration and gliosis occur in the brain and spinal cord, and glial rosettes may be found in the cortex and basal ganglia. Status spongiosus may also be observed in the cortex and in the central gray matter. In the rapidly fatal form described by Heidenhain,[11] the occipital cortex is especially involved and the basal ganglia are spared.

The evidence that a slow virus infection may cause kuru[12] has stimulated the search for an infectious agent in other progressive neurological diseases. Recent attempts to transmit Creutzfeldt-Jakob disease to primates have been successful,[13-15] and this disease now appears to be another of the erstwhile "degenerative" conditions that may really be infectious.

References

1. Creutzfeldt HG: Über eine eigenartige herdf: mige Erkankung des Zentralnervensystems. Z G Neurol Psychiat **57**:1-18, 1920.
2. Creutzfeldt HG: Über eine eigenartige herdf(mige Erkrankung des Zentralnervensystems, : Nissel F, Alzheimer A (eds): *Histologische u histopathologische Arbeiten über die Grosshirnrind* Jena, Germany, Gustav Fischer, 1921, pp 1-48.
3. Hassin GB: Neuropathology: An historic: sketch. *J Neuropath Exp Neurol* **9**:1-17, 1950.
4. Jakob A: Über eigenartige Erkrankungen de: Zentralnervensystems mit bemerkenswertem ana tomischem Befunde (spastische Pseudsklerose-En cephalomyelopathie mit disseminierten Degenera tionsherden). *Deutsch Z Nervenheilk* **70**:132-146, 1921.
5. Jakob A: Über eigenartige Erkrankungen de: Zentralnervensystems mit bemerkenswertem ana tomischen Befunde (Spastische Pseudsklerose-En cephalomyelopathie mit disseminierten Degenera tionsherden). *Z Ges Neurol Psychiat* **64**:147-228, 1921.
6. Jakob A: Über eine der multiplen Sklerose klinisch nahestehende Erkrankung des Centralner vensystems (spastische Pseudsklerose) mit bemer kenswertem anatomischem Befunde: Mitteilung eines vierten Falles. *Med Klin* **17**:372-376, 1921.
7. Jakob A: *Die extrapyramidalen Erkrankungen mit besonderer Berücksichtigung der pathologischen Anatomie und Histologie und der Pathophysiologie der Bewegungsstörungen.* Berlin, Julius Springer, 1923, pp 215-245.
8. Jacob H: Alfons Jakob (1884-1931), in Haymaker W, Schiller F (eds): *The Founders of Neurology*, ed 2. Springfield, Ill, Charles C Thomas Publisher, 1970, pp 338-342.
9. May WW: Creutzfeldt-Jakob disease: 1. Survey of the literature and clinical diagnosis. *Acta Neurol Scand* **44**:1-32, 1968.
10. Kirschbaum WR: *Jakob-Creutzfeldt Disease (Spastic Pseudosclerosis, A. Jakob; Heidenhain Syndrome; Subacute Spongiform Encephalopathy).* New York, American Elsevier Publishing Co, 1968.
11. Heidenhain A: Klinische und anatomische Untersuchungen über eine eigenartige organische Erkrankung des Zentralnervensystems im Praesenium. *Z Ges Neurol Psychiat* **118**:49-114, 1929.
12. Johnson RT, Johnson KP: Slow and chronic virus infections of the nervous system, in Plum F (ed): *Recent Advances in Neurology.* Philadelphia, FA Davis Co, 1969, pp 33-78.
13. Gibbs CJ Jr, Gajdusek DC, Asher DM, et al: Creutzfeldt-Jakob disease (spongiform encephalopathy): Transmission to the chimpanzee. *Science* **161**:388-389, 1968.
14. Beck E, Daniel PM, Matthews WB, et al: Creutzfeldt-Jakob disease: The neuropathology of a transmission experiment. *Brain* **92**:699-716, 1969.
15. Gibbs CJ Jr, Gajdusek DC: Infection as the etiology of spongiform encephalopathy (Creutzfeldt-Jakob disease). *Science* **165**:1023-1025, 1969.

Concerning a Unique Disease of the Central Nervous System
with Noteworthy Anatomical Findings[*][1]
(Spastic Pseudosclerosis—Encephalomyelopathy with Disseminated Foci of Degeneration)

by

A. Jakob

(From the Anatomical Laboratory of the University Psychiatric Clinic and
State Hospital of Hamburg—Friedrichsberg [Prof. Dr. Weygandt])

[Creutzfeldt's case is reviewed, but Jakob's three cases are presented in detail]

. . . . We are dealing with an illness of middle and advanced age . . . that begins with slowly progressive motor and sensory symptoms. The patients complain of weakness and pain in the extremities, especially the legs, which become stiff. The legs often give way during walking, causing the patient to fall. Objective findings are usually minimal, but spasticity and an early diminution in the abdominal reflexes may be present. It should be emphasized that the motor disturbances have a functional quality early in the disease, and the symptoms fluctuate in severity. Gradually, however, more distinct disturbances of movement appear, which often exhibit a peculiar mixture of spastic and striatal signs that are difficult to analyze. Without showing demonstrable weakness, the patient's locomotion is strikingly incoordinated . . . , and finally standing and walking become impossible. . . .

Speech is slow and monotonous, and is often . . . dysarthric. Tendon reflexes are usually increased, but may be normal or even absent. The Babinski sign is present in certain phases of the illness. The abdominal reflexes are diminished or absent. The eyegrounds are always normal. Examinations of blood and spinal fluid are negative as a rule.

After the neurological symptoms develop, they are joined by pronounced psychic disturbances consisting of apathy, negativism, and anxious, delirious, hallucinatory confusion. . . . Finally, signs of cerebral irritability come to the fore, and the illness is often terminated with a high fever coincident with bulbar dysfunction, stupor and epileptiform seizures. . . . The duration of the illness varies between several weeks and a year from the onset of the severe symptoms.

. . . . It is easy to differentiate this disease clinically from Westphal-Strümpel's pseudosclerosis and Wilson' disease, since spasticity is dominant, and the purely striatal signs recede. Also the corneal ring and signs of liver disease are absent. . . . The disease involves older individuals, and severe psychic symptoms are prominent. It may be difficult to differentiate from multiple sclerosis . . . but there are no ocular signs, pronounced intention ataxia, or staccato speech. Also, the eyegrounds are normal. . . .

In addition to its clinical individuality, the disease has a very characteristic anatomical substrate. The macroscopic findings are minimal. . . , with atrophy of the brain and thickening of the pia. . . . Microscopically, there is a diffuse parenchymal degeneration, with small focal lesions that indicate the sites of most severe involvement. . . . There is prominent involvement of the entire pyramidal system, the striatal system, and the ventromedial nucleus of the thalamus. . . .

The marked changes in the gray matter, suggesting a selective necrosis of ganglion cells, point to a primary affection of the gray matter. Other histological characteristics, such as the scattering of glial rosettes in the white matter, can be attributed to the same primary process. . . .

In closing, I must say that the foregoing statements and descriptions still have numerous gaps. . . . Nevertheless, I believe I have demonstrated that we have here a unique disease which cannot be denied a nosological niche.

Supplement: . . . I have been able to investigate one further case, which corroborates the foregoing statements. It will be reported in Med. Klin., 1921.

---

[*]Translation of: Über eigenartige Erkrankungen des Zentralnervensystems mit bemerkenswertem anatomischen Befunde (Spastische Pseudosklerose—Encephalomyelopathie mit disseminierten Degenerationsherden.) *Zeitschrift für die gesamte Neurologie und Psychiatrie* **64**:147-228, 1921.

1. Presented as an abstract at the meeting of German neurologists in Leipzig, 1920 (Congress Report).

XLI Parinaud's Syndrome

HENRI PARINAUD (1844 to 1905) had an unusual opportunity to study disorders of eye movement since he served as ophthalmologist to Charcot's neurological service at the Salpêtrière.[1] As a result of this experience, Parinaud became one of the first to distinguish between central and peripheral ocular paralyses.

Among the types of central paralysis that he described was paralysis of ocular convergence accompanied by paralysis of vertical eye movements.[2-5] Parinaud postulated that the lesion accounting for this form of paralysis might affect the corpora quadrigemina instead of directly involving the oculomotor nuclei, and this hypothesis has subsequently been confirmed. However, he failed to mention a useful physical sign of a supranuclear lesion, the preservation of the vestibuloocular reflexes, or "doll's head" movements, which tend to be abolished with nuclear and peripheral lesions.

Parinaud's syndrome, now defined as a paralysis of conjugate vertical eye movements (especially upgaze), with varying degrees of paralysis of convergence and pupillary constriction and usually with preservation of doll's head movements, has been observed in association with a number of different pathological processes directly involving the tectum.[6,7] However, the syndrome characteristically results from compression of the tectum by a neighboring pineal tumor.[8,9]

References

1. H. Parinaud (1844-1905). *Ann Oculist* 133:321-337, 1905.
2. Parinaud H: Paralysie des mouvements associés des yeux. *Arch Neurol* 5:145-172, 1883.
3. Parinaud H: Paralysie de la convergence. *Bull Mem Soc Franc Ophthal* 4:23-33, 1886.
4. Parinaud H: Paralysie de la convergence. *Ann Oculist* 95:205-206, 1886.
5. Parinaud H: Paralysis of the movement of convergence of the eyes. *Brain* 9:330-341, 1886.
6. Cogan DG: *Neurology of the Ocular Muscles*, ed 2. Springfield, Ill, Charles C Thomas Publisher, 1956, pp 123, 124.
7. Walsh FB, Hoyt WF: *Clinical Neuro-Ophthalmology*. Baltimore, Williams & Wilkins Co, 1969, vol 1, pp 228-232.
8. Posner M, Horrax G: Eye signs in pineal tumors. *J Neurosurg* 3:15-24, 1946.
9. Poppen JL, Marino R Jr: Pinealomas and tumors of the posterior portion of the third ventricle. *J Neurosurg* 28:357-364, 1968.

PARALYSIS OF THE MOVEMENT OF CONVERGENCE OF THE EYES.*

BY H. PARINAUD, M.D. (PARIS)

(Translated from the French MS. by HENRY JULER, F.R.C.S.)

THE paralyses of the muscles of the eye,[1] as of those of other parts of the body, arise either from central or peripheral causes. Until the last few years this fact appears to have been ignored, for the descriptions are devoted almost exclusively to the paralyses of the third pair of nerves, and the symptomatology is exactly deduced from the distribution of these nerves and from the action of each muscle. Several works, however, have been published on this question, notably those on conjugate paralysis, paralysis of the sixth pair, and Hutchinson's ophthalmoplegia.

I may here be permitted to remark that in several publications, of which the first appeared in 1877, I have endeavoured to establish the distinction between peripheral and central paralyses. Hitherto these subjects have not seriously occupied the attention of oculists, but at the present time, thanks to the efforts of Prof. Mauthner, this gap in the literature of ophthalmology is becoming filled up. . . .

Associated paralyses, *i.e.* those referring to similar binocular movements, are central paralyses *par excellence*. . . . Amongst other forms of associated paralysis that I have studied, I have signalised the *Paralysis of Convergence*, of which I desire to delineate the characteristic features.

*Reprinted from *Brain* 9:330-341, 1886.

[1]The cases on which this paper was written were observed, either in Dr. Parinaud's ophthalmic clinique or in the Salpêtrière, where the author fills the post of Ophthalmologist to the Neurological Department of Prof. Charcot. . . .

It is hardly necessary to remark that this central paralysis of convergence is distinct from the insufficiency of the internal recti muscles, with which we are familiar in connection with myopia, with peculiar arrangement of the cranial bones, and from a congenital muscular insufficiency.

The deficient converging power observed in exophthalmic goitre[2] by Möbius has always seemed to me to be in relation with the ocular protrusion. In certain cases it is true this symptom may appear before the latter is very manifest. But, though the disease be primarily of nervous origin, the loss of convergence in Basedow's disease must be referred to a mechanical cause, as Möbius suggests, and must not be taken for a paralysis strictly so called. . . .

These are two forms of paralysis of convergence arising from central causes. The one may be called *essential* and the other *combined*; combined, because it coincides with paralysis of elevation and depression.

A.—ESSENTIAL PARALYSIS OF CONVERGENCE

The vision of a near object is accompanied by three distinct muscular acts; the *convergence* of the eyes towards the object looked at, the effort of *accommodation*, and the *contraction of the pupil*. These three acts are concerned in the typical forms of essential paralysis of convergence.

(*a.*) Paralysis of the movement of convergence is indicated by two principal symptoms: the objectively appreciable defect of convergence and a peculiar diplopia.

In order to recognise the defect of convergence, we proceed in the same manner as for insufficiency of the internal recti. If the patient be told to fix the finger as it rapidly approaches his face, the eyes remain immovable; if the movement be performed, it is incomplete, the patient cannot continue to look at the object with both eyes, but one of the eyes turns outwards and he squints. Lastly, in making him fix a near object alternately with either eye, the eye which has been momentarily excluded from vision executes a movement of readjustment, in order to fix the object. . . .

On the other hand, in the lateral movements the internal recti contract normally. In a word, the innervation of the internal recti is only concerned [impaired—ed.] in the movement of convergence; it remains normal for adduction in displace-

---

[2]'Centralblatt für Nervenheilkunde,' 1886.

ments where the visual axes are parallel. The *diplopia* appears in the median plane at a variable distance from the subject; *it is crossed, and there is moderate separation of the images which persist without notable modification in all directions of looking.* The separation is not sensibly increased when the candle is moved laterally, sometimes it diminishes, a character which distinguishes this diplopia from that of all ordinary paralyses of the internal recti. The images not infrequently become fused at four or five metres from the patient, a distance at which but little convergence is exercised, but cases do occur in which the diplopia persists at all ranges; this may be explained either by the degree of paralysis, or by the individual differences in the static condition of the eyes. There are subjects in whom, during absolute repose, the globes have such a tendency to diverge, that the maintenance of parallelism necessitates the intervention of converging force.

If the patient does not complain of diplopia when a coloured glass is employed, a prism, placed base upwards, before one of the eyes will generally cause the double vision to appear, and so allow its characters to be studied.

(*b.*) Accommodation is involved in this form of paralysis in various ways. In certain cases there is absolute paralysis in both eyes; in others there is more or less notable reduction of its amplitude: whilst in a third class the accommodation is normal.

Accommodation remains defective in monocular as well as in binocular vision. . . . The double paralysis of accommodation is not accompanied by mydriasis from paralysis of the sphincter, which distinguishes it from certain facts of double paralysis belonging to ophthalmoplegia interna and derived from another process. . . .

(*c.*) If in this form of paralysis there be no paralytic mydriasis, the pupillary reflexes are nevertheless modified, and mostly in a very characteristic manner. *The reflex is abolished for convergence and retained for light,* thus constituting a modification exactly inverse to that pointed out by Argyll Robertson as occurring in tabes. The reflex is equally defective when the patient is made to fix a near object with one eye only. In certain cases the pupil, though not dilated, will not react to any excitation. . . .

B.—COMBINED PARALYSIS OF CONVERGENCE

In this form of paralysis, the defect of convergence is accompanied by paralysis of elevation, and of depression in both eyes, with retention of lateral movements.

This paralysis appears to be very rare in its typical and complete form. I have seen one case where the visual trouble, which had come on suddenly in a polyuric patient, was clearly characterised. The following is a résumé of the observations, reported more fully in my memoir on *Associated Paralyses.*[3]

OBSERVATION VII.—*Paralysis of Convergence with Paralysis of Elevation and Depression in both Eyes. Retention of Lateral Movements.* M. Sey-, aet. 67.

Movements of elevation and depression almost nil in both eyes.

Complete paralysis of convergence.

The internal recti contract normally for adduction in lateral movements.

The diplopia is crossed or homonymous, according to the distance of the candle. The image of the right eye always remains rather the lower.

The elevators of the lids are intact.

No paralysis of iris; there is, on the contrary, slight myosis with abolition of reflexes.

The amplitude of accommodation is almost nil, but, knowing the patient's age, one cannot ascertain whether this be paralysed.

The paralysis appeared suddenly on the night of Feb. 8, 1881. Since that date there has been a tendency to fall to the left. Polyuria recurring in crisis, with heaviness of the head, from which the patient suffered before the development of the ocular trouble. Pulse 52. . . .

This form of paralysis may be incomplete. With paralysis of convergence we may have only paralysis of elevation (Observation V. in my memoir), or paralysis of depression (Observation by Priestley Smith[4]).

These symptoms correspond exactly to those of paralysis by lesion of the nuclei of the 3rd pair, as we take it to be along with integrity of the nuclei of the 6th pair, which are well known to innervate the external rectus of the same side and the internal rectus of the opposite side, but only for the lateral movements.

The extension of the paralysis to both eyes may be explained by the alteration of the two nuclei which are sufficiently near to each other to be simultaneously attacked by the same lesion. Moreover it is not impossible that the lesion of a single nucleus may produce bilateral results. This hypothesis has already been advanced to explain certain cases of labio glosso-pharyngeal paralysis. . . .

Finally, it is not impossible that the lesion, instead of directly attacking the bulbo-pontal nuclei, is situated in a neighbouring centre, which acts immediately upon them, and it appears that this centre may be the tubercula quadrigemina. This appears to be the result of Wernicke's observation (paralysis of elevation in each eye, with conservation of lateral movements), where the autopsy proved a lesion of the *right corpora quadrigemina,* and of another by Hénoch[5] in which the paralysis of elevation in each eye was connected with a well-defined tubercular lesion of the *left posterior quadrigeminal body.*

It has been long known that connections exist between the oculo-motor centres and the quadrigeminal bodies. In this direction we shall bear in mind the recent experiences of Darkchewitch,[6] who confirms and delineates the existence of these connections.

---

[3] ['Archives de Neurologie,' March 1883—ed.]

[4] 'Ophth. Hosp. Reports,' 1876.

[5] 'Berlin. Klin. Wochensch.,' 1864, No. 13.

[6] 'Neurolog. Centralblatt,' 1885.

Appendix of Additional References

A. General Reference Sources

BAILEY, H., AND BISHOP, W. J.: *Notable Names in Medicine and Surgery.* London: H. K. Lewis and Co., 3rd. Ed., 1959.

DURHAM, R. H.: *Encyclopedia of Medical Syndromes.* New York: Hoeber, 1960.

JABLONSKI, S.: *Illustrated Dictionary of Eponymic Syndromes and Diseases and Their Synonyms.* Philadelphia: W. B. Saunders, 1969.

KELLY, E. C.: *Encyclopedia of Medical Sources.* Baltimore: Williams & Wilkins, 1948.

MAGALINI, S. I.: *Dictionary of Medical Syndromes.* Philadelphia: J. B. Lippincott, 1971.

MORTON, L. T.: *A Medical Bibliography (Garrison and Morton). An Annotated Check-List of Texts Illustrating the History of Medicine.* Philadelphia: J. B. Lippincott Co., 3rd Ed., 1970.

SCHMIDT, J. E.: *Medical Discoveries. Who and When.* Springfield, Illinois: Charles C. Thomas, 1959.

TALBOTT, J. H.: *A Biographical History of Medicine: Excerpts and Essays on the Men and Their Work.* New York: Grune & Stratton, 1970.

THORNTON, J. L.: *A Select Bibliography of Medical Biography.* London: The Library Association, 2nd Ed., 1970.

B. General Works Concerning the History of Neurology

ACKERKNECHT, E. H.: Experiment und Klinik in der Geschichte der Neurologie. *Bull. Schweiz. Akad. Med. Wiss. 21*: 51-56, 1965.

ALPER, L.: The History of Neurology During the Nineteenth Century. *Bull. Univ. Miami Sch. Med. 14*: 75-81, 1960.

BARROWS, H. S.: Neurological Eponyms. *Arch. Neurol. 3*: 91-97, 1960.

BELING, C. A.: Neurology, Neurosurgery, and Psychiatry in New Jersey. *Bull. Acad. Med. N. J. 11*: 19-27, 1965.

BHATIA, S. L.: History of Certain Aspects of Neurology. *Neurol. India 15*: 90-98, 1967.

BRAIN, R.: Neurology: Past, Present, and Future. *Br. Med. J. 1*: 355-360, 1958.

BRAIN, R.: The Neurological Tradition of the London Hospital or the Importance of Being Thirty. *Lancet 2*: 575-581, 1959.

COBB, S.: One Hundred Years of Progress in Neurology, Psychiatry and Neurosurgery. *Arch. Neurol. Psychiat. 59*: 63-98, 1948.

CRITCHLEY, M.: Hughlings Jackson, the Man; and the Early Days of the National Hospital. *Proc. R. Soc. Med. 53*: 613-618, 1960.

CRITCHLEY, M.: "The Beginnings of the National Hospital, Queen Square (1859-1860)," in *The Black Hole and Other Essays,* London: Pitman Medical Publishing Co., Ltd., 1964, pp. 155-173.

DEJONG, R. N.: The Founding of the American Neurological Association and Its Relationship to Neurology as a Specialty in 1875. *Trans. Am. Neurol. Assoc. 90*: 3-11, 1965.

GARRISON, F. H.: "History of Neurology," in C. L. Dana (ed.): *Textbook of Nervous Diseases for the Use of Students and Practitioners of Medicine.* New York: W. Wood & Co., 10th Ed., 1925, pp. xv-lvi.

GIBSON, W. C.: The Undergraduate Activities of Some Contributors to Neurological Science. *Yale J. Biol. Med. 28*: 273-284, 1955-56.

GIBSON, W. C.: *Young Endeavour. Contributions to Science by Medical Students of the Past Four Centuries.* Springfield, Illinois: Charles C. Thomas, 1958, pp. 184-235.

GREEN, J. R.: "The Origins of Neurological Institutes," in Barrow Neurological Institute of St. Joseph's Hospital, Phoenix, Arizona: *Horizons in Neurological Education and Research.* Springfield, Illinois: Charles C. Thomas, 1965, pp. 125-199.

GUTHRIE, L. G.: *Contributions to the Study of Precocity in Children: The History of Neurology.* London: Eric G. Millar, 1921, pp. 71-160.

HAYMAKER, W., AND SCHILLER, F.: *The Founders of Neurology. One Hundred and Forty-Six Biographical Sketches by Eighty-Eight Authors.* Springfield, Illinois: Charles C. Thomas, 2nd Ed., 1970.

HOLMES, G.: *The National Hospital, Queen Square, 1860-1948.* Edinburgh: E. & S. Livingstone, Ltd., 1954.

KESERT, B. H.: An Historical Review of Neurology. *Proc. Inst. Med. Chic. 24*: 284-290, 1963.

KOLLE, K.: *Grosse Nervenärzte; Lebensbilder.* Stuttgart: Georg Thieme, 3 Vols., 1956, 1959, 1963.

KOLLE, K.: Genealogie der Nervenärzte des deutschen Sprachgebietes. *Fortschr. Neurol. Psychiatr. 32*: 512-538, 1964.

LEVINSON, A.: "Notes on the History of Pediatric Neurology," in S. R. Kagan (ed.): *Victor Robinson Memorial Volume. Essays on the History of Medicine.* New York: Froben Press, Inc., 1948, pp. 225-240.

MACKAY, R. P.: The History of Neurology in Chicago. *J. Int. Coll. Surg. 40*: 191-205, 1963.

MACKAY, R. P.: The History of Neurology in Chicago. *Ill. Med. J. 125*: 51-58, 142-146, 256-259, 341-344, 539-544, 636-640; *126*: 60-64, 1964.

MACNALTY, A.: Some Pioneers of the Past in Neurology. *Med. Hist. 9*: 249-259, 1965.

McHENRY, L. C., JR.: *Garrison's History of Neurology.* Springfield, Illinois: Charles C. Thomas, 1969.

McMENEMEY, W. H.: Neurological Investigation in Britain from 1800 to the Founding of The National Hospital. *Proc. R. Soc. Med. 53*: 605-612, 1960.

PETERMAN, M. G.: Pediatric Contributions to Neurology. *JAMA 165*: 2161-2162, 1957.

PETTE, H.: Stand und Entwicklung der Neurologie. *Internist (Berlin) 4*: 258-266, 1963.

RIESE, W.: History and Principles of classification of Nervous Diseases: A Short History of the Doctrines of Nervous Function Under Pathological Conditions and a General Scheme of Classification of Nervous Diseases According to Function. *Bull. Hist. Med. 18*: 465-512, 1945.

RIESE, W.: *A History of Neurology.* New York: M D Publications, Inc., 1959.

RIESE, W.: "Dynamic Aspects in the History of Neurology," in L. Halpern (ed.): *Problems of Dynamic Neurology.* Jerusalem: Hebrew Univ., 1963, pp. 1-29.

RILEY, H. A.: The Neurological Institute of New York. The First Hospital in the Western Hemisphere for the Treatment of Disorders of the Nervous System. The Intermediate Years. *Bull. N. Y. Acad. Med. 42*: 654-678, 1966.

RITTER, G.: Zur Entwicklungsgeschichte der neurologischen Semiologie. *Nervenarzt 37*: 507-513, 1966.

RITTER, G.: Zur Entwicklungsgeschichte der Neurologie. Die altägyptischen Papryi. *Nervenarzt 39*: 541-546, 1968.

RITTER, G.: Die Neurologie in der hippokratischen Medizin. Versuch eines Überblicks. *Nervenarzt 40*: 327-333, 1969.

SOMERS, J.: A Short History of Neurology. *Univ. Mich. Med. Bull. 22*: 467-481, 1956.

STOOKEY, B.: Historical Background of the Neurological Institute and the Neurological Societies. *Bull. N. Y. Acad. Med. 35*: 707-729, 1959.

STOOKEY, B.: What is Past is Prologue. *Arch. Neurol. 1*: 467-474, 1959.

STOOKEY, B.: The Neurological Institute and Early Neurosurgery in New York. *J. Neurosurg. 17*: 801-814, 1960.

STOOKEY, B.: A Lost Neurological Society With Great Expectations. *J. Hist. Med. 16*: 280-291, 1961.

TILNEY, F., AND JELLIFFE, S. E.: *Semi-Centennial Anniversary Volume of the American Neurological Association 1875-1924.* Albany, N. Y.: American Neurological Association, 1924.

VIETS, H. R.: Fifty Years of the Boston Society of Neurology and Psychiatry. *N. Engl. J. Med. 203*: 914-917, 1930.

VIETS, H. R.: Neurology—Past and Present. JAMA 109: 399-402, 1937.

Viets, H. R.: The History of Neurology in the Last One Hundred Years. *Bull. N. Y. Acad. Med. 24*: 772-783, 1948.

WARTENBERG, R.: On Neurologic Terminology, Eponyms and the Lasègue Sign. *Neurology (Minneap.) 6*: 853-858, 1956.

WECHSLER, I. S.: "Introduction to the History of Neurology," in I. S. Wechsler: Clinical Neurology With an Introduction to the History of Neurology. Philadelphia: W. B. Saunders Co., 9th Ed., 1963, pp. 641-675.

C. References Related to the Specific Neurological Classics Reprinted in This Volume

1. Huntington's Chorea

DEJONG, R. N.: George Huntington, and His Relationship to the Earlier Descriptions of Chronic Hereditary Chorea. *Ann. Med. Hist. 9*: 201-210, 1937.

GIBSON, W. C.: The Undergraduate Activities of Some Contributors to Neurological Science. *Yale J. Biol. Med. 28*: 273-284, 1955-56.

GIBSON, W. C.: *Young Endeavour. Contributions to Science by Medical Students of the Past Four Centuries.* Springfield, Illinois: Charles C. Thomas, 1958, pp. 216-219.

HANS, M. B., AND GILMORE, T. H.: Huntington's Chorea and Genealogical Credibility. *J. Nerv. Ment. Dis. 148*: 5-13, 1969.

HUNTINGTON, G.: Recollections of Huntington's Chorea as I Saw It at East Hampton, Long Island, During My Boyhood. *J. Nerv. Ment. Dis. 37*: 255-257, 1910.

LEWY, F. H.: Historical Introduction: The Basal Ganglia and Their Diseases. *Res. Publ. Assoc. Res. Nerv. Ment. Dis. 21*: 1-20, 1942.

MALTSBERGER, T.: Even Unto the Twelfth Generation — Huntington's Chorea. *J. Hist. Med. 16*: 1-17, 1961.

MYRIANTHOPOULOS, N. C.: Huntington's Chorea. *J. Med. Genet. 3*: 298-314, 1966.

2. Babinski's Sign

BAILEY, P.: Joseph Babinski (1857-1932). The Man and His Works. *World Neurol. 2*: 134-140, 1961.

GUTRECHT, J. A., ESPINOSA, R. E., AND DYCK, P. J.: Early Descriptions of Common Neurologic Signs. *Mayo Clin. Proc. 43*: 807-814, 1968.

LISTA, G. A.: El Signo de Babinski. *Prensa Med. Argent. 53*: 1874-1880, 1966.

RITTER, G.: Historische Bemerkungen zum sogenannten Babinskischen Phänomen. *J. Neurol. Sci. 5*: 1-7, 1967.

TOURNAY, A.: *La Vie de Joseph Babinski.* Amsterdam: Elsevier Publishing Co., 1967.

3. Charcot-Marie-Tooth Disease

ALAJOUANINE, T.: "Pierre Marie (1853-1940)," in Kolle, K. (ed.): *Grosse Nervenärzte*, Stuttgart: Georg Thieme, 1959, Vol. 2, pp. 153-161.

BEESON, B. B.: Jean Martin Charcot. A Summary of His Life and Works. *Ann. Med. Hist. 10*: 126-132, 1928.

CRITCHLEY, M.: "Pierre Marie, 1853-1940," in *The Black Hole and Other Essays*, London: Pitman Medical Publishing Co., Ltd., 1964, pp. 146-154.

ELLENBERGER, H. F.: Charcot and the Salpêtrière School. *Am. J. Psychother. 19*: 253-267, 1965.

4. Encephalitis Lethargica

HUARD, P., THÉODORIDÈS, J., AND VETTER, T.: A Propos du Cinquantenaire de la Découverte de l'Encéphalite Léthargique par C. Von Economo (1917). *Hist. Sci. Méd. 2*: 95-104, 1968.

LEBENSOHN, J. E.: *An Anthology of Ophthalmic Classics.* Baltimore: Williams & Wilkins, 1969, pp. 367-372.

MACNALTY, A.: Some Pioneers of the Past in Neurology. *Med. Hist. 9*: 249-259, 1965.

STRANSKY, E.: "Constantin von Economo (1876-1931)," in Kolle, K. (ed.): *Grosse Nervenärzte,* Stuttgart: Georg Thieme, 1959, Vol. 2, pp. 180-185.

THÉODORIDÈS, J.: Constantin von Economo (1876-1931): Savant, Humaniste, Homme d'Action. in: *C. R. XIXe Congr. Int. Histoire de la Médecine, Basel, 1964,* Basel: Karger, 1966, pp. 624-636.

VETTER, T., AND THÉODORIDÈS, J.: A Propos du Cinquantenaire de la Découverte de l'Encéphalite Léthargique par C. von Economo. *Episteme 3*: 45-57, 1969.

5. Guillain-Barré-Strohl Syndrome

GREEN, D.: Infectious Polyneuritis and Professor André Strohl — A Historical Note. *N. Engl. J. Med. 267*: 821-822, 1962.

7. Adie's Syndrome

HARRIMAN, D. G. F., AND GARLAND, H.: The Pathology of Adie's Syndrome. *Brain 91*: 401-418, 1968.

LEBENSOHN, J. E.: *An Anthology of Ophthalmic Classics.* Baltimore: Williams & Wilkins, 1969, pp. 373-378.

8. Romberg's Sign

FINKE, J.: Zur Geschichte neurologischer Untersuchungsmethoden. *Dtsch. Med. Wochenschr. 91*: 2226-2230, 1966.

VIETS, H. R.: The History of Neurology in the Last One Hundred Years. *Bull. N. Y. Acad. Med. 24*: 772-783, 1948.

10. Brown-Séquard Syndrome

DAMRAU, F.: *Pioneers in Neurology.* St. Louis: Dios Chemical Co., 1937, pp. 9-17.

11. Argyll Robertson Pupil

LEBENSOHN, J. E.: *An Anthology of Ophthalmic Classics.* Baltimore: Williams & Wilkins, 1969, pp. 354-358.

LOEWENFELD, I. E.: The Argyll Robertson Pupil, 1869-1969. A Critical Survey of the Literature. *Survey Ophthalmol. 14*: 199-299, 1969.

SNYDER, C.: *Our Ophthalmic Heritage.* London: J. & A. Churchill, Ltd., 1967, pp. 145-148.

THORNTON, S. P.: *Ophthalmic Eponyms.* Bir-

mingham, Alabama: Aesculapius Publishing Co., 1967, pp. 12-13.

12. Horner's Syndrome

LEAKE, C. D.: Historical Aspects of the Autonomic Nervous System. *Anesthesiology 29*: 623-624, 1968.

TALBOTT, J. H.: Johann Friedrich Horner (1831-1886): "A Form of Ptosis." *JAMA 208*: 1899-1900, 1969.

13. Duchenne's Muscular Dystrophy

BICK, E. M.: The Classic. *Clin. Orthop. 39*: 3-5, 1965.

DAMRAU, F.: *Pioneers in Neurology.* St. Louis: Dios Chemical Co., 1937, pp. 3-8.

JOKL, E.: Guillaume Benjamin Amand Duchenne de Boulogne et la Physiologie des Mouvements. *Episteme 1*: 273-283, 1967.

KAPLAN, E. B.: "Duchenne of Boulogne and the Physiologie des Mouvements," in S. R. Kagan (ed.): *Victor Robinson Memorial Volume. Essays on the History of Medicine.* New York: Froben Press, Inc., 1948, pp. 177-192.

MOYA, G.: Evolución de las Ideas en Patología Neuromuscular. *Arch. Neurobiol. (Madrid) 32*: 347-385, 1969.

14. Tay-Sachs' Disease

LEBENSOHN, J. E.: *An Anthology of Ophthalmic Classics.* Baltimore: Williams & Wilkins, 1969, pp. 282-287.

TAY, W.: A Fourth Instance of Symmetrical Changes in the Yellow-Spot Region of an Infant, Closely Resembling Those of Embolism. *Trans. Ophthalmol. Soc. U. K. 12*: 125-126, 1892.

TOWER, D. B.: Origins and Development of Neurochemistry. *Neurol. (Minneap.) 8*(Suppl. 1): 3-31, 1958.

15. Little's Disease

BICK, E. M.: The Classic. *Clin. Orthop. 46*: 7-22, 1966.

16. Sydenham's Chorea

LEVINSON, A.: "Notes on the History of Pediatric Neurology," in S. R. Kagan (ed.): *Victor Robinson Memorial Volume. Essays on the History of Medicine.* New York: Froben Press, Inc., 1948, pp. 225-240.

TRAIL, R. R.: Sydenham's Impact on English Medicine. *Med. Hist. 9*: 356-364, 1965.

17. Parkinson's Syndrome

BARBEAU, A.: The Understanding of Involuntary Movements: An Historical Approach. *J. Nerv. Ment. Dis. 127*: 469-489, 1958.

GREENFIELD, J. G.: Historical Landmarks in the Pathology of Involuntary Movements. *J. Neuropathol. Exp. Neurol. 15*: 5-11, 1956.

HOEHN, M. M., AND YAHR, M. D.: Parkinsonism:

Onset, Progression, and Mortality. *Neurology (Minneap)* 17: 427-442, 1967.

LEWY, F. H.: Historical Introduction: The Basal Ganglia and Their Diseases. *Res. Publ. Assoc. Res. Nerv. Ment. Dis. 21*: 1-20, 1942.

MONES, R. J.: Parkinson's Disease. *N. Y. State J. Med. 70*: 2687-2691, 2822-2828, 1970.

TALBOTT, J. H.: Parkinson—Physician, Oryctologist, and Social Reformer. *JAMA 184*: 58-59, 1963.

19. Raynaud's Phenomenon

GIBSON, W. C.: *Young Endeavour. Contributions to Science by Medical Students of the Past Four Centuries.* Springfield, Illinois: Charles C. Thomas, 1958, pp. 60-61.

MACCARTY, C. S.: "Surgical Procedures on the Smypathetic Nervous System for Peripheral Vascular Disease," in Allen, E. V., Barker, N. W., and Hines, E. A., Jr. (eds.): *Peripheral Vascular Diseases.* Philadelphia: W. B. Saunders Co., 1955, 2nd Ed., pp. 665-678.

20. Alzheimer's Disease

MCMENEMEY, W. H.: "Alois Alzheimer and His Disease," in Wolstenholme, G. E. W. and O'Connor, M. (eds.): *Alzheimer's Disease and Related Conditions,* London: J. & A. Churchill, 1970, pp. 5-9.

TALBOTT, J. H.: Franz Nissl (1860-1919): Neuropathologist. *JAMA 205*: 208-209, 1968.

TALBOTT, J. H.: Alois Alzheimer (1864-1915): Neurohistopathologist. *JAMA 208*: 1017-1018, 1969.

21. The Signs of Kernig and Brudzinski

GUTRECHT, J. A., ESPINOSA, R. E., AND DYCK, P. J.: Early Descriptions of Common Neurologic Signs. *Mayo Clin. Proc. 43*: 807-814, 1968.

22. Lasègue's Sign

COTURRI, E.: La Malattia Sciatica e l'Importanza nella Storia della sua Conoscenza sia Anatomo-Patologica che Patogenetica del "de Ischiade Nervosa" di Domenico Cotugno. *Pagine Storia della Med. 9*: 11-15, 1965.

RANG, M.: *Anthology of Orthopaedics.* Edinburgh: E. & S. Livingstone, Ltd., 1966, pp. 59-64, 150-151.

23. Lhermitte's Sign

REIDER, N.: Sensation of Electric Shock Following Head Injury. *Arch. Neurol. Psychiat. 56*: 30-41, 1946.

24. Erb's Palsy

BAILEY, H., AND BISHOP, W. J.: *Notable Names in Medicine and Surgery.* London: H. K. Lewis & Co., 3rd Ed., 1959, pp. 130-131, 168-169.

BRIM, C. J.: Paralysis in the Old Testament. A Treatise on Some of the Neurological Observations Recorded in the Bible by the Ancient Hebrew Prophets. *J. Nerv. Ment. Dis. 97*: 656-665, 1943.

DUCHENNE, G. B. A.: *De l'Électrisation Localisée et de Son Application à la Pathologie et à la Thérapeutique.* Paris: J. B. Baillière, 3rd Ed., 1872, p. 357.

JOHNSON, E. W., JR.: Brachial Palsy at Birth. *Int. Abstr. Surg. 111*: 409-416, 1960.

RANG, M.: *Anthology of Orthopaedics.* Edinburgh: E. & S. Livingstone, Ltd., 1966, pp. 52-56.

VIETS, H. R.: The History of Neurology in the Last One Hundred Years. *Bull. N. Y. Acad. Med. 24*: 772-783, 1948.

VOGEL, P.: Die Heidelberger neurologische Schule. *Heidelb. Jahrb. 14*: 73-84, 1970.

25. Sturge-Weber Syndrome

AITA, J. A.: *Neurocutaneous Diseases.* Springfield, Illinois: Charles C. Thomas, 1966, p. 7.

GELLIS, S. S., AND FEINGOLD, M.: *Atlas of Mental Retardation Syndromes. Visual Diagnosis of Facies and Physical Findings.* Washington, D. C.: U. S. Government Printing Office, 1968, pp. 146-147.

SMITH, D. W.: *Recognizable Patterns of Human Malformation. Genetic, Embryologic, and Clinical Aspects.* Philadelphia. W. B. Saunders Co., 1970, pp. 156-157.

26. Bell's Palsy and Bell's Phenomenon

BELL, J. W.: The Bells of Edinburgh. *Surgery 38*: 794-805, 1955.

GUTHRIE, L. G.: *Contributions to the Study of Precocity in Children: The History of Neurology.* London: Eric G. Millar, 1921, pp. 71-160.

KINDLER, W.: Die Fazialislähmungen in der darstellenden Kunst seit mehr als 4 Jahrtausenden. *Z. Laryngol. Rhinol. Otol. 48*: 135-139, 1969; *49*: 1-5, 1970.

MCMENEMEY, W. H.: Neurological Investigation in Britain from 1800 to the Founding of The National Hospital. *Proc. R. Soc. Med. 53*: 605-612, 1960.

POWER, D 'A.: *A Mirror for Surgeons. Selected Readings in Surgery.* Boston: Little, Brown & Co., 1939, pp. 128-132.

27. Causalgia

GOLDNER, J. C.: S. Weir Mitchell: Nerves, Peripheral and Otherwise. *Mayo Clin. Proc. 46*: 274-281, 1971.

28. Jacksonian Epilepsy

CRITCHLEY, M.: "The Contribution of Hughlings Jackson to Neurology," in *The Black Hole and Other Essays,* London: Pitman Medical Publishing Co., Ltd., 1964, pp. 133-136.

DOOSE, H.: Aus der Geschichte der Epilepsie. *Munch. Med. Wochenschr. 107*: 189-196, 1965.

FULTON, J. F.: Clifford Allbutt's Description of Psychomotor Seizures. *J. Hist. Med. 12*: 75-77, 1957.

LENNOX, W. G.: The Centenary of Bromides. *N.*

Engl. J. Med. 256: 887-890, 1957.

MABERLY, A.: Epilepsy—A Brief Historical Review, or Fits—Then and Now. *Alberta Med. Bull. 29*: 65-72, 1964.

MARGERISON, J. H.: Epilepsy — Historical Perspective. *St. Barth. Hosp. J. 73*: 424-428, 1969.

TEMKIN, O.: The Doctrine of Epilepsy in the Hippocratic Writings. *Bull. Inst. Hist. Med. 1*: 277-322, 1933.

TEMKIN, O.: Galen's "Advice for an Epileptic Boy." *Bull. Inst. Hist. Med. 2*: 179-189, 1934.

TEMKIN, O.: Epilepsy in an Anonymous Greek Work on Acute and Chronic Diseases. *Bull. Inst. Hist. Med. 4*: 137-144, 1936.

TEMKIN, O.: Research Before Hughlings Jackson. *Res. Publ. Assoc. Res. Nerv. Ment. Dis. 26*: 3-7, 1947.

TEMKIN, O.: *The Falling Sickness. A History of Epilepsy From the Greeks to the Beginnings of Modern Neurology.* Baltimore: The Johns Hopkins Press, 2nd Ed., 1971.

TEMKIN, O., AND TEMKIN, C. L.: Subjective Experiences in Temporal Lobe Epilepsy: An Anonymous Report of 1825. *Bull. Hist. Med. 42*: 566-568, 1968.

VOEGELE, G. E., AND DIETZE, H. J.: An Historical Reflection on the Medico-Social Aspects of Epilepsy. *Del. Med. J. 36*: 131-136, 1964.

29. Wernicke's Sensory Aphasia

BAY, E.: "The History of Aphasia and the Principles of Cerebral Localization," in Schaltenbrand, G., and Woolsey, C. N. (eds.): *Cerebral Localization and Organization.* Madison: Univ. of Wisconsin Press, 1964, pp. 43-52.

BENTON, A. L.: Contributions to Aphasia Before Broca. *Cortex 1*: 314-327, 1964.

BENTON, A. L.: Johann A. P. Gesner on Aphasia. *Med. Hist. 9*: 54-60, 1965.

BENTON, A. L., AND JOYNT, R. J.: Early Descriptions of Aphasia. *Arch. Neurol 3*: 205-222, 1960.

BENTON, A. L., AND JOYNT, R. J.: Three Pioneers in the Study of Aphasia. *J. Hist. Med. 18*: 381-383, 1963.

CRITCHLEY, M.: "The Study of Language-Disorder: Past, Present, and Future," in J. T. Culbertson (ed.): *The Centennial Lectures Commemorating the One Hundredth Anniversary of E. R. Squibb & Sons.* New York: G. P. Putnam's Sons, 1959, pp. 269-292.

CRITCHLEY, M.: Jacksonian Ideas and the Future, With Special Reference to Aphasia. *Br. Med. J. 2*: 6-12, 1960.

CRITCHLEY, M.: "Broca's Contribution to Aphasia Reviewed a Century Later," in H. Garland (ed.): *Scientific Aspects of Neurology.* Baltimore: Williams & Wilkins Co., 1961, pp. 131-141.

CRITCHLEY, M.: The Origins of Aphasiology. *Scott Med. J. 9*: 231-242, 1964.

CRITCHLEY, M.: Dax's Law. *Int. J. Neurol. 4*: 199-206, 1964.

CRITCHLEY, M.: *Aphasiology and Other Aspects of Language.* London: Edward Arnold, Ltd., 1970.

ELIASBERG, W. G.: A Contribution to the Prehistory of Aphasia. *J. Hist. Med. 5*: 96-101, 1950.

GREENBLATT, S. H.: Hughlings Jackson's First Encounter with the Work of Paul Broca: The Physiological and Psychological Background. *Bull Hist. Med. 44*: 555-570, 1970.

HEAD, H.: Hughlings Jackson on Aphasia and Kindred Affections of Speech. *Brain 38*: 1-190, 1915.

HEAD, H.: *Aphasia and Kindred Disorders of Speech.* Cambridge, England: University Press, 1926, Vol. 1, pp. 1-141.

JOYNT, R. J.: Centenary of Patient "Tan." His Contribution to the Problem of Aphasia. *Arch. Intern. Med. 108*: 953-956, 1961.

JOYNT, R. J.: Paul Pierre Broca: His Contribution to the Knowledge of Aphasia. *Cortex 1*: 206-213, 1964.

JOYNT, R. J., AND BENTON, A. L.: The Memoir of Marc Dax on Aphasia. *Neurology (Minneap.) 14*: 851-854, 1964.

MARX, O. M.: Freud and Aphasia: An Historical Analysis. *Am. J. Psychiatry. 124*: 815-825, 1967.

RIESE, W.: The Early History of Aphasia. *Bull. Hist. Med. 21*: 322-334, 1947.

RIESE, W.: Auto-Observation of Aphasia. Reported by an Eminent Nineteenth Century Medical Scientist. *Bull. Hist. Med. 28*: 237-242, 1954.

RIESE, W.: Hughlings Jackson's Doctrine of Aphasia and Its Significance Today. *J. Nerv. Ment. Dis. 122*: 1-13, 1955.

RIESE, W.: The Sources of Hughlings Jackson's View on Aphasia. *Brain 88*: 811-822, 1965.

SCHILLER, F.: Leborgne—In Memoriam. *Med. Hist. 7*: 79-81, 1963.

STENDER, A.: Über die Forschungstätigkeit von Eduard Hitzig (1838-1907) und Carl Wernicke (1848-1905) in Berlin. *Dtsch. Med. J. 19*: 335-339, 1968.

STOOKEY, B.: Jean-Baptiste Bouillaud and Ernest Auburtin. Early Studies on Cerebral Localization and the Speech Center. *JAMA 184*: 1024-1029, 1963.

30. Wallenberg's Syndrome

CURRIER, R. D.: "Syndromes of the Medulla Oblongata," in P. J. Vinken, G. W. Bruyn, and A. Biemond (eds.): *Handbook of Clinical Neurology,* Amsterdam: North-Holland Publishing Co., 1969, Vol. 2, pp. 217-237.

WOLF, J. K.: *The Classical Brain Stem Syndromes. Translations of the Original Papers with Notes on the Evolution of Clinical Neuroanatomy.* Springfield, Illinois: Charles C. Thomas, 1971, pp. 113-136.

32. Von Recklinghausen's Neurofibromatosis

CROWE, F. W., SCHULL, W. J., AND NEEL, J. V.: *A Clinical, Pathological, and Genetic Study of Multiple Neurofibromatosis.* Springfield, Illinois: Charles C. Thomas, 1956.

TALBOTT, J. H.: Friedrich von Recklinghausen (1833-1910): German Pathologist. *JAMA 205*: 640-641, 1968.

33. Gerstmann's Syndrome

GERSTMANN, J.: Some Posthumous Notes on the Gerstmann Syndrome. *Wien. Z. Nervenheilkd. 28*: 12-19, 1970.

36. Wilson's Disease

ASAO, H., AND OJI, K.: *Hepatocerebral Degeneration.* Springfield, Illinois: Charles C. Thomas, 1968.

TALBOTT, J. H.: S. A. Kinnier Wilson (1878-1937): Lenticular-Hepatic Degeneration. *JAMA 205*: 871-872, 1968.

37. Infantile Spinal Muscular Atrophy

VOGEL, P.: Die Heidelberger neurologische Schule. *Heidelb. Jahrb. 14*: 73-84, 1970.

39. Lindau's Disease

WILKINS, R. H.: "Genetic Factors Related to the Induction and Hereditary Transmission of Primary Intracranial Neoplasms," in W. M. Kirsch, E. Grossi-Paoletti, and P. Paoletti (eds.): *The Experimental Biology of Brain Tumors.* Springfield, Illinois: Charles C. Thomas, 1972, pp. 551-560.

40. Creutzfeldt-Jakob Disease

MACCHI, G., AND LECHI, A.: Le Syndrome de Creutzfeldt-Jakob. *Excerpta Med., Int. Congr. Series 100*: 576-579, 1965.

WARICK, L. H., AND BARROWS, H. S.: The Creutzfeldt-Jakob syndrome. Clinicopathologic Study of a Case Diagnosed by Biopsy with a Review of the Literature. *Bull. Los Angeles Neurol. Soc. 28*: 56-69, 1963.

41. Parinaud's Syndrome

WOLF, J. K.: *The Classical Brain Stem Syndromes, Translations of the Original Papers with Notes on the Evolution of Clinical Neuroanatomy.* Springfield, Illinois: Charles C. Thomas, 1971, pp. 85-100.

D. English Translations of Other Classic Works in Neurology

ATKINSON, M.: Menière's Original Papers. Reprinted with an English Translation Together with Commentaries and Biographical Sketch. *Acta Otolaryngol. [Suppl.] (Stockh.) 162*, 1961.

CHARCOT, [J. M.]: Sclerosis in Scattered Patches. T. Oliver (transl.) *Edinburgh Med. J. 21: 720-726, 1010-1020; 22: 50-56, 117-125, 322-327, 414-421, 1876.

CHARCOT, J. M.: *Lectures on the Diseases of the Nervous System.* Second Series, G. Sigerson (transl. and ed.), New York: Hafner Publishing Company, 1962.

DUCHENNE, G. B. A.: *Selections From the Clinical Works of Dr. Duchenne (de Boulogne).* G. V. Poore (transl. and ed.), London: New Sydenham Society, 1883.

DUCHENNE, G. B. A.: *Physiology of Motion Demonstrated by Means of Electrical Stimulation and Clinical Observation and Applied to the Study of Paralysis and Deformities.* E. B.

Kaplan (transl. and ed.), Philadelphia: W. B. Saunders, 1959.

EMMERSON, J. S.: *Translations of Medical Classics. A List.* Newcastle Upon Tyne, England: University Library, 1965.

GLOOR, P.: Hans Berger on the Electroencephalogram of Man. The Fourteen Original Reports on the Human Electroencephalogram. *Electroencephalogr. Clin. Neurophysiol.* Suppl. *28*, 1969.

MEDIN, O.: An Epidemic of Infantile Paralysis. *Clin. Orthop. 45*: 5-11, 1966.

VICTOR, M., AND YAKOVLEV, P. I.: S. S. Korsakoff's Psychic Disorder in Conjunction with Peripheral Neuritis. A Translation of Korsakoff's Original Article with Brief Comments on the Author and His Contribution to Clinical Medicine. *Neurology (Minneap.) 5*: 394-406, 1955.

WILKINS, R. H.: Neurosurgical Classics, I-XXXVIII. *J. Neurosurg. 19*: 700-710, 1962, et seq.

WILKINS, R. H.: *Neurosurgical Classics.* New York: Johnson Reprint Corporation, 1965.

WOLF, J. K.: *The Classical Brain Stem Syndromes: Translations of the Original Papers with Notes on the Evolution of Clinical Neuroanatomy.* Springfield, Illinois: Charles C. Thomas, Publisher, 1971.

E. Historical References Concerning Other Neurological Diseases

ADLER, A.: The Work of Paul Schilder. *Bull N. Y. Acad. Med. 41*: 841-853, 1965.

ALAJOUANINE, T., AND BOURGUIGNON, A.: La Première Description de la Myasthénie. *Presse Med. 62*: 519-520, 1954.

AMELI, N. O.: Avicenna and Trigeminal Neuralgia. *J. Neurol. Sci. 2*: 105-107, 1965.

BARBEAU, A.: The Understanding of Involuntary Movements: An Historical Approach. *J. Nerv. Ment. Dis. 127*: 469-489, 1958.

BRIM, C. J.: Paralysis in the Old Testament. A Treatise on Some of the Neurological Observations Recorded in the Bible by the Ancient Hebrew Prophets. *J. Nerv. Ment. Dis. 97*: 656-665, 1943.

CLARKE, E.: Apoplexy in the Hippocratic Writings. *Bull. Hist. Med. 37*: 301-314, 1963.

DAVEY, L. M., AND GERMAN, W. J.: Ménière's Disease. A Centennial Historical Note. *J. Neurosurg. 19*: 82-83, 1962.

DEJONG, R. N.: Migraine. Personal Observations by Physicians Subject to the Disorder. *Ann. Med. Hist. 4*: 276-283, 1942.

GLASSCOCK, M. E., III: History of the Diagnosis and Treatment of Acoustic Neuroma. *Arch. Otolaryngol. 88*: 578-585, 1968.

GLOBUS, J. H.: Brain Tumor: Its Contribution to Neurology in the Remote and Recent Past. *J. Neuropathol. Exp. Neurol. 5*: 85-105, 1946.

GOULD, G. M.: The History and Etiology of "Migraine." *JAMA 42*: 168-172, 239-244, 1904.

GRADY, F. J.: Some Early American Reports on

Meningitis. *J. Hist. Med. 20*: 27-32, 1965.

GREENFIELD, J. G.: Historical Landmarks in the Pathology of Involuntary Movements. *J. Neuropathol. Exp. Neurol. 15*: 5-11, 1956.

HEPPNER, F.: Zur Geschichte des Hydrocephalus und seiner Behandlung. *Wien. Med. Wochenschr. 116*: 1046-1048, 1966.

HERRMANN, C., JR.: Myasthenia Gravis—The First Three Centuries—or "The Default of the Explosive Copula." *Bull. Los Angeles Neurol. Soc. 32*: 131-140, 1967.

JOHNSON, J.: Thomsen and Myotonia Congenita. *Med. Hist. 12*: 190-194, 1968.

KEYNES, G.: The History of Myasthenia Gravis. *Med. Hist. 5*: 313-326, 1961.

LEWY, F. H.: Historical Introduction: The Basal Ganglia and Their Diseases. *Res. Publ. Assoc. Res. Nerv. Ment. Dis. 21*: 1-20, 1942.

LOESER, J. D.: History of Skeletal Traction in the Treatment of Cervical Spine Injuries. *J. Neurosurg. 33*: 54-59, 1970.

MAXWELL, H.: Migraine—A Note on Its History. *Hist. Med. 2*: 5-8, 1970.

MCMURTRY, J. G., III: The History of Medical and Surgical Interests in Facial Pain. *Headache 9*: 1-6, 1969.

MOYA, G.: Evolución de las Ideas en Patología Neuromuscular. *Arch. Neurobiol. (Madrid) 32*: 347-385, 1969.

MÜLLENER, E.-R.: Six Geneva Physicians on Meningitis. *J. Hist. Med. 20*: 1-26, 1965.

PATEL, A. N.: Birth of the Subclavian Steal Syndrome. *Neurol. India 16*: 14-16, 1968.

PAUL, J. R.: *A History of Poliomyelitis.* New Haven: Yale University Press, 1971.

POSER, C. M., AND VAN BOGAERT, L.: Natural History and Evolution of the Concept of Schilder's Diffuse Sclerosis. *Acta Psychiatr. Neurol. 31*: 285-331, 1956.

SCHILLER, F.: Concepts of Stroke Before and After Virchow. *Med. Hist. 14*: 115-131, 1970.

SCHNEIDER, R. C.: Cervical Traction, with Evaluation of Methods, and Treatment of Complications. *Int. Abstr. Surg. 104*: 521-529, 1957.

SHERWIN, A. L.: Multiple Sclerosis in Historical Perspective. *McGill Med. J. 26*: 39-48, 1957.

VAN LIERE, E. J.: Dr. John H. Watson and the Subclavian Steal. *Arch. Intern. Med. 118*: 245-248, 1966.

VIETS, H. R.: History of Peripheral Neuritis as a Clinical Entity. *Arch. Neurol. Psychiat. 32*: 377-394, 1934.

VIETS, H. R.: A Historical Review of Myasthenia Gravis From 1672 to 1900. *JAMA 153*: 1273-1280, 1953.

VIETS, H.: The Miracle at St. Alfege's. *Med. Hist. 9*: 184-185, 1965.

VOZZA, J. A.: Historiographical Commentary Concerning the Knowledge of the Acoustic Tumours. *Rev. Laryngol. Otol. Rhinol. (Bord.) 86*: 253-261, 1965.

WILKINS, R. H.: *Neurosurgical Classics.* New York: Johnson Reprint Corp., 1965.

WILKINS, R. H., AND WOODHALL, B.: "Introduction and Historical Background," in W. M. Kirsch, E. Grossi-Paoletti, and P. Paoletti (eds.): *The Experimental Biology of Brain Tumors.* Springfield, Illinois: Charles C. Thomas, 1972, pp. 3-16.

WILSON, T. G.: Historical Aspects of Meniere's Disease. *Laryngoscope 75*: 1491-1496, 1965.

F. Historical References Concerning Neurological Diagnostic Techniques

ABRAMS, H. L.: "Introduction and Historical Notes," in H. L. Abrams: *Angiography.* Boston: Little, Brown & Co., 2nd Ed., 1971, Vol. 1, pp. 3-13.

BENDHEIM, O. L.: On the History of Hoffmann's Sign. *Bull. Inst. Hist. Med. 5*: 684-686, 1937.

BRUWER, A. J.: *Classic Descriptions in Diagnostic Roentgenology.* Springfield, Illinois: Charles C. Thomas, 1964. (Ventriculography, Encephalography, Myelography, Cerebral Angiography).

BULL, J.: Myelography. *Neuroradiology 2*: 1-2, 1971.

BULL, J. W. D.: History of Neuroradiology. *Br. J. Radiol. 34*: 69-84, 1961.

BULL, J. W. D.: The History of Neuroradiology. *Proc. R. Soc. Med. 63*: 637-643, 1970.

DAVIDOFF, L. M.: Neuroradiology: Reflections of a Neurosurgeon. *Radiol. Clin. North Am. 4*: 3-9, 1966.

DAVIS, L.: Neurological Surgery, So to Speak, Out of Roentgenology. Hickey Lecture, 1956. *Am. J. Roentgenol. Radium Ther. Nucl. Med. 76*: 217-225, 1956.

FINKE, J.: Zur Geschichte neurologischer Untersuchungsmethoden. *Dtsch. Med. Wochenschr. 91*: 2226-2230, 1966.

GIBBS, F. A., AND GIBBS, E. L.: *Atlas of Electroencephalography.* Cambridge, Mass.: L. A. Cummings Co., 1941, pp. 2, 4, 6, 8.

GINZBERG, R.: Three Years with Hans Berger. A Contribution to His Biography. *J. Hist. Med. 4*: 361-371, 1949.

GUTRECHT, J. A., ESPINOSA, R. E., AND DYCK, P. J.: Early Descriptions of Common Neurologic Signs. *Mayo Clin. Proc. 43*: 807-814, 1968.

HALL, G. W.: Neurologic Signs and Their Discoverers. *JAMA 95*: 703-707, 1930.

KOLLE, K.: Die Geschichte der Neuroradiologie. *Fortschr. Neurol. Psychiatr. 33*: 145-157, 1965.

LICHT, S.: The History of Electrodiagnosis. *Bull. Hist. Med. 16*: 450-467, 1944.

LICHT, S.: "History of Electrodiagnosis," in S. Licht (ed.): *Electrodiagnosis and Electromyography.* New Haven, Conn.: E. Licht, 1961, pp. 1-23.

MARK, H. H.: The First Ophthalmoscope? Adolf Kussmaul 1845. *Arch. Ophthalmol. 84*: 520-521, 1970.

PETERSON, H. O.: Myelography. Past and Present (1935-1968). *Minn. Med. 52*: 1881-1887, 1969.

SCHILLER, F.: The Reflex Hammer: In Memoriam Robert Wartenberg (1887-1956). *Med. Hist. 11*: 75-85, 1967.

SCHRENK, M.: Hans Bergers Idee von der "psychischen Energie." Zur ersten Publikation "Über das Elektrenkephalogramm des Menschen" vor 40 Jahren. *Nervenarzt 41*: 263-273, 1970.

SCHWEITZER, N. M. J.: History of Ophthalmoscopy. *Bibl. Ophthalmol. 72*: 2-10, 1967.

SHAPIRO, R.: *Myelography.* Chicago: Year Book Medical Publishers, Inc., 2nd Ed., 1968, pp. 11-13.

WENZEL, E.: Luigi Galvani—Alexander von Humboldt—Hans Berger. (Aus der Geschichte der Elektroenzephalographie). *Munch. Med. Wochenschr. 104*: 1146-1150, 1962.

WHITE, D. N.: Ultrasonic Encephalography. *Acta Radiol. [Diagn.] (Stockh.) 9*: 671-674, 1969.

WILKINS, R. H.: *Neurosurgical Classics.* New York: Johnson Reprint Corp. 1965, pp. 242-317. (Ophthalmoscope and Papilledema, Pineal Shift, Lumbar Puncture, Queckenstedt Test, Myelography, Cerebral Arteriography, Pneumoencephalography, Pneumoventriculography).

G. Historical References Concerning Neuroanatomy, Neurophysiology, and Neuropathology

1. Cerebral Localization

ASK-UPMARK, E.: Swedenborg as a Pioneer in Cerebral Localization. *JAMA 183*: 805-806, 1963.

BAKAN, D.: The Influence of Phrenology on American Psychology. *J. Hist. Behav. Sci. 2*: 200-220, 1966.

BRAZIER, M. A. B.: The History of the Electrical Activity of the Brain as a Method for Localizing Sensory Function. *Med. Hist. 7*: 199-211, 1963.

CRITCHLEY, M.: Neurology's Debt to F. J. Gall (1758-1828). *Br. Med. J. 2*: 775-781, 1965.

GIBSON, W. C.: Pioneers in Localization of Function in the Brain. *JAMA 180*: 944-951, 1962.

GIBSON, W. C.: "The Early History of Localization in the Nervous System," in P. J. Vinken and G. W. Bruyn (eds.): *Handbook of Clinical Neurology* Amsterdam: North-Holland Publishing Co., Vol. 2, 1969, pp. 4-14.

HERRNSTEIN, R. J., AND BORING, E. G.: "Cerebral Localization," in *A Source Book in The History of Psychology.* Cambridge, Mass.: Harvard Univ. Press, 1965, pp. 204-252.

HOLLANDER, B.: The Centenary of Francis Joseph Gall, 1758-1828. *Med. Life 35*: 373-380, 1928.

JASPER, H. H.: Evolution of Conceptions of Cerebral Localization Since Hughlings Jackson. *World Neurol. 1*: 97-112, 1960.

JEFFERSON, G.: The Prodromes to Cortical Localization. *J. Neurol. Neurosurg. Psychiatry 16*: 59-72, 1953.

JEFFERSON, G.: Variations on a Neurological Theme—Cortical Localization. *Br. Med. J. 2*: 1405-1408, 1955.

KLINGLER, M.: Zur cerebralen Lokalisationslehre. Betrachtungen zur Geschichte einer Hypothese. *Schweiz. Med. Wochenschr. 97*: 725-731, 1967.

KOSHTOYANTS, K. S.: The History of the Problem of Brain Cortex Excitability. *Actes VIII Congrès Int. d'Histoire des Sciences 2*: 862-864, 1956.

LESKY, E.: Structure and Function in Gall. *Bull. Hist. Med. 44*: 297-314. 1970.

LEVINSON, A.: Early Studies of Cerebral Function. *Bull. Soc. Med. Hist. Chic. 3*: 116-121, 1923.

RIEGEL, R. E.: Early Phrenology in the United States. *Med. Life 37*: 361-376, 1930.

RIESE, W.: Changing Concepts of Cerebral Localization. *Clio Med. 2*: 189-230, 1967.

RIESE, W.: Cerebral Dominance: Its Origin, Its History and Its Nature. *Clio. Med. 5*: 319-326, 1970.

RIESE, W., AND HOFF, E. C.: A History of the Doctrine of Cerebral Localization. Sources, Anticipations, and Basic Reasoning. *J. Hist. Med. 5*: 50-71, 1950.

RIESE, W., AND HOFF, E. C.: A History of the Doctrine of Cerebral Localization. Second Part: Methods and Main Results. *J. Hist. Med. 6*: 439-470, 1951.

SCHALTENBRAND, G., AND WOOLSEY, C. N.: *Cerebral Localization and Organization.* Madison: Univ. of Wisconsin Press, 1964.

STOOKEY, B.: A Note on the Early History of Cerebral Localization. *Bull. N. Y. Acad Med. 30*: 559-578, 1954.

SWAZEY, J. P.: Action Propre and Action Commune: The Localization of Cerebral Function. *J. Hist. Biol. 3*: 213-234, 1970.

TEMKIN, O.: Gall and the Phrenological Movement. *Bull. Hist. Med. 21*: 275-321, 1947.

TIZARD, B.: Theories of Brain Localization from Flourens to Lashley. *Med. Hist. 3*: 132-145, 1959.

WALKER, A. E.: The Development of the Concept of Cerebral Localization in the Nineteenth Century. *Bull. Hist. Med. 31*: 99-121, 1957.

WALKER, A. E.: Stimulation and Ablation. Their Role in the History of Cerebral Physiology. *J. Neurophysiol. 20*: 435-449, 1957.

WALSHE, F.: An Attempted Correlation of the Diverse Hypotheses of Functional Localization in the Cerebral Cortex. *J. Neurol Sci. 1*: 111-128, 1964.

YOUNG, R. M.: The Functions of the Brain: Gall to Ferrier (1808-1886). *Isis 59*: 251-268, 1968.

YOUNG, R. M.: *Mind, Brain and Adaptation in the Nineteenth Century.* Oxford: Clarendon Press, 1970.

2. Other Subjects

ADRIAN, [E. D.]: Progress in Brain Physiology in the Present Century. *Acta Biol. Exp. (Warsz)* 29: 229-237, 1969.

BARNES, C. D., AND KIRCHER, C.: *Readings in Neurophysiology.* New York: John Wiley & Sons, Inc., 1968.

BEACH, E. L., JR.: The Historical Significance of Pavlov's Experiments on Conditional Reflexes. *Cond. Reflex 1*: 281-287, 1966.

BEST, A. E.: Pourfour du Petit's Experiments on the Origin of the Sympathetic Nerve. *Med. Hist 13*: 154-174, 1969.

BEST, A. E.: Reflections on Joseph Lister's Edinburgh Experiments on Vaso-Motor Control. *Med. Hist. 14*: 10-30, 1970.

BLACKWOOD, W.: The National Hospital, Queen Square, and the Development of Neuropathology. *World Neurol. 2*: 331-335, 1961.

BRAZIER, M. A. B.: Rise of Neurophysiology in the 19th Century. *J. Neurophysiol. 20*: 212-226, 1957.

BRAZIER, M. A. B.: The Development of Concepts Relating to the Electrical Activity of the Brain. *J. Nerv. Ment. Dis. 126*: 303-321, 1958.

BRAZIER, M. A. B.: "The Historical Development of Neurophysiology," in J. Field (ed.): *Handbook of Physiology. A Critical, Comprehensive Presentation of Physiological Knowledge and Concepts.* Washington, D. C.: American Physiological Society, 1959, Sect. 1, *1*, pp. 1-58.

BRAZIER, M. A. B.: *A History of the Electrical Activity of the Brain. The First Half-Century.* London: Pitman Medical Publishing Co., 1961.

BRAZIER, M. A. B.: "Historical Introduction. The Discoverers of the Steady Potentials of the Brain: Caton and Beck," in M. A. B. Brazier (ed.): *Brain Function. Proceedings of the First Conference, 1961. Cortical Excitability and Steady Potentials. Relations of Basic Research to Space Biology.* Berkeley and Los Angeles: Univ. of California Press, 1963, pp. 1-13.

BRAZIER, M. A. B.: The Growth of Concepts Relating to Brain Mechanisms. *J. Hist. Behav Sci. 1*: 218-234, 1965.

BRAZIER, M. A. B.: The Growth of Concepts Relating to Brain Mechanisms. *Int. J. Psychiatry 3*: 40-52, 1967.

BUCKLEY, R. E.: Three Basic Brain Models of the Last Three Centuries. *Minn. Med. 52*: 235-241, 1969.

BURDACH, K. F.: *Vom Baue und Leben des Gehirns.* Leipzig: Dyk'sche Buchhdl., 3 Vols., 1819, 1822, 1826.

CLARKE, E.: The Early History of the Cerebral Ventricles. *Trans. Coll. Physicians Philad 30*: 85-89, 1962.

CLARKE, E.: Aristotelian Concepts of the Form and Function of the Brain. *Bull. Hist. Med. 37*: 1-14, 1963.

CLARKE, E., AND BEARN, J. G.: The Brain "Glands" of Malpighi Elucidated by Practical History. *J. Hist. Med 23*: 309-330, 1968.

CLARKE, E., AND O'MALLEY, C. D.: *The Human Brain and Spinal Cord. A Historical Study Illustrated by Writings From Antiquity to the Twentieth Century.* Berkeley, California: Univ. of California Press, 1968.

CLARKE, E., AND STANNARD, J.: Aristotle on the Anatomy of the Brain. *J. Hist. Med. 18*: 130-148, 1963.

CUMMING, W. J. K.: An Anatomical Review of the Corpus Callosum. *Cortex 6*: 1-18, 1970.

DOHRMANN, G. J.: The Choroid Plexus: A Historical Review. *Brain Res. 18*: 197-218, 1970.

ECCLES, J. C.: "The Development of Ideas On The Synapse," in C. McC. Brooks and P. F. Cranefield (eds.): *The Historical Development of Physiological Thought.* New York: Hafner Pub. Co., 1959, pp. 39-66.

FAULL, R. L. M., TAYLOR, D. W., AND CARMAN, J. B.: Soemmerring and the Substantia Nigra. *Med. Hist. 12*: 297-299, 1968.

FEARING, F.: *Reflex Action A Study in the History of Physiological Psychology.* Baltimore: Williams & Wilkins Co., 1930.

FLAMM, E. S.: Historical Observations on the Cranial Nerves. *J. Neurosurg. 27*: 285-297, 1967.

FRENCH, R.: The Origins of the Sympathetic Nervous System From Vesalius to Riolan. *Med. Hist. 15*: 45-54, 1971.

FRENCH, R. D.: Some Concepts of Nerve Structure and Function in Britain, 1875-1885: Background to Sir Charles Sherrington and the Synapse Concept. *Med. Hist. 14*: 154-165, 1970.

FULTON, J. F.: A Note on Francesco Gennari and the Early History of Cytoarchitectural Studies of the Cerebral Cortex. *Bull. Inst. Hist. Med. 5*: 895-913, 1937.

FULTON, J. F.: Introduction: Historical Résumé. *Res. Publ. Assoc. Res. Nerv. Ment. Dis. 20*: xiii-xxx, 1940.

FULTON, J. F.: Notes on the History of the Postural Reflexes. *Folia Psychiatr. 56*: 455-459, 1953.

FULTON, J. F.: Contemporary Concepts of the Hypothalamus and Their Origin. *Q. Bull. Northw. Univ. Med. Sch 28*: 10-16, 1954.

FULTON, J. F.: "Historical Reflections on the Backgrounds of Neurophysiology: Inhibition, Excitation, and Integration of Activity," in C. McC. Brooks and P. F. Cranefield (eds.): *The Historical Development of Physiological Thought.* New York: Hafner Pub. Co., 1959, pp. 67-79.

FULTON, J. F.: *Selected Readings in the History of Physiology.* Springfield, Illinois: Charles C. Thomas, 1966.

GIBSON, W. C.: The History of the Neurone Theory. *Clio Med. 5*: 249-253, 1970.

GOSS, C. M.: On Anatomy of Nerves by Galen of Pergamon. *Am. J. Anat. 118*: 327-336, 1966.

HASSIN, G. B.: Neuropathology: An Historical Sketch. *J. Neuropathol. Exp. Neurol. 9*: 1-17, 1950.

HASSLER, R.: Die Entwicklung der Architektonik seit Brodmann und ihre Bedeutung für die moderne Hirnforschung. *Dtsch. Med. Wochenschr. 87*: 1180-1185, 1962.

HOFF, H. E.: Vagal Stimulation Before the Webers. *Ann. Med. Hist. 8*: 138-144, 1936.

HOFF, H. E.: The History of Vagal Inhibition. *Bull. Hist. Med. 8*: 461-496, 1940.

HOFF, H. E., AND KELLAWAY, P.: The Early History of the Reflex. *J. Hist. Med. 7*: 211-249, 1952.

HOME, R. W.: Electricity and the Nervous Fluid. *J. Hist. Biol. 3*: 235-251, 1970.

JACKSON, S. W.: Force and Kindred Notions in Eighteenth-Century Neurophysiology and Medical Psychology. *Bull. Hist. Med. 44*: 397-410, 539-554, 1970.

JANDOLO, M.: Il Concetto di "Impulso Nervoso" (Dai Primordi ai Nobel per la Medicina 1963). *Riv. Stor. Med. 8*: 151-158, 1964.

KAUFMANN, J. C. E.: Neuropathology in the Bible. *S. Afr. Med. J. 38*: 748-750, 788-789, 805-808, 1964.

KUNTZ, A.: *The Autonomic Nervous System.* Philadelphia: Lea & Febiger, 4th Ed., 1953, pp. 15-20, 491-543.

LACHMAN, S. J.: *History and Methods of Physiological Psychology. A Brief Overview.* Detroit: Hamilton Press, 1963.

LEAKE, C. D.: Historical Aspects of the Autonomic Nervous System. *Anesthesiology 29*: 623-624, 1968.

LIDDELL, E. G. T.: *The Discovery of Reflexes.* Oxford: Clarendon Press, 1960.

LINDSLEY, D., AND MAGOUN, H. W.: *The History of Russian Neurophysiology.* Washington: The American Institute of Biological Sciences, 1964.

LYONS, J. B.: The Advent of Neurophysiology. *J. Ir. Med. Assoc. 52*: 55-61, 1963.

MAGOUN, H. W.: "Development of Ideas Relating the Mind with the Brain," in C. McC. Brooks and P. F. Cranefield (eds.): *The Historical Development of Physiological Thought.* New York: Hafner Publishing Co., 1959, pp. 81-89.

MAGOUN, H. W.: "Development of Ideas Relating the Mind and Brain," in J. T. Culbertson (ed.): *The Centennial Lectures Commemorating the One Hundredth Anniversary of E. R. Squibb & Sons.* New York: G. P. Putnam's Sons, 1959, pp. 247-267.

MEYER, A.: Marcello Malpighi and the Dawn of Neurohistology. *J. Neurol. Sci. 4*: 185-193, 1967.

MEYER, A.: Karl Friedrich Burdach and his Place in the History of Neuroanatomy. *J. Neurol. Neurosurg. Psychiatry 33*: 553-561, 1970.

MEYER, A.: *Historical Aspects of Cerebral Anatomy.* London: Oxford Univ. Press, 1971.

MEYER, A., AND HIERONS, R.: Observations on the History of the "Circle of Willis." *Med. Hist. 6*: 119-139, 1962.

MEYER, A., AND HIERONS, R.: A Note on Thomas Willis' Views on the Corpus Striatum and the Internal Capsule. *J.*

Neurol. Sci. 1: 547-554, 1964..

MEYER, A., AND HIERONS, R.: On Thomas Willis' Concepts of Neurophysiology. *Med. Hist. 9*: 1-15, 142-155, 1965.

MEYER, A. W.: The Gasser of the Gasserian Ganglion. *Ann. Med. Hist. 8*: 118-123, 1936.

MISHKIN, S.: The Interdependence of Clinical Neurology and Neurophysiology. An Historical Review of the Vestibulo-Ocular Reflex. *McGill Med. J. 33*: 80-97, 1964.

DE MORSIER, G.: Leonard De Vinci et l'Anatomie du Cerveau Humain. *Physis. Riv. Stor. Sci. 6*: 335-346, 1964.

NEUBUERGER, K. T.: "The History of Neuropathology," in J. Minckler (ed.): *Pathology of the Nervous System.* New York: McGraw-Hill, 1969, pp. 1-14.

NEUBURGER, M.: *Die historische Entwicklung der experimentellen Gehirn und Rückenmarksphysiologie vor Flourens.* Stuttgart: Enke, 1897.

O'MALLEY, C. D.: Gabriele Falloppia's Account of the Cranial Nerves. *Sudhoffs Arch. 7*: 132-137, 1966.

O'NEILL, Y. V.: William of Conches and the Cerebral Membranes. *Clio Med. 2*: 13-21, 1967.

PAVLOV, I. P.: *Conditioned Reflexes: An Investigation of the Physiological Activities of the Cerebral Cortex.* G. V. Anrep (transl.), New York: Dover Publications, Inc., 1960.

PHILLIPS, E. D.: The Brain and Nervous Phenomena in the Hippocratic Writings. *Ir. J. Med. Sci. 6*: 377-390, 1957.

POLYAK, S.: *The Vertebrate Visual System.* H. Klüver (ed.). Chicago: Univ. of Chicago Press, 1957, pp. 9-203, 1059-1358.

POYNTER, F. N. L.: *The History and Philosophy of Knowledge of The Brain and Its Functions. An Anglo-American Symposium. London, July 15th – 17th, 1957.* Springfield, Illinois: Charles C. Thomas, 1958.

RASMUSSEN, A. T.: *Some Trends in Neuroanatomy.* Dubuque, Iowa: W. C. Brown Co., 1947.

RATH, G.: Neural Pathology. A Pathogenetic Concept of the 18th and 19th Centuries. *Bull. Hist. Med. 33*: 526-541, 1959.

ROIZIN, L.: Essay on the Origin and Evolution of Neuropathology. Some Fundamental Neuropathologic Contributions to Psychiatry. *Psychiatr. Quart. 31*: 531-555, 1957.

RUCKER, C. W.: History of the Numbering of the Cranial Nerves. *Mayo Clin. Proc. 41*: 453-461, 1966.

SCHILLER, F.: The Rise of the "Enteroid Processes" in the 19th Century: Some Landmarks in Cerebral Nomenclature. *Bull. Hist. Med. 39*: 326-338, 1965.

SCHILLER, F.: The Vicissitudes of the Basal Ganglia (Further Landmarks in Cerebral Nomenclature). *Bull. Hist. Med. 41*: 515-538, 1967.

SCHILLER, F.: Stilling's Nuclei – Turning Point in Basic Neurology. *Bull. Hist. Med. 43*: 67-84, 1969.

SCHULTE, B. P. M.: Vesalius on the Anatomy of the Brain. *Janus 53*: 40-49, 1966.

SECHENOV, I.: *Reflexes of the Brain.* K. Koshtoyants, S. Belsky, G. Gibbons, and S. Gellerstein (transl. and eds.), Cambridge, Mass.: The M. I. T. Press, 1965.

SHARP, J. A.: Alexander Monro Secundus and the Interventricular Foramen. *Med. Hist. 5:* 83-89, 1961.

SHEEHAN, D.: Discovery of the Autonomic Nervous System. *Arch. Neurol. Psychiatry 35:* 1081-1115, 1936.

SHEER, D. E.: "Brain and Behavior: The Background of Interdisciplinary Research," in D. E. Sheer (ed.): *Electrical Stimulation of the Brain. An Interdisciplinary Survey of Neurobehavioral Integrative Systems.* Austin: Univ. of Texas Press, 1961, pp. 3-21.

SIMOWITZ, F. M.: Some Historical Notes on the Brain and Its Functions. *Univ. Mich. Med. Cent. J. 35:* 41-43, 1969.

SINGER, C.: Brain Dissection Before Vesalius. *J. Hist. Med. 11:* 261-274, 1956.

SOLMSEN, F.: Greek Philosophy and the Discovery of the Nerves. *Mus. Helveticum 18:* 150-197, 1961.

SOURY, J.: *Le Système Nerveux Central. Structure et Fonctions. Histoire Critique des Théories et des Doctrines.* Paris: Georges Carré et C. Naud, Éditeurs, 1899.

SWISHER, C. N.: The Centripetal and Centrifugal History of The Circle of Willis. *McGill Med. J. 33:* 110-124, 1964.

SYMONDS, C.: The Circle of Willis. *Br. Med. J. 1:* 119-124, 1955.

THOMAS, H. M.: Decussation of the Pyramids — An Historical Inquiry. *Johns Hopkins Hosp. Bull. 21:* 304-311, 1910.

TIMME, W.: The Vegetative Nervous System: Historical Retrospect. *Res. Publ. Assoc. Res. Nerv. Ment. Dis. 9:* 1-11, 1930.

VAN DER LOOS, H.: "The History of the Neuron," in H. Hydén (ed.): *The Neuron.* Amsterdam: Elsevier Publishing Co., 1967, pp. 1-47.

WANG, G. H.: Johann Paul Karplus (1866-1936) and Alois Kreidl, (1864-1928): Two Pioneers in the Study of Central Mechanisms of Vegetative Function. *Bull. Hist. Med. 39:* 529-539, 1965.

WARTENBERG, R.: Studies in Reflexes. History, Physiology, Synthesis and Nomenclature. *Arch. Neurol. Psychiatry 51:* 113-133, 414; *52:* 341-358, 359-382, 1944.

WHITE, J. C., SMITHWICK, R. H., AND SIMEONE, F. A.: *The Autonomic Nervous System: Anatomy, Physiology, and Surgical Application.* New York: Macmillan Co., Publishers, 3rd Ed., 1952, pp. 3-15.

WILLIS, T.: *The Anatomy of the Brain and Nerves.* W. Feindel (ed.), Montreal: McGill Univ. Press, 1965.

Index